美国针灸立法汇编

美国西南部地区针灸立法汇编

Collection of Acupuncture Laws in the Southwestern United States of America

（汉英对照）

总顾问

刘保延　沈远东

主　编

桑　珍　杨宇洋　宋欣阳　张博源

上海科学技术出版社

内 容 提 要

　　针灸于19世纪上半叶传入美国,在20世纪70年代"针灸热"的影响之下,开始在美国流行。针灸在美国流行的五十年间,经历了三次热潮,完成了法律本土化、教育本土化、职业本土化和医学属性本土化四个层次的本土化,广泛应用于变态反应性疾病、糖尿病、艾滋病、肿瘤、高血压、肥胖症、戒毒、戒酒、戒烟、化疗或手术后发生的恶心和呕吐等领域。美国47个州及华盛顿特区都在州议会法中专章规定了针灸师执业法律制度,广泛涉及针灸与东方医学的概念、针灸师的准入条件、教育培训、执业规范、行业组织管理和惩戒规则等内容。

　　本书为美国西南部六州针灸立法汇编,包括阿拉斯加州、俄克拉何马州、得克萨斯州、夏威夷州、新墨西哥州、亚利桑那州六州,从针灸人员的法律地位、准入与注册、日常管理机构、职业道德、惩戒报告等方面展开介绍。希望本书的出版能为中医药政策和法律的制定者、中医药政策和法制研究者以及高等院校、科研机构中医药学科的研习者们提供参考和借鉴。

图书在版编目（CIP）数据

　　美国西南部地区针灸立法汇编 = Collection of Acupuncture Laws in the Southwestern United States of America : 汉英对照 / 桑珍等主编；刘保延,沈远东总顾问. -- 上海 : 上海科学技术出版社, 2025.2
　　（美国针灸立法汇编）
　　ISBN 978-7-5478-6593-4

　　Ⅰ. ①美… Ⅱ. ①桑… ②刘… ③沈… Ⅲ. ①针灸学－立法－汇编－美国－汉、英 Ⅳ. ①D937.122.16

　　中国国家版本馆CIP数据核字(2024)第071783号

美国西南部地区针灸立法汇编：Collection of Acupuncture Laws in the Southwestern United States of America（汉英对照）
总顾问　刘保延　沈远东
主　编　桑　珍　杨宇洋　宋欣阳　张博源

上海世纪出版(集团)有限公司
上海科学技术出版社　出版、发行
(上海市闵行区号景路159弄A座9F－10F)
邮政编码 201101　　　www.sstp.cn
上海颛辉印刷厂有限公司印刷
开本 787×1092　1/16　印张 20.75
字数 400千字
2025年2月第1版　2025年2月第1次印刷
ISBN 978－7－5478－6593－4/R·2994
定价：188.00元

编委会名单

丛 书 前 言

　　针灸是我国历代劳动人民及医学家在长期与疾病作斗争中创造和发展起来的一种医学,具有悠久的历史。它是以中医理论为指导,运用针刺和艾灸防治疾病的一门临床学科。针灸具有适应证广、疗效明显、操作方便、经济安全等优点,数千年来深受广大劳动人民的欢迎,对中华民族的繁衍昌盛作出了巨大的贡献。

　　几千年来,针灸不仅对我国人民的保健事业作出重大贡献,而且很早就流传到国外,成为世界医学的重要组成部分,并产生积极而深远的影响。根据世界卫生组织统计,目前有113个成员国认可使用针灸,其中29个成员国设立了相关法律法规,20个成员国将针灸纳入医疗保险体系。针灸的神奇疗效引发全球持续的"针灸热"。针灸推拿等治疗手段成为奥运会运动员们缓解伤痛的新时尚。我国援外医疗队采用针灸、推拿、中药以及中西医结合方法治疗了不少疑难重症,挽救了许多垂危病人的生命,得到受援国政府和人民的充分肯定。不少国家先后对针灸进行了立法,成立了针灸学术团体、针灸教育机构和研究机构。

　　从20世纪70年代开始,世界卫生组织就积极地向全世界推广针灸,在多国设立针灸培训机构,支持创建世界针灸学会联合会,发布了针灸治疗的适宜病症、针灸经穴定位、从业人员培训指南等一系列国际标准,努力推进针灸的国际化与标准化进程。伴随着针灸的全球化应用,针灸针的国际贸易也逐年增长。2011年5月,国际标准化组织/中医药技术委员会(ISO/TC 249)在第二次荷兰海牙年会上,决议成立专门的工作组承担针灸针的国际标准研制工作,由中国专家担任召集人的职位。《ISO 17218:2014 一次性使用无菌针灸针》于2014年2月3日正式出版,成为首个在传统医药领域内由中国主导发布的ISO国际标准。截至目前,ISO/TC 249已发布了7项针灸针的国际标准,为针灸的国际化推广应用作出了积极的贡献。

　　针灸于19世纪上半叶传入美国,在20世纪70年代"针灸热"的影响之下,开始在美国流行。针灸在美国流行的五十年间,经历了三次热潮,完成了法律本土化、教育本土化、职业本土化和医学属性本土化四个层次的本土化。起初,针灸在美国主要用于治疗疼痛症状,后来也广泛应用于变态反应性疾病、糖尿病、艾滋病、各种肿瘤、高血压、肥胖症、戒毒、戒酒、戒烟、化疗或手术后发生的恶心和呕吐、不孕症、性功能不全、神经衰弱、紧张综合征、网球肘、肌纤维组织炎、中风后遗症、骨性关节炎、美容、体外受精、血液病、哮喘等领域。针灸在美国的发展并没有昙花一现，而是入乡随俗，遍地开花。美国的医疗改革给低成本针灸提供了全新的发展契机。中医针灸疗法针对很多病症可以采取非手术的保守疗法，成本低廉，疗效显著。迄今为止，美国 50 个州除了南达科他州、亚拉巴马州、俄克拉何马州 3 个州没有专门的针灸立法之外，其余 47 个州及华盛顿特区都在州议会法中专章规定了针灸师执业法律制度，广泛涉及针灸与东方医学的概念、针灸师的准入条件、教育培训、执业规范、行业组织管理和惩戒规则等内容。

　　"美国针灸立法汇编"丛书编委会经过两年多的信息搜集，资料整理分析，将美国 47 个州针灸法律英文文本进行了收集、翻译、校对和法律评析，重点展示美国各州现行针灸法律制度的全貌。本丛书共 5 册，按照新英格兰地区、中西部地区、西部地区、南部地区、西南部地区划分。每一区域立法均从针灸人员的法律地位、准入与注册、日常管理机构、职业道德、惩戒报告等方面展开介绍。希望本丛书的出版能为中医药政策和法律的制定者、中医药政策和法制研究者以及高等院校、科研机构中医药学科的研习者们提供参考和借鉴。由于时间仓促、经验不足，可能存在不严谨之处，望广大读者朋友不吝指正。

编　者

2023 年 3 月

目　录

阿 拉 斯 加 州

阿拉斯加州针灸法[①]

第 08.06.010 条　禁止无执照从事针灸实践

不得在没有执照的情况下从事针灸实践。

第 08.06.020 条　执照申请

拟从事针灸实践的人员,应当向部门提出书面申请。

第 08.06.030 条　针灸执照

(a) 申请针灸执照应当具备以下条件:

(1) 良好品德。

(2) 至少年满二十一周岁。

(3) 符合以下任意一个条件:

(A) 已完成一项符合经部门批准的与针灸和东方医学审核委员会(ACAOM)核心课程和指导一致的课程。

(B) 在另一个司法管辖区获发针灸执照,该司法管辖区具有和本州同等的针灸执照要求。

(4) 具备国家针灸及东方医学认证委员会(NCCAOM)认证的针灸证书。

(5) 在申请时未处于纪律处分程序中,且不存在未决投诉。

(6) 没有在本州或者其他司法管辖区被吊销或者撤销针灸执照。

(b) 部门应当向合格并且支付适当费用的人员颁发针灸执照。

(c) 根据本章获准从事针灸实践的人员,应当在其从事针灸实践地点的显著位置展示该执照。

第 08.06.040 条　执照续期

除非申请人以部门所确立的方式证明其具备能继续作为针灸师从事针灸实践的能力,否则部门不得为其续期本章所规定的执照。

---

① 根据《阿拉斯加州议会法》注释版第 8 卷第 06 章"针灸"译出。

第 08.06.050 条　披露

（a）从事针灸实践的人员应当披露其在针灸方面的训练和实践：

（1）向每位患者披露。

（2）所有用于针灸并提供给患者或者公众的材料。

（b）未投保医疗事故保险的从事针灸实践的人员,应当向每位患者披露未投保事宜。

第 08.06.060 条　对针灸实践的限制

从事针灸实践的人员不得：

（1）在治疗中给予、开处方或者推荐：

（A）处方药。

（B）管制药物。

（C）毒药。

（2）从事外科手术。

（3）在头衔中使用"医生"一词,除非该人已经获得医生执照。

第 08.06.070 条　实施纪律处分的理由

在听证后,如果部门发现持证人存在下列情形,可以根据本章实施纪律处分：

（1）通过欺骗、欺诈或者故意谎报取得执照的。

（2）在提供专业服务或者从事专业活动过程中,存在欺骗、欺诈或者故意谎报的。

（3）以虚假、误导性的方式宣传专业活动。

（4）被判犯有重罪或者其他影响持证人继续安全实践能力的罪行。

（5）故意或过失从事患者护理,或者允许持证人监督下的人员进行患者护理,该等护理不符合最低专业标准,无论是否对患者造成实际伤害。

（6）未遵守本章、根据本章通过的规则或者部门的命令。

（7）存在如下不适情形,仍然从事针灸实践的：

（A）不称职行为。

（B）未能及时了解当前的专业做法。

（C）酗酒或者严重依赖酒精或者其他损害安全执业能力的药物。

（D）身体或者精神残疾；或者

（8）在为患者提供专业服务中存在淫乱、不道德的行为。

第 08.06.080 条　免责条款

本章不适用于根据《阿拉斯加州议会法》注释版第 8 卷第 36 章或者第 64 章的规定进行针灸的人员。

第 08.06.090 条　处罚

违反本章或者根据本章通过的规则的人员,犯有 B 类轻罪。

第 08.06.100 条　规则

部门为了实施本章规定,可以制定相应的规章制度,包括：

（1）针灸疗法标准。

（2）继续教育培训标准。

（3）针灸职业道德规范。

第 08.06.190 条　定义

本章中：

（1）"针灸"系指从中国传统中医理念中发展出来的一种治疗方式,通过针刺刺激体表或者体表附近的某些穴位,以防止或者改变疼痛的感觉或者使生理功能正常化。

（2）"部门"系指商务、社会和经济发展部。

（3）"针灸疗法"系指在针灸诊断的基础上插入无菌针灸针,并将艾灸应用于人体的特定区域;针灸疗法包括机械、热、电和电磁治疗的辅助疗法,以及推荐膳食指南和治疗性运动。

阿拉斯加州针灸行政法[①]

第 1 节　颁 发 执 照

第 12.AAC 05.100 条　申请要求

（a）针灸执照的申请人应当完成部门提供的申请表格,并且支付《阿拉斯加州行政法典》第 12.AAC 02.108 条规定的申请费。

（b）针灸执照的申请人应当提交符合《阿拉斯加州议会法》注释版第 08.06.030（a）条规定的证明文件：

（1）两封证明申请人良好品德的推荐信。

（2）如果可以,提交一份由经批准的针灸学校出具的成绩单核证副本,以证实申请人所学课程。

（3）由每位申请人持有或者曾经持有针灸执照的司法管辖区直接发给部门的官方证明;该证明含有申请人的纪律处分程序或者尚未解决的控诉信息。

（4）由国家针灸及东方医学认证委员会（NCCAOM）颁发的申请人针灸证书文凭的经验证副本,或者一封 NCCAOM 的信函,以证实申请人有资格获得该针灸证书文凭。

第 12.AAC 05.110 条　经批准的针灸学校

针灸学校必须获得针灸和东方医学院委员会（CCAOM）或者针灸及东方医学教育审核委员会（ACAOM）的认可,才可以获得部门的批准。

第 2 节　执照续期和继续教育

第 12.AAC 05.200 条　执照续期

（a）针灸执照在偶数年的 9 月 30 日到期。

（b）持证人申请执照续期应当：

（1）完成部门提供的续期申请表格。

[①]　根据《阿拉斯加州行政法典》第 12 卷第 1 编第 5 章"针灸"译出。

(2)支付《阿拉斯加州行政法典》第12.AAC 02.108条规定的续期费。

(3)2019年12月25日废止。

(4)按照《阿拉斯加州行政法典》第12.AAC 05.210条要求,应当提交一份在最后许可期内完成的继续教育活动学时的宣示报告书。

第12.AAC 05.210条 继续教育要求

(a)申请针灸执照续期的申请人应当完成以下内容之一:

(1)在整个执照有效期内,具有NCCAOM授予的针灸学位证书;或者

(2)在整个执照有效期内,在NCCAOM规定的核心针灸能力活动中获得了十五个专业拓展活动积分。

(b)申请针灸执照续期的申请人,如获得执照的时长少于十二个月,应当免于适用免除本条规定的要求。

(c)2019年12月25日废止。

第12.AAC 05.220条 经批准的继续教育活动

在《阿拉斯加州行政法典》第12.AAC 05.210(a)(2)条规定下的继续教育活动,应当被国家针灸及东方医学认证委员会(NCCAOM)指定为核心针灸能力专业拓展活动,才能被部门接受。

第12.AAC 05.230条 继续教育要求的审核

(a)部门将根据《阿拉斯加州行政法典》第12.AAC 02.960条的规定审核续期申请,以监督申请人是否符合上述法典第12.AAC 05.210条和第12.AAC 05.220条规定的继续教育要求。

第3节 执 业 标 准

第12.AAC 05.300条 披露

(a)持证人应当通过在患者候诊室张贴显著的通知,以及通过向患者或者公众提供书面材料,向每个患者展示其针灸培训和实践。

(b)未投保医疗事故保险的持证人应当:

(1)在患者候诊室张贴显著的通知,说明持证人没有医疗事故保险;或者

(2)要求每位患者或者患者监护人签署一份声明,确认患者或者患者监护人已被告知持证人未在医疗事故保险范围内。

(c)如果持证人的患者为盲人或者无法阅读本条规定的书面公示,则持证人应当:

(1)在患者初次就诊时向患者或者患者监护人口头说明持证人针灸培训和实践。

(2)如果持证人不在医疗事故保险范围内,应当在患者初次就诊时向患者或者患者监护人口头说明该实施情况,并且至少向患者每年公示一次。

第4节 总 则

第12.AAC 05.990条 定义

除文意另有所指外,在本章以及《阿拉斯加州议会法》注释版第08.06章的下列术语,具

有如下的含义：

（1）"部门"系指商务、社会和经济发展部。

（2）"NCCAOM"系指国家针灸及东方医学认证委员会。

（3）2019 年 12 月 25 日废止。

俄克拉何马州

俄克拉何马州针灸行政法[①]

第 140 – 15 – 10 – 1 条　委员会注册

除非脊椎按摩医师持有由委员会颁发的注册证书,证明该脊医精通针灸和/或经络疗法,否则任何脊医不得向公众声明其是针灸和/或经络疗法的专家。

委员会应当备存一份列出所有获得委员会授权的脊医名单。

此规则不适用于在 2000 年 1 月 1 日及之前从脊医机构毕业,并获得俄克拉何马州脊椎按摩医师执照的脊医。

第 140 – 15 – 10 – 2 条　注册申请;教育要求

(a)各位脊医如果向公众表示其是针灸和/或经络疗法的专家,应当按照委员会制定的申请表格进行申请。

每位脊医应当向委员会提供文件材料,证明其成功完成至少一百学时的针灸和/或经络疗法教育。

此类教育应当为受委员会批准或者已通过委员会批准的教育计划,并且符合以下标准:

(1)由完全认证的脊医学院研究生院、国家针灸与东方医学学院认证委员会及美国针灸与东方医学院校资质委员会认可的针灸学校或者学院,赞助实施和讲授。

(2)要求完成委员会批准的认证考试。

(3)符合委员会认为适当的其他标准。

(b)一旦成功证明这些要求,委员会将把脊医姓名记录在名单中。

---

① 根据《俄克拉何马州行政法典》第 140 卷第 15 章第 10 节"针灸"译出。

得 克 萨 斯 州

得克萨斯州针灸法[①]

第 A 节　一　般　规　定

第 205.001 条　定义

本节中:

(1)"针灸专家"系指根据本法第 205.303 条获得执照的人。

(2)"针灸"系指:

(A)非手术、非刺针和在人体特定部位应当用针灸作为治疗和减轻人体病情的主要治疗方式,包括对病情的评价和评估。

(B)在进行(A)所述治疗的同时,搭配使用热疗或者电疗,或者建议膳食指南、能量流运动,或者膳食或者草药补充剂。

(3)"针灸委员会"系指得克萨斯州针灸审查委员会。

(4)"针灸师"系指从事下列业务者:

(A)针灸执业。

(B)直接或者间接收取执行针灸服务的费用。

(5)"脊椎按摩师"系指由得克萨斯州脊椎按摩审查委员会授权的脊椎按摩治疗从业者。

(6)"行政主管"系指得克萨斯州医学委员会的行政主管。

(7)"医学委员会"系指得克萨斯州医学委员会。

(8)"医生"系指经得克萨斯州医学委员会授权行医的人。

第 205.002 条　2005 年 9 月 1 日,根据 2005 年法案第 79 编第 269 章第 3.35 条废除

第 205.003 条　豁免;限制

(a)本章不适用于根据州另一项议会法获得执照并在许可范围内行事的卫生保健专业人员。

---

① 　根据《得克萨斯州议会法》注释版第 3 卷第 C 编第 205 章"针灸"译出。

（b）本章并不旨在：

（1）限制医生的执业。

（2）允许未经授权者的行医；或者

（3）允许某人分发、管理或者供应管制药物、麻醉品或者危险药品，除非其已获得其他法律的授权。

第 B 节　得克萨斯州针灸考试委员会

第 205.051 条　委员会；委员会成员

（a）得克萨斯州针灸审查委员会由九名成员组成，由州长任命，经参议院的建议和同意如下：

（1）四名针灸师成员，他们在这个州至少有五年的针灸实践经验，但他们不能是医生。

（2）两名有针灸实践经验的医生成员。

（3）三名未获得卫生保健专业执照或者未经培训的普通公众成员。

（b）针灸委员会的任命应当不考虑被任命者的种族、肤色、残疾、性别、宗教、年龄或者国籍。

第 205.052 条　公众成员资格

如果某人或者其配偶存在如下情形，不能被任命为针灸委员会的公众成员：

（1）由卫生保健领域的职业监管机构注册、认证或者颁发执照。

（2）受雇于或者参与由医学委员会规定的商业实体或者其他组织，或者接受医学委员会或者针灸委员会的资金。

（3）直接或者间接拥有或者控制由医学委员会或者针灸委员会管理的商业实体或者其他组织百分之十以上的权益，或者从医学委员会获得资金。

（4）使用或者从医学委员会或者针灸委员会获得大量有形物品、服务或者资金，但法律授权的对针灸委员会成员、出席或者费用的补偿或者报销除外；或者

（5）拥有、经营一所针灸学校或者在该校拥有经济利益。

第 205.053 条　成员和员工的限制

（a）本条的"得克萨斯州行业协会"系指本州商业或行业竞争者自愿加入的合作性全州协会，旨在协助其成员及其行业或者专业人士处理共同的业务或者专业问题，并促进他们的共同利益。

（b）得克萨斯州医疗保健领域行业协会的州长、委员会成员、雇员或者有偿顾问，不得担任针灸委员会的成员或者医学委员会的雇员。他们不受州内职位分类计划的限制，也不得获得总拨款法规定的职位分类工资表第 1 级 A17 工资组的报酬或者高于这一数额的报酬。

（c）某人可能并非针灸委员会的成员，也可能并不具有"真正的行政、管理或者专业能力"（该用语用于确立对 1938 年《联邦公平劳动标准法法案》，《美国法典》第 29 卷第 201 编及后续章节的加班条款的豁免）的医学委员会雇员，如果：

（1）此人是得克萨斯州医疗保健领域行业协会的官员、雇员或者付费顾问；或者

（2）此人的配偶是得克萨斯州医疗保健领域行业协会的官员、管理者或者付费顾问。

（d）如果根据《政府法典》第305章被要求注册为院外游说者，则不得担任针灸委员会的成员、针灸委员会或者医学委员会的总法律顾问，因为该人通过代表某种行业进行有偿行为，与医学委员会或者针灸委员会的运作存在关联。

（e）如果某人拥有、经营针灸学校或者在该校拥有经济利益，则不得在针灸委员会任职。

第 205.054 条　任期；空缺

（a）针灸委员会成员的交错任期为六年。三名成员的任期在每个奇数年的 1 月 31 日到期。

（b）针灸委员会的空缺应当由州长的任命来填补。

第 205.055 条　审裁官

州长应当指定一名针灸委员会的针灸师成员担任审裁官。

审裁官按照州长的意愿任职。

第 205.056 条　免职理由

（a）针灸委员会成员因为如下理由被免职：

（1）在委任时没有具备本法第 205.051 条和第 205.052 条所要求的资格。

（2）在针灸委员会任职期间，不维持本法第 205.051 条和第 205.052 条所要求的资格。

（3）违反了本法第 205.053 条规定的禁令。

（4）在任职的绝大部分时间，因为疾病或者残疾不能履行该成员的职责；或者

（5）该会员在一个日历年内缺席了超过一半的针灸委员会例会。

（b）针灸委员会行动的有效性，不受免职针灸委员会成员的理由时所采取的事实的影响。

（c）如果行政主管知道有可能存在针灸委员会成员的免职理由，其应当将可能出现的情况通知针灸委员会的主席。

主席应当通知州长和司法部部长，可能存在免职的情形。

如果可能的免职理由涉及审裁官，行政主管应当通知针灸委员会的另一名最高负责人，该人应当通知州长和司法部部长，存在可能的免职理由。

第 205.057 条　培训

（a）获得委任并有资格担任针灸委员会成员的人，不得投票、商议或者被作为出席针灸委员会会议的成员，直到此人完成符合本条的培训计划。

（b）培训计划应当向相关人员提供以下信息：

（1）管理针灸委员会运作的法律。

（2）针灸委员会的项目、职能、规则和预算。

（3）针灸委员会规则制定权力的范围和限制。

（4）针灸委员会的规则、解释和执行行动可能通过限制竞争或者影响从事针灸委员会规定的职业或者业务的人收取的价格而涉及联邦反垄断法的规则、解释和执行行动的类型，包括任何规则、解释或者执行行动：

（A）管制针灸委员会监管的职业或者业务人士的执业范围。

（B）限制针灸委员会规定的职业或者业务人士的广告。

（C）影响针灸委员会监管的职业或者业务人士提供的商品或者服务的价格；或者

（D）限制参与针灸委员会规定的职业或者业务。

（5）针灸委员会最近一次正式审计的结果。

（6）要求如下：

（A）有关公开会议、公开信息、行政程序的法律，并且披露利益冲突。

（B）适用于针灸委员会成员履行职责的其他法律。

（7）针灸委员会或者得克萨斯州伦理委员会采用的伦理政策。

（c）根据《一般拨款法案》的规定，被任命为针灸委员会成员的人有权报销参加培训项目所产生的差旅费用，无论参加该项目的时间是在个人有资格就职之前还是之后。

（d）行政主管应当编制一个包括（b）所要求的培训信息手册。

行政主管应当每年向每个针灸委员会成员分发一份培训手册的副本。

每名委员会成员应当签署并向行政主管提交一份声明，确认其已收到并审查了培训手册。

第 205.058 条　行为信息的资格和标准

行政主管或者行政主管的指定人员应当在必要时经常向针灸委员会的成员提供有关他们的信息：

（1）本节规定的任职资格。

（2）在有关州长行为标准的适用法律下的责任。

第 205.059 条　补偿；每日津贴

针灸委员会成员不得因在针灸委员会服务而获得报酬，但有权获得立法拨款规定的每日津贴，用于成员从事针灸委员会业务的每日的交通和相关费用。

第 205.060 条　公开会议；公开记录和行政诉讼法的适用

除本节规定外，针灸委员会受《政府法典》第 551 章、第 552 章和第 2001 章的约束。

第 C 节　针灸委员会和医学委员会的职权

第 205.101 条　针灸委员会的基本权力和职责

（a）经医学委员会的意见和批准，针灸委员会应当：

（1）建立本州针灸师的执业标准。

（2）为针灸委员会制定必要的最低教育和培训要求，以建议医学委员会颁发针灸执照。

（3）管理一项由独立测试专业人员验证的针灸执业执照的考试。

（4）通过对其他州的背书方式颁发执照的要求。

（5）规定针灸执照的申请表。

（6）建议制定执照和其他费用的规则。

（7）为完成至少四十八学期的针灸学生制定辅导课程的要求。

（8）建议使用管理和执行本节所需的其他规则。

（b）针灸委员会没有独立的规则制定权力。

针灸委员会通过的一项规则应当经医学委员会批准。

（c）针灸委员会应当：

（1）审核、批准或者拒绝执照签发或者续期申请。

（2）发放各项执照。

（3）拒绝、吊销或撤销执照，或者以其他方式约束持证人。

第 205.102 条　医学委员会的协助

（a）医学委员会应当根据需要提供行政和文书人员，使针灸委员会能够根据本节进行管理。

（b）根据医学委员会的建议和批准，针灸委员会应当制定和实施政策，明确区分针灸委员会的决策职责、行政主管和医学委员会工作人员的管理职责。

第 205.103 条　费用

医学委员会应当规定和收取合理和必要的费用，以支付管理和执行本节的费用，避免使用医学委员会提供的任何其他资金。

第 205.104 条　限制广告或者竞争性招标的规则

（a）医学委员会不得根据本节采取限制持证人的广告或者竞争性投标的规则，除非禁止虚假、误导或者欺骗行为。

（b）在其禁止虚假、误导或者欺骗行为的规则中，医学委员会不得包括以下规则：

（1）限制使用任何广告媒介。

（2）限制持证人在广告中使用自己的个人形象或者声音。

（3）涉及由持证人发布的广告的规模或者持续时间；或者

（4）限制持证人在商品名称下的广告。

第 205.1041 条　早期参与规则制定过程的指南

（a）针灸委员会应当确定指导方针，以便在规则制定过程中接受对针灸委员会所辖事项有兴趣的个人和团体的意见。

针灸委员会在其向医学委员会提交拟通过的规则之前，应当为个人和组织提供意见的机会。

（b）针灸委员会通过的规则不得以针灸委员会不遵守本条为由进行质疑。

在规则制定过程的早期，如果针灸委员会不能向公众或者受影响的人充分征求意见，应当以书面说明原因。

第 205.1045 条　有关犯罪结果的规则

针灸委员会应当采取符合第 53 章规定的规则和准则。但是，本节比第 53 章的要求更为严格的情形除外。

第 205.105 条　2011 年 7 月 17 日，根据 2011 年法案第 82 编第 1083 章（《附属法例》第 1179 章）第 25（139）条废除

第 205.106 条　技术的使用

经医学委员会的建议和批准，针灸委员会应当执行一项政策，要求针灸委员会使用适当的技术解决方案，以提高针灸委员会的履职能力。

该政策应当确保公众能够在互联网上与针灸委员会进行互动。

第 205.107 条　协商规则制定和替代性争议解决政策

（a）在医学委员会的建议和批准后,针灸委员会应当制定和实施一项政策,以鼓励使用:

（1）根据《政府法典》第 2008 节,通过针灸委员会规则的制定程序。

（2）根据《政府法典》第 2009 节规定的适当替代性争议解决程序,协助解决针灸委员会管辖范围内的内部和外部纠纷。

（b）针灸委员会与替代性争议解决方式有关的程序,应当尽可能符合州行政听证办公室发布的由州机构使用替代争议解决的示范指导方针。

（c）针灸委员会应当指定一名训练有素的人员:

（1）协调（a）规定的政策的实施。

（2）作为执行协商规则制定或者替代性争议解决程序所需的培训资源。

（3）收集有关针灸委员会有效实施这些程序的数据。

第 D 节　公众查阅资料及申诉程序

第 205.151 条　公共利益信息

（a）针灸委员会应当准备符合公众利益的信息,说明针灸委员会的职能,以及向针灸委员会提出申诉并解决申诉的程序。

（b）针灸委员会应当向公众和适当的州政府机构提供这些信息。

第 205.152 条　申诉

（a）针灸委员会应当根据规则规定制定方法,通知消费者和服务接受者的姓名、邮寄地址,以及针灸委员会的电话号码,目的是为了向针灸委员会提出申诉。

针灸委员会可以在以下文件上做出提示:

（1）在受本节规定监管的人员的每份登记表、申请或者书面合同上。

（2）在受本节规定监管的人员的营业地点显著标识上;或者

（3）在受本节规定监管的人员所提供的服务账单上。

（b）针灸委员会应当保存向针灸委员会提交的每份申诉信息。

信息包括:

（1）收到申诉的日期。

（2）申诉人的姓名。

（3）申诉的主要事项。

（4）与申诉有关的所有相关人员的记录。

（5）对申诉书的审查或者调查结果的摘要。

（6）对于针灸委员会没有处理申诉,对申诉未采取行动就结束的原因的解释。

（c）针灸委员会应当保存关于向针灸委员会提交的有权解决的每一份书面申诉的文件。

针灸委员会应当向申诉人和申诉对象提供针灸委员会有关申诉调查和解决的政策和程序。

（d）针灸委员会至少每季度,在申诉的最终处理之前,应当通知申诉人和申诉对象每个申诉的状况,除非该通知会阻碍调查。

第 205.1521 条　调查行为

针灸委员会应当在收到申诉之日起的第三十日内,完成对收到的申诉进行的初步调查。

针灸委员会应当首先确定针灸师是否对公共福利构成持续的威胁。

在初步调查完成后,针灸委员会应当决定是否继续进行申诉。

如针灸委员会未能在本节规定的时间内完成初步调查,则针灸委员会对该申诉的正式调查将被视为于该日开始。

第 205.153 条　公众参与

（a）经医学委员会的建议和批准,针灸委员会应当制定和实施政策,为公众提供面对面接触针灸委员会,并就针灸委员会管辖范围内的问题发表言论的合理机会。

（b）行政主管应当准备并维持一份书面计划,说明如何让不会说英语的人合理地接触到针灸委员会的项目和服务。

第 E 节　执 照 要 求

第 205.201 条　需要执照

除第 205.303 条的规定外,任何人不得在本州从事针灸实践,除非该人持有根据本章颁发的针灸执照。

第 205.202 条　执照颁发

（a）针灸委员会应当向符合本章通过的规则要求的人,颁发在本州从事针灸实践的执照。

（b）针灸委员会可以授权医学委员会员工,根据本章向明确符合所有执照要求的申请人颁发执照。

如果医学委员会员工确定申请人不符合要求,应当向针灸委员会退回该申请。

根据本款颁发的执照不需要针灸委员会的正式批准。

第 205.2025 条　颁发执照的犯罪历史记录信息要求

（a）按照委员会的规定,针灸委员会要求执照申请人提交一套完整的和清晰的指纹,目的是委员会或者公共安全部门能够从公共安全部门和联邦调查局获得有关犯罪历史记录信息。

（b）针灸委员会不得向不符合(a)的人发放执照。

（c）针灸委员会应当使用以下信息对每个执照申请人进行犯罪历史记录信息检查:

（1）根据本条由个人提供。

（2）由公共安全部、联邦调查局和任何其他刑事司法机构根据《政府法典》第 411 章提供给委员会。

（d）针灸委员会可以:

（1）与公共安全部签订协议,管理本条要求的犯罪历史记录信息检查。

（2）授权公共安全部向每个申请人收取公共安全部在进行犯罪历史记录信息检查时所发生的费用。

第 205.203 条　执照考试

（a）申请针灸执照的申请人,应当通过本节规定的针灸考试和经针灸委员会批准的法学考试。

（b）申请人必须具备以下条件,才有资格参加考试：

（1）至少年满二十一周岁。

（2）完成至少六十学时的大学课程,包括针灸委员会决定的基础科学课程。

（3）毕业于针灸学校,其入学要求与教学课程符合本法第205.206条规定的标准。

（c）针灸考试应当对实践和理论针灸以及针灸委员会要求的其他科目进行。

（c-1）对本州针灸专业执业所适用的许可要求和其他法律或者法规进行法学审查。

（d）根据针灸委员会的要求,考试应可以是书面形式,也可以通过实践操作证明申请人的技能,或两者兼而有之。

（e）医学委员会应当向每位申请人通知考试的时间和地点。

（f）针灸委员会应当通过（c-1）规定的法学审查规则：

（1）本考试的发展情况。

（2）申请费用。

（3）负责考试的管理工作。

（4）复审程序。

（5）分级程序。

（6）通知结果。

第205.204条　申请考试

申请考试时,应当是：

（1）以针灸委员会规定的书面形式呈现。

（2）经宣誓书核实。

（3）向行政主管提交的文件。

（4）提交医学委员会规定的费用。

第205.2045条　申请人在针灸委员会出庭

针灸执照的申请人不得在针灸委员会或者针灸委员会内部的理事会露面,除非该申请提出有关以下问题：

（1）申请人的身体或者精神障碍。

（2）申请人犯罪;或者

（3）撤销申请人持有的职业执照。

第205.205条　考试结果

（a）在本节规定执照考试后三十日内,针灸委员会应当将考试结果通知每位考生。如果考试由州测试机构评分或者审查,针灸委员会应当不迟于针灸委员会收到测试结果之日起的第十四日将考试结果通知考生。

（b）州考试服务机构评分或者审核的考试将逾期超过九十日的,针灸委员会应当在考试九十日前将逾期原因通知考生。针灸委员会可能要求考试服务机构通知考生考试结果。

（c）如未通过本节规定的执照考试的人提出书面要求,如果州检测服务机构提供分析报告,针灸委员会应当向患者提供患者在考试中的表现分析报告。

第 205.206 条　针灸学校

（a）一个声誉良好的针灸学校,除了符合针灸委员会制定的标准外,还应当:

（1）维持一个不少于四个月的住院教学课程,一共六次,总共不少于一千八百学时。

（2）为住院医师提供至少两学期的受监督的患者治疗。

（3）开设解剖学方面的教学课程——组织学、细菌学、生理学、症状学、病理学、经络和穴位位置、卫生学和公共卫生。

（4）具备必要的教学力量和设施,以便对必修课程进行适当的教学。

（b）在制定针灸学校的入学要求和课程教学标准时,针灸委员会可以考虑国家针灸和东方医学学校和学院认证委员会(NACSCAOM)制定的标准。

（c）除本节的其他要求外,针灸学校或者学位课程应当经得克萨斯州高等教育协调委员会的批准,除非该学校或者课程符合《教育法典》第 61.303 条规定的豁免条件。

（d）在按照(c)审查针灸学校或者学位课程时,得克萨斯州高等教育协调委员会应当征求针灸委员会的意见,以评估学校或者学位课程能否具备培养个人从事针灸实践的能力。

第 205.207 条　互惠许可

医学委员会在审查了申请人的资历,确定申请人持有的另一个州的执照要求与本州基本相同后,可以免除对申请人的条件限制。

第 205.208 条　临时执照

（a）针灸委员会可以通过行政主管向下列申请人颁发从事针灸实践的临时执照:

（1）以针灸委员会规定的形式提交申请。

（2）已通过针灸委员会认可的与针灸执业有关的州或者其他考试。

（3）支付一定的费用。

（4）如果在其他州有执照,也可获得针灸师资格。

（5）符合本节规定的所有执照资格,但正在等待医学委员会的下一次预定会议,以便颁发执照。

（b）临时执照的有效期为签发日期后的一百日,首发的临时执照到期后只能再延长三十日。

第 F 节　执 照 续 期

第 205.251 条　续期要求

（a）医学委员会应当根据规则规定,每年或者每两年续期一次针灸执照。

（b）医学委员会可以根据规则,在一年中规定不同的执照到期日。对于执照有效期变更的年份,执照费用应当按月按比例分配,以便每位持证人只需支付与执照有效月数相应的那部分执照费用。在新的到期日续期执照时,应当全额支付执照续期费。

第 205.2515 条　续期执照所需的犯罪历史记录

（a）根据本章签发的执照续期的申请人应当提交一套完整、清晰的指纹,以便根据第 205.2025 条的规定对申请人进行犯罪历史记录信息检查。

(b)对不符合(a)要求的人,针灸委员会可以吊销或者拒绝续期执照。

(c)如果持证人之前曾在以下情形提交过指纹,则无须根据本条提交指纹:

(1)根据第205.2025条获得首次执照;或者

(2)本条作为执照事先续期的一部分。

第205.252条　执照到期通知

在个人执照到期前三十日内,医学委员会应当根据记录,向该人最新地址发送执照即将到期的书面通知。

第205.253条　续期程序

(a)拥有其他资格条件续期执照的人,可以在执照到期前向医学委员会支付所需的续期费用,以续期未到期的执照。执照到期人员,在根据本条或者第205.254条续期执照之前,不得从事需要执照方可从事的活动。

(b)个人执照期满九十日或者以下的,可以向医学委员会支付相当于所需续期费用一点五倍的费用来续期执照。

(c)执照到期九十日以上不满一年的,可以向医学委员会支付所需续期费两倍的费用。

(d)执照期满一年以上的,不得续期。该人可以通过提交复审并遵守获得原始执照的要求和程序,获得一份新的执照。

第205.254条　由州外的执业医师执照的续期

(a)医学委员会可在不复审的情况下续期在该州执业的人的执照,如果某人在本州获得了针灸执照,移居到另一州,并且在申请之前的两年内,目前在另一州获得了执照并一直在执业,那么医学委员会可以不经重新审查而为其续期执照。

(b)该人应当向医学委员会支付一笔相当于执照所需续期费的两倍的费用。

第205.255条　继续教育

(a)针灸委员会可以通过规则要求持证人,完成一定数量的针灸委员会批准的继续教育课程,以续期执照。

(a-1)针灸委员会应当制定授予继续教育学分的书面指导原则,具体规定如下:

(1)程序要求。

(2)被认为是继续教育首选提供者所需的资格。

(3)课程内容要求。

(b)针灸委员会应当考虑批准一门由以下人员主持的课程:

(1)一位有知识背景的保健提供者;或者

(2)一所有信誉的学校、州或者专业组织。

(c)在根据(a-1)制定准则后,针灸委员会应当授权医学委员会雇员对明确符合准则的课程申请进行审批。医学委员会雇员应当将任何不明显符合准则的课程提交给针灸委员会审查和批准。

第205.256条　违反委员会命令而被拒绝

如果持证人违反了针灸委员会的命令,针灸委员会可以拒绝续期根据本章颁发的执照。

第 G 节　持证人的实践

第 205.301 条　需要其他卫生保健从业者的转诊

（a）持证人只有在以下情况下才可以对某人做针灸治疗：

（1）在实施针灸之前的六个月内,由医生或者牙医对所治疗的疾病进行评估;或者

（2）在实施针灸之前的三十日内,由脊椎按摩师转诊。

（b）根据（a）（1）行事的持证人应当获得合理的文件,证明已经进行了所需的评估。如果持证人不能确定已经进行了评估,持证人应当获得一份由当事人在针灸委员会规定的表格上签字的书面声明,说明当事人已经在规定时间内接受了医生或者牙医的评估。该表格必须包含一项明确声明,即该人应当由医生或者牙医对持证人所治疗的疾病进行评估。

（c）根据（a）（2）行事的持证人,在针灸二十次或者三十日后（以先发生者为准）,如果该人的病情没有发生实质性改善,应当将其转诊给其他医生。

（d）医学委员会在征求针灸委员会的意见后,可以通过规则修改如下内容：

（1）根据（a）（1）规定的评估范围。

（2）根据（a）（1）或者（a）（2）应当开始治疗的时期;或者

（3）根据（c）要求转诊给医生之前的治疗次数或者天数。

第 205.302 条　无转诊的授权执业

（a）经过通知和公开听证后,医学委员会应当通过规则确定针灸师是否可以在没有医生、牙医或者按摩师转诊的情况下为患者治疗酒精中毒或者慢性疼痛。

医学委员会应当根据临床证据和医学委员会确定的符合受影响患者的最佳利益来做出决定。

（b）尽管有第 205.301 条的规定,持证人可以在没有医生、牙医或者脊椎医生转诊的情况下,为以下的个人进行针灸治疗：

（1）吸烟成瘾。

（2）减肥;或者

（3）药物滥用,在医学委员会规定的范围内。

第 205.303 条　针灸戒毒专家

（a）医学委员会可以根据本条规定,将某人认证为针灸戒毒专家,如果该人：

（1）向医疗委员会提供其文件。

（A）是持证社会工作者、持证专业咨询师、持证心理学家、持证化学药物依赖咨询师、持证职业护士,或者持证注册护士。

（B）已经顺利完成了符合医学委员会批准的准则的针灸戒毒培训课程。

（2）支付由医学委员会规定的认证费。

（b）针灸戒毒专家只可以在以下情况下从事针灸实践：

（1）在医学委员会通过的治疗酒精中毒、药物滥用或者化学药物依赖的规则允许的范围内。

（2）在持证针灸师或者医生的监督下。

（c）包括针灸戒毒专家服务的项目应当：

（1）通知该项目的每个参与者其针灸戒毒专家的资质以及向医学委员会申诉针灸戒毒专家的程序。

（2）记录每个客户的姓名，客户接受针灸戒毒专家服务的日期，以及针灸戒毒专家的姓名、签名和认证号码。

（d）医学委员会可以根据本节规定每年续期针灸戒毒专家的认证，如果该人：

（1）向医学委员会提供以下文件：

（A）根据（a）（1）（A）要求的证书或者执照是有效的。

（B）该人已成功达到医学委员会根据（e）规定的继续教育要求。

（2）支付医学委员会规定的金额的认证续期费。

（e）医学委员会应当制定针灸戒毒专家的继续教育要求，至少包括六学时的针灸实践教育和一门关于洁针技术或者通用感染控制预防程序的课程。

第 205.304 条　专业审查法

第 160.002 条、第 160.003 条、第 160.006 条、第 160.007（d）条、第 160.013 条、第 160.014 条和第 160.015 条的规定，适用于与针灸师或者针灸师学员的针灸实践有关的专业审查法。

第 205.305 条　持证人的信息

（a）每位持证人都应当向针灸委员会备案以下信息：

（1）持证人的邮寄地址。

（2）持证人的居住地址。

（3）持证人的各办公室的通信地址。

（4）持证人的各办公室的实际地址，如果该办公室的实际地址与通信地址不同。

（b）持证人应当：

（1）通知针灸委员会其居住地址或者工作地址的变更。

（2）在地址变更后的三十日内，向针灸委员会提供持证人的新地址。

第 H 节　纪律处分程序

第 205.351 条　拒绝颁发执照或者纪律处分的依据

（a）在下列情况下，可以拒绝颁发针灸执业执照，或者在通知和听证之后，根据第 205.352 条对持证人实施纪律处分：

（1）滥用药物或者醉酒，以至于委员会认为可能危及患者的生命。

（2）以欺诈或者欺骗的方式获得或者试图获得执照。

（3）被法院判定为精神不健全的。

（4）有精神或者身体状况，使其不能安全地履行针灸师的职责。

（5）未能以符合公众健康和福利的可接受的方式从事针灸实践。

（6）违反本节规定或者根据本节通过的规则。

（7）曾被判定犯有涉及道德败坏的罪行或者重罪，或者因此类罪行被延期判决或者审前改造。

（8）以医生或者外科医生或者这些术语的任何组合或者衍生物的身份出现,除非该人也获得了医疗委员会的医生或者外科医生执照。

（9）欺诈性或者欺骗性地使用执照。

（10）从事违反职业道德或者不光彩的行为,有可能欺骗、欺诈或者伤害公众成员。

（11）犯有违反州法律的行为,如果该行为与该人的针灸师实践有关。

（12）未对在持证人监督下活动的人的活动进行充分监督的。

（13）直接或者间接地帮助或者教唆任何未获针灸委员会颁发针灸执照的人从事针灸实践。

（14）因疾病、醉酒或者过度使用药物、麻醉品、化学品或者任何其他类型的材料,或者因任何精神或者身体状况,无法以合理的技能安全地对患者从事针灸实践。

（15）在针灸委员会看来,多次或者反复出现有价值的医疗责任索赔,证明其专业能力不足,可能会伤害公众。

（16）曾被其他州吊销、撤销或者限制针灸执业资格,或者受到其他州或者美国军警部门有关针灸师执业的其他纪律处分;或者

（17）通过持证人的针灸师执业行为对他人进行性虐待或者剥削。

（b）如果针灸委员会提议吊销、撤销或者拒绝续期某人的执照,该人有权要求由州行政听证办公室进行听证。

（c）根据（a）（11）提起的诉讼,不需要对违法行为的申诉、起诉或者定罪。

证明在针灸实践中或者以针灸实践为幌子而实施的行为,足以让针灸委员会采取行动。

（d）就（a）（16）而言,州或者美国军警部门采取行动的记录的认证副本是该行动的决定性证据。

第 205.352 条　针灸委员会的纪律处分权力

（a）在发现有理由拒绝颁发执照或者对持证人采取纪律处分时,针灸委员会可以通过命令:

（1）拒绝该人的针灸执照、执照续期或者证书的申请,或者撤销该人的针灸执照或者证书。

（2）要求该人接受针灸委员会指定的卫生保健从业者的护理、咨询或者治疗,以此作为颁发、延续或者续期针灸执照或者证书的条件。

（3）要求接受针灸委员会规定的教育或者咨询。

（4）暂停、限制该人的针灸执照或者证书,包括将该人的执业活动限制在或者排除在一项或者多项特定的针灸活动之外,或者规定由针灸委员会定期审查。

（5）要求该人在针灸委员会指定的针灸师指导下执业一段时间。

（6）依照第 J 节的规定对被执行人作出行政处罚。

（7）要求该人从事针灸委员会认为适当的公共服务。

（8）暂停执行命令,将当事人列入察看状态,针灸委员会保留撤销察看的权利,并对不遵守察看条款的行为执行原命令,或者实施本条授权的各种其他补救措施或者制裁。

（9）要求该人继续接受或者复习专业教育,直到其在第（8）款规定的察看期的基础上达到针灸委员会满意的技能程度。

（10）要求该人定期向针灸委员会报告作为第（8）款规定的察看基础的事项；或者

（11）进行公开训斥。

（b）针灸委员会可以恢复或者重新颁发执照，或者取消针灸委员会根据本规条定采取的各种纪律处分或者补救措施。

第 205.3522 条 注销执照

（a）针灸委员会可以接受自愿注销执照。

（b）除非针灸委员会根据针灸委员会的规则确定原持证人有能力恢复执业，否则不得将注销的执照归还给持证人。

（c）针灸委员会应当向医学委员会建议确定前持证人恢复执业能力的规则。

第 205.3523 条 身体或者精神检查

（a）针灸委员会应当与本条有关或者受本条影响的人员共同制定准则，使委员会能够评估针灸师或者申请人在何种情况下可能被要求就精神或者身体健康状况、酗酒和药物滥用或者专业行为问题接受检查。

（b）针灸委员会应当将有身体或者精神健康问题的针灸师或者申请人转诊至最适当的医疗专家。除非有相关医学指征表明，否则针灸委员会不得要求针灸师或者申请人接受委员会指定的专科医生的检查。针灸委员会不得要求针灸师或者申请人在距离其居住地或者营业地点不合理的距离接受检查，除非针灸师或者申请人居住和工作的地区能够进行适当检查的医生数量有限。

（c）根据本条通过的准则并不损害或者取消针灸委员会作出独立颁发执照决定的权力。

第 205.353 条 2005 年 9 月 1 日，根据 2005 年法案第 79 编第 269 章第 3.35 条废除

第 205.354 条 纪律处分程序规则

医学委员会根据《政府法典》第 2001.004 条通过的适用于纪律处分程序的实践规则，不得与国家行政听证办公室通过的规则相冲突。

第 205.3541 条 非正式程序

（a）针灸委员会应当通过规则来管理以下程序：

（1）根据《政府法典》第 2001.056 条对有争议的案件进行非正式处理。

（2）根据《政府法典》第 2001.054 条规定进行的非正式程序。

（b）根据本条通过的规则应当规定：

（1）根据《政府法典》第 2001.054 条的规定，非正式会议应当在向针灸委员会提出申诉之日起一百八十日内安排，除非针灸委员会有充分理由在该日期之后安排非正式会议。

（2）针灸委员会不迟于会议召开前三十日将会议的时间、地点通知持证人。

（3）给予申诉人和持证人申诉的机会。

（4）作为小组成员参加非正式会议的针灸委员会成员至少有一名是代表公众的成员。

（5）针灸委员会的法律顾问或者总检察长的代表出席会议，为针灸委员会或者医学委员会的工作人员提供建议。

（6）医学委员会的一名雇员应出席会议，向针灸委员会代表陈述医学委员会工作人员合理地认为可以通过合格的证据或者合格的证人在听证会上证明的事实。

（c）受影响的针灸师有权以口头或者书面的方式：

（1）对工作人员的陈述作出答复。

（2）在听证会上提出针灸师合理地认为可以通过合格的证据或者合格的证人证明的事实。

（d）在给予充分的陈述时间后，针灸委员会小组应当建议结束调查，或者尝试对有争议的事项进行调解，并根据有关争议案件的适用法律，在没有听证的情况下，就案件的处理提出建议。

（e）如果持证人曾经受过针灸委员会的纪律处分，针灸委员会应当在可行的情况下尽快安排非正式会议，但不得迟于（b）（1）规定的最后期限。

第 205.3542 条　针灸委员会在非正式诉讼中的代理权

（a）在根据本法第 205.3541 条进行的非正式程序中，应当至少任命两名专家小组成员，以确定非正式处理是否适当。

（b）尽管有（a）和第 205.3541（b）（4）条的规定，如果涉案针灸师放弃至少由两名小组医生进行非正式程序的要求，则可以由一名小组医生进行非正式程序。如果针灸师放弃了这个要求，小组成员可以是针灸委员会的任何成员。

（c）（a）所述的专家组要求适用于针灸委员会根据第 205.3541 条进行的非正式程序，包括针对以下目的的程序：

（1）审议违纪案件，确定是否发生违纪行为；或者

（2）请求变更或者终止命令。

（d）（a）所述的专家组要求不适用于针灸委员会根据第 205.3541 条为表明对针灸委员会命令的遵守而进行的非正式程序。

第 205.3543 条　非正式程序参与者的角色和责任

（a）针灸委员会成员在第 205.3541 条规定的非正式会议上担任小组成员，应当就申诉或者指控的处理提出建议。该成员可以随时请求医学委员会雇员的协助。

（b）医学委员会雇员应当就针对受影响针灸师的指控，以及雇员合理地认为可以在正式听证中得到适当证据证明的与该指控有关的事实，提交摘要。

（c）尽管（e）另有规定，针灸委员会或者医学委员会的律师应当担任小组的律师，并应当在非正式会议和小组讨论期间出席，就程序中出现的法律问题向小组提供意见。律师可以在非正式会议中向与会者提问，以澄清与会者所作的陈述。律师应当向小组提供针灸委员会或者医学委员会出现过的具有可比性的案例的历史观点，使诉讼程序聚焦于正在讨论的案件，并确保医学委员会的雇员和受影响的针灸师有机会陈述与案件相关的信息。在小组审议期间，律师只能就法律问题向小组提供咨询意见，并就针灸委员会或者医学委员会审理过的类似案件提供资料。

（d）小组和医学委员会雇员应当为受影响的针灸师和针灸师的授权代表提供机会，以答复委员会雇员的陈述，并提出针灸师和代表合理地认为可以在正式听证会上有足够证据证明的口头和书面陈述以及事实。

（e）参与陈述指控或者在调查申诉中收集资料的医学委员会雇员、受影响的针灸师、针

灸师的授权代表、申诉人、证人和公众人士不得出席小组的讨论。只有专家组成员和担任专家组律师的律师可以在审议过程中出席。

（f）专家小组应当建议驳回申诉或者指控，或者如果专家小组确定受影响的针灸师违反了法规或者针灸委员会规则，专家小组可以建议委员会采取行动和非正式解决案件的条款。

（g）小组根据(f)提出的建议应当以书面形式提出，并提交给受影响的针灸师及其授权代表。针灸师可以以小组在非正式会议上确定的时间内接受提议的解决方案。如果针灸师拒绝拟议的解决方案或者未在规定时间内采取行动，针灸委员会可以向州行政听证办公室提出正式申诉。

第 205.3544 条　调查文件查阅限制

针灸委员会应当按照第 164.007(c)条规定的方式，禁止或者限制在非正式程序中查阅与持证人有关的调查文件。

第 205.355 条　未获得转诊的必要纪律处分

除第 205.301(a)(2)条的规定外，如果申请人或者持证人违反了第 205.301(a)(1)条的规定，则应当拒绝颁发针灸执照，或者经通知和听证后吊销执照。

第 205.356 条　康复令

（a）针灸委员会可以通过一项商定的命令或者在一项有争议的程序后，对申请人或者持证人发出非纪律处分性质的康复令，作为颁发执照的先决条件，其理由如下：

（1）由医生提供的医疗护理或者治疗引起的习惯或者成瘾直接造成的过度使用药品或者酒精。

（2）该人在报告日期之前的五年内过度使用药物或者酒精，而可能对该人安全从事针灸实践的能力产生不利影响，如果该人：

（A）曾报告其有过度使用历史。

（B）针灸委员会此前并未发出与药物滥用有关的命令。

（C）未因药物或酒精损害而违反治疗标准。

（3）法院作出该人精神不健全的判决；或者

（4）精神或者身体检查的结果，或者该人的承认，表明该人由于疾病或者任何身体或者精神状况的原因而遭受潜在危险的限制或者无法以合理的技能和安全的方式从事针灸实践。

（b）如果针灸委员会在该人签署拟议的命令之前收到该人过度使用药物或者酒精并影响治疗标准的有效申诉，则该委员会不得根据本条规定发布康复令。

（c）在根据本条规定下达命令之前，针灸委员会应当确定个人是否违反了本条(a)(2)所述的治疗标准。

（d）针灸委员会只能根据第 205.3562 条的规定向当地或者全州的私人针灸协会披露康复令。

第 205.3561 条　免疫专家

协助针灸委员会工作的专家，在协助委员会实施纪律处分的过程中，在没有欺诈或者恶意的情况下进行的任何调查、报告、建议、陈述、评估、发现或者其他行动，可以免于起诉和判决，也不得受到损害赔偿的起诉。

总检察长应当在专家为针灸委员会真诚提供的服务所引起的任何诉讼中代表专家。

第 205.3562 条　私人协会的职责

（a）如果根据第 205.356 条规定的康复令要求持证人参加当地或者全州私人针灸协会提供的活动或者项目,针灸委员会应当将持证人在康复令下的职责告知该协会。根据本条规定提供的信息应当包括具体的指导,以使该协会能够遵守各项必要的要求,协助针灸师复权。

（b）针灸委员会可以向协会提供委员会认为必要的各种信息,包括康复令的副本。协会收到的任何信息都是保密的,不受证据、传票或者其他法律强制手段的约束,并且只能向针灸委员会披露。

第 205.357 条　康复令的影响

（a）根据第 205.356 条施加的康复令是一项非纪律处分性的私人命令。如果是通过协议达成的,则该命令为民事诉讼目的而达成的协议处理或者和解协议,不受公开记录法的约束。

（b）根据第 205.356 条作出的康复令应当包含事实调查结果和法律结论。该命令可以撤销、取消、吊销、列入察看期或者限制期,或者本节授权或者针灸委员会和受命令人同意的各种其他期限。

（c）违反康复令可以根据本节的规定对有争议的事项或者商定的命令的条款实施纪律处分。

（d）违反康复令可以根据下列理由实施纪律处分:

（1）违反职业道德或者不光彩的行为;或者

（2）本节中适用于导致违规的行为的各项规定。

第 205.358 条　康复令的审核

（a）针灸委员会应当将根据第 205.356 条实施的康复令保存在一个保密档案中。该档案应当接受单独审计,以确保只有合格的持证人才受到康复令的约束。审计工作应当由州审计师或者与针灸委员会签约的私人审计师进行。

（b）在针灸委员会的指导下,可以在任何时候进行审计。针灸委员会应当确保在每三年内至少进行一次审计。

（c）审计结果属于公共记录,并且应当以维护每个受康复令约束的持证人的保密的方式进行报告。

第 205.359 条　传票

（a）医学委员会行政主管或者针灸委员会审裁官可以以针灸委员会的名义发出传票:

（1）为了与下列情况有关的调查或者有争议的程序:

（A）指控针灸师的不端行为;或者

（B）指控违反本节规定或者与针灸师执业有关的其他法律,或者在本节授权下提供医疗保健服务。

（2）决定是否:

（A）颁发、吊销、限制、撤销或者取消本节授权的执照;或者

（B）拒绝或者批准根据本节规定提出的执照申请。

（b）未能及时遵守根据本节规定发出的传票可作为以下理由之一：

（1）由针灸委员会或者任何其他对被传唤的个人或者单位有管辖权的执照或者监管机构实施纪律处分。

（2）拒绝执照申请。

第205.360条　特定申诉处理的授权

（a）针灸委员会可以授权医学委员会雇员对不直接涉及患者护理或者只涉及行政违规的申诉进行驳回或者达成协议解决。该委员会决定的处理方式应当由针灸委员会在公开会议上批准。

（b）在下列情况下，根据本条授权的申诉应当根据第205.3541条提交非正式程序：

（1）雇员委员会决定不应当驳回申诉或者进行和解。

（2）委员会无法达成一致的解决方案；或者

（3）受影响的针灸师要求将该申诉转为非正式程序。

第205.361条　暂时吊销

（a）针灸委员会主席经该委员会批准，应当任命一个由针灸委员会成员组成的三人纪律处分小组，以决定是否应当暂时吊销某人的针灸执照。

（b）如果纪律处分小组根据提交给小组的资料确定，获发针灸师执照的人若继续从事针灸师实践，将对公众福利构成持续威胁，则纪律处分小组应当暂时吊销该人的执照。

（c）在下列情况下，可以根据本条的规定吊销执照，无须通知或者就申诉举行听证会：

（1）在暂时吊销的同时提请针灸委员会听证。

（2）根据《政府法典》第2001节以及本节规定尽快举行听证。

（d）尽管有《政府法典》第551节的规定，如果纪律处分小组需要立即采取行动，而在一个地点召开纪律处分小组会议对任何纪律处分小组成员都不方便，则纪律处分小组可以通过电话会议的方式举行会议。

第205.362条　终止和禁止令

（a）如果针灸委员会认为没有根据本节获得执照的人正在违反本节规定、根据本节通过的规则，或者与针灸实践有关的其他州的法规或者规则，委员会在通知并有机会进行听证后，可以发出终止和禁止令，禁止该人从事该活动。

（b）违反本条规定的命令构成根据第205.352条实施行政处罚的理由。

第205.363条　退款

（a）在遵守（b）的规定的前提下，针灸委员会可以命令持证人按照非正式和解会议达成的协议规定，向消费者支付退款，而不是根据本节的规定进行行政处罚，或者将其作为补充。

（b）根据（a）要求的退款金额，不得超过消费者为本节规定的服务向持证人支付的金额。针灸委员会不得在退款命令中要求支付其他损失或者预估伤害。

第205.364条　行政法法官对调查结果或者裁决的修改

只有在针灸委员会做出《政府法典》第2001.058（e）条所要求的决定时，针灸委员会才可以改变事实认定或者法律结论，或者撤销或者修改行政法法官的命令。

第 I 节　刑事处罚和其他强制性条款

第 205.401 条　刑事处罚

（a）除第 205.303 条规定的情况外，如果某人在本州没有根据本节获发执照而从事针灸实践，则构成犯罪行为。

（b）违反（a）的规定而每日从事针灸实践的人，构成单独的犯罪。

（c）（a）规定的犯罪行为是三级重罪。

第 205.402 条　禁令救济；民事处罚

（a）针灸委员会、总检察长，或者地区或者县检察官可以提起民事诉讼，以强制遵守本节规定或者执行根据本章通过的规则。

（b）除禁令救济或者法律规定的各种其他补救措施外，违反本章规定或者根据本节通过的规则的人应向国家承担民事罚款，每次罚款金额不超过两千美元。

（c）就实施民事处罚而言，违法行为持续或者发生的每一日都是一个单独的违法行为。

（d）总检察长在针灸委员会的要求下，或者在总检察长的倡议下，可以提起民事诉讼，收取民事罚款。

第 J 节　行　政　处　罚

第 205.451 条　行政处罚的实施

针灸委员会可以通过命令对违反本节规定获发执照或者规定的人，或者对违反本节通过的规则或者命令的人实施行政处罚。

第 205.452 条　行政处罚的程序

（a）针灸委员会应当按照规则规定其可以施加行政处罚的程序。

（b）本分节规定的诉讼应当受《政府法典》2001 节的约束。

第 205.453 条　罚款金额

（a）每项违法行为的行政处罚金额不得超过五千美元。违法行为持续或者发生的每一日都是一个单独的违法行为，以便进行处罚。

（b）罚款金额应当根据以下情况而定：

（1）违法行为的严重性，包括：

（A）任何被禁止行为的性质、情况、范围和严重性。

（B）对公众健康、安全或者经济福利造成的危害或者潜在危害。

（2）违法行为对财产或者环境造成的经济损害。

（3）既往违规史。

（4）阻止未来违法行为所需的金额。

（5）为纠正违法行为所做的努力。

（6）司法可能要求的任何其他事项。

第 205.454 条　违规和处罚通知书

（a）如果针灸委员会通过命令确定发生了违规行为并进行了行政处罚，则针灸委员会应当将委员会的命令通知受影响的人。

（b）该通知应当包括该人对该命令进行司法审查的权利声明。

第 205.455 条　选择以下决定：缴纳罚款或者提出上诉

（a）不迟于针灸委员会的行政处罚决定书生效后的第三十日，当事人应当：

（1）缴纳罚款。

（2）缴纳罚款，并就违法行为的发生、罚款金额或者两者提出司法审查申请；或者

（3）在不支付罚款的情况下，就违法行为的发生、罚款金额或者两者提出司法审查申请。

（b）在三十日的期限内，根据（a）（3）行事的人可以：

（1）通过以下方式停止执行处罚：

（A）向法院支付罚款，并将其存入代管账户；或者

（B）向法院提交一份由法院批准的超额保证金，金额为处罚金额，该保证金在针灸委员会命令的所有司法审查结束前有效；或者

（2）通过以下方式请求法院停止执行该处罚：

（A）向法院提交一份该人的宣誓书，说明该人在经济上无力支付罚款，也无力提供超额保证金。

（B）将宣誓书的副本以挂号信的方式上交给针灸委员会的审裁官。

（c）如果针灸委员会审裁官收到（b）（2）规定的宣誓书副本，则其可在收到副本后的第五日内向法院提交对宣誓书的异议。

（d）法院应在可行的情况下尽快就宣誓书中指控的事实举行听证会，并在认定指控的事实属实后暂缓当事人执行处罚。提交宣誓书的人有责任证明其在经济上无力支付罚款和超额保证金。

第 205.456 条　收取罚款

如果当事人不支付行政处罚的罚款，且处罚的执行未被中止，则针灸委员会的审裁官可以将该事项提交给总检察长，以收取罚款。

第 205.457 条　法院裁决

（a）如果法院在上诉时维持对发生违法行为的裁定，法院可以维持或者减少行政处罚的金额，并命令该人支付全额或者减少的罚款。

（b）如果法院不维持发生违法行为的裁定，法院应下令不予罚款。

第 205.458 条　罚息汇付

（a）经司法审查，行政处罚减轻或者不予行政处罚的，判决终结后，法院应当：

（1）已缴纳罚款的，责令将适当金额和应计利息汇给该人；或者

（2）不予行政处罚的，责令全额发还保证金；已提交超额保证金的，责令在该人缴纳罚款后发还保证金。

（b）根据（a）（1）支付的利息，为纽约联邦储备银行向存款机构收取的贷款利率。利息的支付时间从支付罚款之日起至汇出罚款之日止。

得克萨斯州针灸行政法[①]

第 183.1 条　目的

（a）这些规则是根据《医疗服务法案》（即得克萨斯州《职业法典》第 3 卷 B 编）和《针灸法案》（即得克萨斯州《职业法典》第 205 章）的规定颁布，旨在为本州从事针灸实践者的培训、教育、许可和纪律处分事宜制定程序和标准，从而建立一个以保护公众健康、安全和福利的方式，规范针灸执业的有序制度。

（b）针灸委员会的职能包括但不限于以下内容：

（1）建立针灸的实践标准。

（2）通过针灸执照和纪律处分来规范针灸的执业。

（3）向针灸师和公众解释《针灸法案》和《针灸委员会规则》，确保专业人员、其他相关的卫生保健专业人员和消费者的知情权。

（4）接受投诉并调查可能违反《针灸法案》和《针灸委员会规则》的行为。

（5）通过适当的法律行动来执行针灸法案和针灸委员会的规则。

（6）为关于针灸法案和针灸委员会规则提供公众评论的机制。

（7）经医学委员会批准，在必要和适当时，审查和修改针灸委员会的规则。

（8）检查并许可合格的申请人在得克萨斯州进行针灸实践，以确保符合行业标准。

（9）向立法机关提供关于针灸法案的适当变化的建议，以确保该法案有效，并适用于不断变化的需求和执业活动。

（10）提供有关持证人的非正式公共信息。

（11）保存有关针灸实践的数据。

第 183.2 条　定义

除非另有说明，本章使用的术语具有下列含义：

（1）英语沟通能力——符合本卷第 183.4（a）（8）条（有关执照）要求的申请人。

（2）可接受的获批针灸学校——1996 年 1 月 1 日生效，并符合得克萨斯州《职业法典》第 205.206 条的要求。

（A）位于美国或者加拿大的针灸学院，在申请人毕业时，是针灸及东方医学教育审核委员会（ACAOM）或者得克萨斯州高等教育协调委员会认可的其他认证机构的认证候选人，提供认证的课程申请人的毕业相当于认证的课程，提供硕士学位或者专业证书或者文凭毕业后，并有一千八百学时的课程，其中至少四百五十学时的中药研究当包括以下内容：

（i）基本中药学，包括识别、命名、功效、性味、禁忌证和配伍。

（ii）方剂学，包括传统方剂及其基于传统中药治疗方法的配伍加减或者变化。

（iii）专利中药，包括更常见的专利中药的名称及其用途。

[①]　根据《得克萨斯州行政法典》第 22 卷第 9 编第 183 章"针灸"译出。

（iv）强调中药使用的临床培训；或者

（B）位于美国或者加拿大的针灸学院，在申请人毕业时获得针灸及东方医学审核委员会或者得克萨斯高等教育协调委员会认可的其他认证机构，毕业后提供硕士学位或者专业证书或者文凭，课程时间为一千八百学时，至少有四百五十学时的中药学习，至少包括以下内容：

（i）基本中药学，包括中药识别、命名、功效、性味、禁忌证和配伍。

（ii）方剂学，包括传统方剂及其基于传统中药治疗方法的配伍加减或者变化。

（iii）专利中药学，包括更常见的专利中药的名称及其用途。

（iv）中药应用临床培训；或者

（C）位于美国或者加拿大境外的针灸学校，由委员会确定为基本上相当于得克萨斯州的针灸学校或者本条（B）中定义的学校。美国大学注册和录取管理者协会（AACRAO）的评估或者委员会要求的评估可用于进行实质性等价性的确定。

（3）针灸法案或者"法案"——《得克萨斯州职业法》第 205 章。

（4）针灸

（A）将针灸针和将针灸应当用于人体特定部位作为治疗和减轻人体病情的主要治疗方式，包括对病情的评价和评估。

（B）与（A）所述的治疗同时配合使用饮食指南、能量流功法、膳食或者草药补充剂。

（5）针灸委员会或者"委员会"——得克萨斯州针灸审查委员会。

（6）针灸师——获得针灸委员会颁发的针灸执照的持证人，直接或者间接地对提供针灸服务收取费用。

（7）机构——得克萨斯州医疗委员会、得克萨斯州医师助理委员会和得克萨斯州针灸审查委员会所述的处室、部门和雇员。

（8）APA——《行政程序法案》，即《政府法典》第 2001.001 条。

（9）申请人——向委员会申请执照的一方。

（10）申请——申请是完成申请人的执照申请所需的所有文件和信息，包括以下内容：

（A）由委员会提供，由申请人填写的申请表：

（i）所有需要书面答复的表格和附录都应当用墨水印刷或者打印出来。

（ii）照片应当符合美国政府的护照标准。

（B）由针灸委员会提供的指纹卡，由申请人填写，可以供得克萨斯州公共安全部完整读取。

（C）本标题第 183.4（c）条下要求的所有文件（关于执照文件）。

（D）所需的费用，通过一家美国银行以支票支付。

（11）助理审裁官——由针灸委员会选出的针灸委员会成员，在审裁官无行为能力或者缺席时履行审裁官的职责，或者根据新修订的《罗伯特议事规则》或者委员会规则主持的正式合格的继承者。

（12）委员会成员——针灸委员会的成员之一，根据该法案的第 205.051 条至第 205.053 条被任命和获得资格。

（13）脊椎按摩师——获得得克萨斯州脊椎按摩审查委员会的执照。

（14）争议案件——一种诉讼程序，包括但不限于许可，其中当事人的合法权利、义务或者特权将由委员会在进行裁决听证后决定。

（15）文件——在许可程序中向医疗委员会或者针灸委员会提交的申请书、呈请书、申诉书、动议书、抗议书、答复书、答辩书、通知书或者其他书面文书。

（16）有资格在毕业国家获得法律执业/执照——在学校所在国家完成所有针灸法律执业要求/执照要求的申请人，但任何公民身份要求除外。

（17）行政主管——本机构的行政主管或者行政主管的授权指定人。

（18）完全有效——在另一司法管辖区拥有执照的执照申请人应当拥有完全有效的资格，且不限制、取消、吊销或者撤销。拥有完全有效执照的针灸师可能包括在另一个司法管辖区没有现行有效的年度执照的针灸师，因为该司法管辖区要求针灸师在年度执照生效之前在该司法管辖区执业。

（19）完整的 NCCAOM 考试——国家针灸与东方医学认证委员会考试，包括以下内容：

（A）在 2004 年 6 月 1 日前参加：综合笔试（CWE）、洁针技术考试（CNTP）、点位技能实践考试（PEPLS）以及中草药学考试；或者

（B）在 2004 年 6 月 1 日或者之后参加：NCCAOM 的东方医学基础模块、针灸模块、点位技能模块、中草药学模块和生物医学模块。

（20）良好的职业品格——申请执照的申请人不得违反或者实施了该法案第 205.351 条中所述的任何行为。

（21）行政法官（ALJ）——根据《行政程序法》被任命主持行政听证的个人。

（22）执照——包括法律要求的任何委员会执照、证书、批准、注册或者类似形式的许可的全部或者部分；具体来说，执照和注册。

（23）执照——包括医疗委员会和针灸委员会关于执照的授予、拒绝、续期、撤销、暂停、取消、撤回或者修改的程序。

（24）医学委员会，得克萨斯州医学委员会。

（25）涉及道德败坏的轻罪——以欺诈、不诚实或者欺骗为基本要素的任何轻罪；入室盗窃；抢劫；性犯罪；盗窃；猥亵儿童；药物转移或者药物滥用；在私人社会责任中涉及对他人或社会的一般的卑鄙、堕落的犯罪行为；或者明知而无视正义的罪行。

（26）政党——针灸委员会和个人在 SOAH 听证会上指定或者承认的政党或者有争议的案件。

（27）个人——任何个人、合伙企业、公司、协会、政府部门，或者任何性质的公共或者私人组织。

（28）医生——获得医疗委员会颁发的执照的持证人。

（29）抗辩——当事人就其各自的索赔提出的书面文件。

（30）审裁官——由州长委任的针灸委员会成员，或者根据新修订的《罗伯特议事规则》或者委员会规则，审裁官的正式合格的继承人。

（31）注册——得克萨斯州的注册。

（32）规则——任何实施、解释或者规定法律或者政策，或者描述本委员会的程序或者

执业要求的具有一般适用性的机构声明。该术语包括前一节修订或者废除的条款,但不包括仅涉及任何机构的内部管理或者组织和不影响私人权利或者程序的声明。这一定义包括实质性的条例。

(33)秘书——针灸委员会的财务秘书。

(34)实质上等同于得克萨斯州的针灸学校——一种针灸学校或者学院,它是一所旨在选拔和教育针灸学生的高等教育机构;通过培训为学生提供获得良好针灸基础教育的机会;开发针灸教育项目,培养针灸从业者、教师和研究人员;并为研究生和继续医学教育提供机会。学校应当提供包括教师和设施在内的充足资源,支持以知识讲授和临床实践为基础的课程,使该项目能够满足相关的标准。学校的教职工应当积极促进新知识的发展和传播。针灸学院应当通过包括研究在内的学术活动,增进师生的知识并提升其学术能力。针灸学校应当包括但不限于以下特点:

(A)教学和临床培训设施(即实验室、医院、图书馆等)应当足以确保有接受适当教育的机会。

(B)招生标准应当与得克萨斯州的针灸学校基本同等。

(C)基础课程应当包括与申请人毕业时针灸及东方医学教育审核委员会(ACAOM)核心课程基本同等的课程。

(D)课程期限至少为一千八百学时。

(35)现役军人——正在服役的人员。

(36)军人配偶——与现役军人结婚的人员。

(37)退伍军人——服完现役后退役或者退伍的人员。

(38)现役——根据《政府法典》第437.001条或者其他州类似的兵役的定义,目前在美国武装部队担任全职服役或者在得克萨斯州军队服役的人。

(39)美国的武装部队——陆军、海军、空军、海岸警卫队或者海军陆战队,或者这些武装部队的一个分支的后备部队。

第183.3条 会议

(a)针灸委员会每年最多可以召开四次会议来执行该法案的授权。

(b)特别会议可以由针灸委员会审裁官召集,或者由针灸委员会决议召集,或者由至少三名委员向针灸委员会审裁官提出书面申请。

(c)针灸委员会和委员会会议应当尽可能按照新修订的《罗伯特议事规则》进行,除非针灸委员会根据规则采用不同的程序。

(d)所有选举和任何其他需要针灸委员会投票的问题,应当由出席会议的成员的简单多数决定。针灸委员会处理任何事务的法定人数应当是会议召开时针灸委员会成员的半数以上。如有两名以上的候选人参加选举,或者没有候选人在第一次选票中获得多数选票,则应当在得票数最多的两名候选人之间进行第二次投票。

(e)针灸委员会在定期会议或者特别会议上,可从其成员中选出一名助理审裁官和一名财务秘书,任期一年或者由针灸委员会多数票确定的固定任期。

(f)针灸委员会在定期会议或者特别会议上,经出席会议成员的多数投票,可罢免助理审裁官或者财务秘书。

（g）针灸委员会的常设和永久性委员会。除执行委员会以外,每个委员会应当至少包含一名获得医生执照的委员会成员、一名获得针灸执照的委员会成员以及一名公众委员会成员。如果一个委员会没有一个或者多个这些团体的代表,审裁官应当指定必要的额外成员,以维持该组成。执行委员会应当包括审裁官、助理审裁官和财务秘书,以及其他成员,使得委员会至少由两名获得针灸执照的成员(一名获得医生执照的成员和一名公众委员会成员)组成。这些委员会的职责和权力,除了包括下述内容之外,还包括针灸委员会可能临时委托的其他职责和权力。

（1）执照委员会:

（A）起草和审查有关执照的拟议规则,并就规则修订或者实施向针灸委员会提出建议。

（B）起草和审查建议的执照申请表格,并就这些规则的改变或者实施向针灸委员会提出建议。

（C）监督办理执照的申请流程。

（D）接收和审核执照申请。

（E）确定申请人的资格,提交审查结果,并就发放执照事宜向针灸委员会提出建议。

（F）监督并就考试过程向针灸委员会提出建议。包括批准适当的执照考试、考试管理,以及核实所有执照申请人分数。

（G）起草和审查有关审查的建议规则。

（H）与得克萨斯州针灸学校保持沟通。

（I）就提请执照委员会注意的事项向针灸委员会提出建议。

（2）纪律处分与伦理委员会:

（A）起草和审查关于针灸师的学科和该法案第 H 分节的执行的拟议规则。

（B）监督纪律处分程序,并指导针灸委员会和工作人员如何改进纪律处分程序的方法,更有效地执行的得克萨斯州针灸法第 H 节的规定。

（C）监督纪律处分程序的有效性、适当性和及时性。

（D）就具体案件的解决和处理提出建议,并批准、通过、修改或者拒绝针灸委员会的工作人员或者代表就对待决案件采取的行动提出的建议。批准驳回投诉和结束调查。

（E）起草和审查所提出的关于针灸实践的伦理准则和规则,并就采用该等伦理准则和规则向针灸委员会提出建议。

（F）就政策、优先次序、预算和执行相关的任何其他事项向针灸委员会和工作人员提出建议。

（G）就引起纪律处分和伦理委员会注意的问题,向针灸委员会提出建议。

（3）教育委员会:

（A）起草并提出关于在得克萨斯州获得执照的教育要求的规则,并就修订或者实施规则向针灸委员会提出建议。

（B）起草并提出有关得克萨斯州执照所需培训的规则,并就修订或者实施规则向针灸委员会提出建议。

（C）起草并提出关于更新得克萨斯州执照的继续教育要求的规则，并就修订或者实施规则向针灸委员会提出建议。

（D）与得克萨斯州高等教育协调委员会商讨有关针灸学校的教育要求、每个实体的监督责任、针灸学校可能提供的学位。

（E）与针灸学校保持沟通。

（F）计划并按一定的时间间隔访问针灸学校，以促进与学生见面的机会，使他们能够了解委员会及其职能。

（G）在课程、师资、设施、学术资源和毕业生表现等方面开发有关外国针灸学校的信息。

（H）起草并拟议针灸学位课程要求的规则。

（I）协助处理委员会职权范围内可能出现的与针灸学校的有关问题。

（J）协助执照委员会确定外国针灸学校的毕业生是否有资格获得执照。

（K）研究和核实外国针灸学校的记录并提出建议。

（L）就提请教育委员会注意的问题，向针灸委员会提出建议。

（4）执行委员会：

（A）审查委员会会议的议程。

（B）确保保存委员会所有行动的记录。

（C）审查公众对针灸的要求，并就有关针灸的问题发言。

（D）审查有关政策或者行政程序的查询。

（E）委托其他委员会委派任务。

（F）就委员会会议之间可能出现的紧急事项采取行动。

（G）协助医疗委员会组织、准备和向立法机构和立法机构的委员会提供信息和证词。

（H）就委员会未来的目标和目标，以及确定优先事项和实现方法，制定并向委员会提出建议。

（I）研究并向委员会提出关于委员会办公室和委员会的作用和责任的建议。

（J）根据《职业法典》第 205.102（b）条，研究如何提高委员会管理的效率和有效性，并向委员会提出建议。

（K）就提请执行委员会注意的事项向委员会提出建议。

（h）针灸委员会及其委员会的会议对公众开放，除非这些会议是根据《公开会议法案》和本法案召开的执行会议。为了使委员会会议安全、高效、有序地进行，公众委员会成员在任何时候都不得吸烟或者使用烟草制品、进食或者阅读报纸和杂志。公众委员会成员应当不得从事干扰委员会议事程序的破坏性活动，包括但不限于在会议室内的过度活动、喧哗或者大声说话，以及将脚搁放在桌椅上。公众应当留在委员会办公室中指定为向公众开放的区域内。公众委员会成员不得在会议期间向委员会成员讲话或者提问，除非委员会审裁官公布的议程项目得到认可。

（i）记者与其他公众成员一样，有权参加在公开会议上举行的针灸委员会会议，并受（h）所述的行为规则的约束。委员会会议的记录员可以在公开会议上进行录音或者视频记录，但应当受下列限制：针灸委员会的审裁官可定期要求摄像师关闭人工照明灯，使过多的热量消散;摄像师不得在委员会开会、营业期间拆装其设备;放置麦克风录音委员会程序的工作人员不得扰乱会议或者干扰与会者;记者可在针灸委员会办公室的接待区进行采访,或者在休会或者休会后,由针灸委员会的审裁官酌情决定在会议室进行采访;不得在委员会办公室的走廊上进行采访;针灸委员会审裁官可以将任何受到适当警告后仍坚持本款和(h)款所述行为的人逐出会议。

(j)针灸委员会的助理审裁官在审裁官缺席或者无法履行职责的情况下,应当承担审裁官的职责。

(k)在审裁官和助理审裁官均缺席或者无工作能力时,财务秘书应当承担审裁官的职责。

(l)如审裁官、助理审裁官及财务秘书缺席或者无法履行职责时,针灸委员会成员可选举另一名成员担任委员会会议的审裁官,或者选举一名临时审裁官,直至州长委任另一名审裁官为止。

(m)在助理审裁官或者财务秘书死亡、辞职或者永久丧失工作能力时,针灸委员会应当从其成员中选择一名官员来填补空缺职位。该选举应当在切实可行范围内尽快在针灸委员会的定期或者特别会议上进行。

(n)委员会的会议记录应当由全体委员会批准,出席会议的委员会成员应当达到法定人数,才能投票批准会议记录。

第183.4条　针灸执照

(a)申请资格。

申请人应当向针灸委员会提供充分证据,证明申请人符合以下要求:

(1)至少年满二十一周岁。

(2)具有本章第183.2条中定义的良好的职业品格(有关定义)。

(3)除针灸学校课程外,已顺利完成六十学时的大学普通学术课程,这些课程不属于补习课程,且在美国境内的两年制或者四年制高等教育机构完成课程后可获得学分,该院校获得高等教育协调委员会或者其他州的同等地区认证机构的认可。

如果针灸委员会认为,作为针灸或东方医学学位课程的一部分而完成的课程实质上与大学普通学术水平课程所要求的学时基本同等,则针灸委员会可以接受这些课程。

(4)毕业于已获批的针灸学校。

(5)在五次考试机会内通过了国家针灸与东方医学认证委员会(NCCAOM)考试的各个模块:

(A)如果申请人在2004年6月1日之前或者之后对一项模块进行多次考试,考试次数应当根据测试的主题合并计算。

(B)如果申请人在五次考试机会中未能通过NCCAOM考试的各个模块,若申请人具有下列情形的,可获准申请人在委员会的执照委员会面前出庭重新考虑其申请资格:

(i)被NCCAOM允许进行第六次考试。

(ii)在第六次考试时通过。

(iii)向委员会提出符合要求的证明,说明申请人为什么需要额外的考试尝试,并证明有充分理由重新考虑申请人对不符合资格的决定。

（C）根据（B）的规定,重新考虑申请人资格欠缺的决定,应当由委员会酌情决定。

（6）已经通过了针灸和东方医学学院委员会（CCAOM）洁针技术（CNT）课程和实践考试。

（7）已参加并通过了法学考试（"JP考试"）,该考试应当依据本州针灸专业的许可要求和其他法律、法规或者法规进行。

法学考试的组织和管理方式如下：

（A）有关法学考试的问题,应当由机构工作人员根据针灸委员会的意见回复,机构工作人员应当安排申请人参加考试。

（B）申请人的成绩达到七十五分或者以上,即通过JP考试。

（C）除考官允许外,考生不得携带医学书籍、汇编、笔记、医学期刊、计算器或者其他帮助进入考场,不得未经考官允许与其他考生相互交流,不得离开考场。

（D）考试过程中的违规行为,如提供或者获取未经授权的信息或者协助,如观察或者随后的统计分析证明,应当足以导致申请人终止参加考试,使申请人的考试结果无效,或者采取其他适当行为。

（E）除委员会特殊要求外,已通过法学考试者不得被要求重新参加其他或者类似执照的考试。

（8）能够用英语进行交流,如以下内容之一所述：

（A）通过NCCAOM考试,考试语言为英语；

（B）通过托福考试（TOEFL）,阅读和听力部分的成绩至少达到"中级",口语和写作部分的成绩至少达到"普通",或者纸质考试（PBT）的成绩为五百五十分或者以上。

（C）通过英语口语测试（TSE）,成绩为四十五分或者以上。

（D）通过托业考试（TOEIC）,成绩为五百分或者以上。

（E）从位于美国或者加拿大的可接受的获批针灸学校毕业；或者

（F）在针灸委员会的决定下,通过任何其他类似的、有效考试,测试英语能力的测试服务,其结果应直接报告给针灸委员会,或者通过测试服务和针灸委员会之间的直接联系来验证结果。

（9）申请人可以通过积极的针灸实践,证明当前具备的执业能力：

（A）所有执照申请人应当向委员会提供足够的文件,证明申请人在收到执照申请之前的两年内,曾全职积极治疗过患者,在可接受的获批针灸学校学习,或者在可接受的获批针灸学校担任教师。

（B）就本条而言,"全职工作"一词系指在某一年内执业四十周,每周至少工作二十小时。

（C）不符合（A）和（B）要求的申请人,根据行政主管或者委员会的裁量,申请人可以获得符合以下条件或者限制的无限制执照或者有限制执照：

（i）申请人的执业,仅限于针灸执业的特定部分/排除针灸实践的特定部分；或者

（ii）补习教育,包括但不限于以学生身份入学,并在可接受的获批针灸学校或者委员会

批准的其他结构化课程中成功完成二百四十学时的临床实践。

（10）现役军人、退伍军人和军人配偶的替代执照程序。

（A）申请人如果现役是军人、退伍军人或者军人配偶，可能有资格获得某些执照要求的替代能力证明。除非本款特别允许，否则申请人应当符合本节规定的执照要求。

（B）申请人应当是现役军人、退伍军人或者军人配偶，并符合下列条件之一：

（i）持有由另一个州颁发的不受限制的针灸执照，其执照要求基本上相当于得克萨斯州针灸执照的要求；或者

（ii）在申请日期前的五年内，在该州持有针灸执照。

（C）行政主管在审查了申请人的资格证书后，可放弃获得本款所述的申请人执照的任何先决条件。

（D）符合本款要求的，应当由委员会的执照部门加速申请。

（E）允许进行其他的能力展示。

符合本款规定的申请人：

（i）不要求遵守本款（c）（1）的规定。

（ii）尽管本款（b）（1）（B）规定了一年期限，但在申请失效前允许额外六个月完成申请。

（iii）尽管本款（b）（1）（G）的截止期限为六十日，仍然可以在委员会会议前五日内考虑获得永久执照。

（F）有军队服役经历的申请人。

（i）对于2014年3月1日或者之后提交的申请，对于本章第183.2条定义的军人或者退伍军人的申请人，委员会应当将核实的军事服务、培训或者教育计入委员会颁发的执照要求，而不是考试要求。

（ii）本条不适用于下列申请人：

（I）被其他州或者加拿大省吊销针灸执照的。

（II）持有另一州或者加拿大某省颁发的针灸执照，该执照受到限制、纪律处分措施令或者察看令的约束；或者

（III）有一段不可接受的犯罪历史。

（b）执照申请人的程序规则。

下列规定应当适用于所有执照申请人。

（1）执照申请人应当：

（A）申请人证件上显示的姓名与申请时使用的姓名不符，则必须提供姓名更改的证明。

（B）已向委员会提交的申请超过一年将被视为到期。

除非本卷第175.5条另有规定（有关费用提交或者罚款），否则先前随该申请一起提交的任何费用将被没收。任何进一步的执照申请都需要重新提交申请，并附上当前的执照费。在某些情况下，可以批准延长申请期限，包括：

（i）委员会工作人员延迟处理申请。

（ii）申请需要许可委员会在完成所有其他手续后进行审查，并将在下次例会前到期。

（iii）执照委员会要求申请人满足的具体额外要求，并且申请将在委员会规定的截止日期前到期。

（iv）申请人在完成所有其他要求并努力提供所需材料后，要求有一段合理的、有限的额外时间来获得文件。

（v）申请人因意外的军事任务、医疗原因或者灾难性事件而被延误。

（C）以任何方式伪造申请的，可能被要求到针灸委员会出庭。申请人是否会获得得克萨斯州针灸执照，将由针灸委员会裁量决定。

（D）针灸委员会若收到申请人的负面信息，可能要求该申请人到针灸委员会出庭。针灸委员会将决定该申请人是否将获得得克萨斯州执照。

（E）应当遵守针灸委员会的规则和条例，这些规则和条例在申请人向委员会提交完整的申请表和费用时有效。

（F）在针灸委员会认为对确定申请人能力很有必要时，申请人可能被要求参加额外的口头、书面或者实践考试或者演示。

（G）应当在针灸委员会会议召开前六十日完成执照申请，并且每个细节都清晰可辨，除非针灸委员会根据充分理由另行决定。

（2）希望因残疾而申请合理便利的执照申请人，应当在提交申请时提交要求。

（3）已在其他州、省或者城市获得执照的申请人，应当就以下内容填写经公证的宣誓书或者其他经核实的宣誓声明：

（A）该执照、证书或者执业权限，是否曾鉴于某些针对申请人的事由而因故限制、因故废止、因故暂停，或者吊销执照、撤销其在该州、省或者城市的执业资格。如果存在上述情形，这些法律程序的当前状态如何。

（B）是否有任何司法管辖区正在对申请人进行调查，或者有任何州、联邦、城市、地方或者省级法院对申请人提起诉讼，指控其犯有根据得克萨斯州法律属于重罪的任何罪行。如有，请说明起诉或调查的原因。

（4）执照申请人不得被要求在针灸委员会或者其任何委员会出庭，除非存在对申请人的下列疑问：

（A）身体或者精神障碍。

（B）刑事定罪；或者

（C）吊销职业执照。

（c）执照文件：

（1）原始文件/面试。

根据要求，任何申请人应当到委员会办公室进行个人面试，并向委员会代表出示原始文件以供检查。原始文件可包括但不限于本款（2）所列的文件。

（2）所需文件。

所有执照申请人需要提交的文件应当包括以下内容：

（A）出生证明和年龄证明。

每位执照申请人应当提供一份出生证明的副本，必要时应当提供翻译版本，以证明申请人至少年满二十一周岁。在没有出生证明的情况下,申请人应当提供护照副本或者其他合适的替代文件。

(B)变更姓名。

任何申请人提交的文件显示申请人所申请的姓名以外的姓名,应当提供结婚证、离婚法令或者法院命令说明更改姓名的副本。申请人因入籍而变更姓名的,应当凭专人送达或者挂号信将入籍证明原件提交委员会办公室检查。

(C)考试成绩。

每位执照申请人应当向针灸委员会提交由相关考试服务机构直接出具的经核证的成绩单,以证明其参加了在得克萨斯州举行的所有考试,并获得了得克萨斯州执照。

(D)院长认证。

每位执照申请人应当有一份毕业证书,该证书由针灸学院直接以针灸委员会提供的表格提交。申请人应当在表格上附上一张符合美国政府护照标准的近期照片,然后再提交给针灸学校。学校应当由院长或者指定的指定人在表格上签字,证明表格上的信息,并在照片上加盖学校印章。

(E)文凭或者证书。

所有执照申请人应当提交一份文凭或者毕业证书的副本。

(F)评估。

所有申请人应当根据针灸委员会提供的表格,提供其过去十年或者从针灸学校毕业后的专业关系评估,以最新的时间为准。

(G)针灸学校预科成绩单。

每位申请人必须由相应的一所或多所学校直接向针灸委员会提交一份其本科教育记录的副本。成绩单应当显示所修的课程和所取得的成绩。

如确定申请人提交的文件不足以证明其完成了针灸学校以外的六十学时的大学课程,申请人应当向针灸委员会提交文件以确定教育的充分性,或者向美国境内的两年制或四年制高等教育机构提交文件以获得课程验证。该机构应当得到委员会行政主管的预先批准,并得到由得克萨斯州高等教育协调委员会或者其他州同等机构认可的地区认证机构的认可。

(H)针灸学院的成绩单。

每个申请人应当让他或者她的针灸学校直接向针灸委员会提交课程和成绩的成绩单。成绩单应当清楚地证明完成了一千八百学时的教学,至少四百五十学时的草药研究。

(I)指纹卡。

每个申请人应当按照委员会规定的程序提交其指纹。

(J)其他验证。

如有正当理由,经针灸委员会批准,可以本款未另有规定的方式,对本款所规定的任何资料进行核实。

(3)其他文档。

申请人可能需要提交其他文件,包括但不限于以下内容:

（A）翻译文件。

任何使用英语以外语言的文件的准确核证翻译，应当连同原始文件或者已翻译的原始文件的核证副本一起提交。

（B）逮捕记录。

如果申请人曾被逮捕，逮捕当局的逮捕和逮捕处置的副本，应当由该当局直接提交给针灸委员会。

（C）医疗事故。

申请人曾在向任何责任承运人提出的医疗事故索赔中被点名的，或者申请人曾在医疗事故诉讼中被点名的，申请人应当提交下列文件：

（i）针灸委员会就针对申请人保险的每项索赔提供的完整的责任承保人表格。

（ii）对于每一项成为医疗事故诉讼的索赔，由代表申请人的律师直接向本委员会发出一封信，说明指控、指控日期和诉讼的当前状态。

如果诉讼已经结案，律师应当说明诉讼的处理方式，如果支付了任何款项，也应当说明和解的金额，除非法律或者有管辖权的法院的命令禁止公布此类信息。如果没有该信函，申请人将被要求提供一份经公证的宣誓书，说明无法提供该信函的原因。

（iii）由申请人组成的陈述，解释与患者治疗有关的情况，以为指控辩护。

（D）因酒精/药物滥用或者精神疾病的住院治疗。

在过去五年内，每一位因酒精/药物滥用或者精神疾病接受入院治疗的申请人应当提交以下文件：

（i）申请人对住院治疗情况的解释说明。

（ii）直接从住院机构提交的入院和出院小结。

（iii）申请人的主治医生/心理治疗师关于诊断、预后、处方药物和建议的后续治疗的声明。

（iv）与任何许可机构签署的任何合同或者协议的副本。

（E）对酒精/药物滥用或者精神疾病的门诊治疗。

在过去五年内，每一位因酒精/药物滥用或者精神疾病接受门诊治疗的申请人应当提交以下文件：

（i）申请人对门诊治疗情况的说明。

（ii）申请人的主治医生/心理治疗师关于诊断、预后、处方药物和建议的后续治疗的声明。

（iii）与任何许可机构签署的任何合同或者协议的副本。

（F）附加文件。

被认为需要协助调查任何执照申请的附加文件。

（G）DD214。

DD214 的复制件表明申请人从美国军队某部门离职。

（H）其他验证。

如有正当理由，经针灸委员会批准，可以本款未另有规定的方式，对本款所规定的任何资料进行核实。

（I）虚假文件。

伪造任何宣誓书或者提交虚假信息以获得执照,可能会使针灸师被拒发执照或者根据该法第205.351条受到纪律处分。

（4）替代文件/证明。

如果申请人已尽一切努力提供所需文件,针灸委员会可酌情允许其提供替代文件。这些例外情况将由针灸委员会、委员会或者委员会的行政主管根据具体情况进行审查。

（d）临时执照。

（1）颁发。

针灸委员会可通过该机构的行政主管,向以下执照申请人发放临时执照:

（A）符合该法案下的针灸执照的所有资格,但正在等待针灸委员会的下次预定会议进行审查和颁发执照;或者

（B）没有全职从事本款(a)(9)定义的针灸师,但是符合所有其他许可要求。

（2）续期。

临时执照自颁发之日起有效一百日,自初始临时执照到期之日起仅可再延长三十日。临时执照的颁发可以受行政主管自主裁量,且不得被视为对针灸委员会批准或者拒绝永久执照申请的决定具有决定作用。

（e）特聘教授临时执照。

（1）颁发。

针灸委员会可向以下针灸师颁发特聘教授临时执照:

（A）持有在其他州、省或者城市从事针灸工作的基本同等的执照、证书或者权力。

（B）同意并仅限于本州的任何针灸实践,为针灸学生/教师提供演示或者教学目的的针灸实践,并与已通过针灸及东方医学教育审核委员会(ACAOM)进行认证的针灸学校有直接联系,学生在该学校接受培训/教师进行教学。

（C）同意并仅限于持有本州无限制针灸执照的得克萨斯州执业针灸师的直接监督下进行示范或指导。

（D）支付颁发专聘教授临时执照所需的任何费用。

（E）通过本条(a)(7)中规定的法学考试。

（2）有效期。

特聘教授临时执照有效期为一年;但是,执照可在委员会认为必要的时候撤销。特聘教授临时执照自颁发之日起一年后自动到期。特聘教授的临时执照不得续期或者补发。

（3）纪律处分措施。

特聘教授临时执照,可以因当事人违反针灸委员会规则或者得克萨斯州针灸法第H节而被拒绝、终止、取消、吊销或者撤销。

（f）重新获得执照。

如果针灸执照已到期满一年,则认为该执照已被取消,针灸师不得续期执照。针灸师可以重新提交申请,并且应当遵守获得初始执照的要求和程序。

第 183.5 条　执照续期每 2 年 1 次

（a）根据得克萨斯州针灸法获得执照的针灸师,应当每两年续期一次执照并支付相关费用。针灸师可以提交所需的表格,并且在执照期满日前向针灸委员会支付所需的续期费以续期尚未到期的执照。费用应随附书面申请。申请应当清楚列明持证人的姓名、邮寄地址、持证人从事针灸实践的地址,以及针灸委员会规定的其他必要信息。

（b）伪造申请书或者提交虚假信息以获得执照续期的针灸师,应受到执照续期被驳回的处罚或者根据得克萨斯州针灸法第 205.351 条予以纪律处分。

（c）如果在到期日或者之前未收到续期费或者完整的申请表,则应当按照本卷第 175.3（3）条（与罚款有关）所述征收罚款。

（d）如果针灸执照已到期九十日或不满九十日,针灸师可以通过向委员会提交一份根据本卷第 175.2（3）条（有关注册申请以及续期费）规定的完整的执照申请、注册费,并且提交本卷第 175.3（3）（A）条规定的罚款,以获得新执照。

（e）如果针灸师的执照已经到期超过九十日,但未满一年,针灸师可以通过向委员会提交一份根据本卷第 175.2（3）条（有关注册申请以及续期费）规定的完整的执照申请、注册费,并且提交本卷第 175.3（3）（B）条规定的罚款,以获得新执照。

（f）如果针灸执照已经到期一年或以上,则针灸执照应当自动注销,除非正在进行调查,在此期间针灸师不能申请新执照。

（g）针灸执照根据本条（c）的规定到期后,在未申请获得新执照的情况下从事针灸实践,视同无证从事针灸实践,均应当受到纪律处分。

（h）持有得克萨斯州针灸执照的军人,享有两年的额外期限完成与军人执照续期的相关事宜。

第 183.6 条　拒绝颁发执照；持证人的纪律处分

（a）执照申请者,适用根据《得克萨斯州针灸法》第 205.351 条拒绝颁发执照的规定。

（b）根据上述法案持有执照的针灸师,应当受到该法案第 205.351 条的约束,包括撤销执照。

（c）针灸委员会根据《得克萨斯州针灸法》第 205.351 条拒绝颁发执照或者采取纪律处分,应当符合该法、本卷第 187 和 190 章（有关程序规则和纪律处分指导原则）、《行政程序法》以及州行政听证会办公室条例的规定。

本卷第 187 章和第 190 章（有关程序规则和纪律处分指导）应当在适当的范围内适用于针灸师。如果这两章的规定与《得克萨斯州针灸法》或者相关规则相互矛盾,则应当以本章的法案和规则为准。

（d）纪律处分指导原则。

（1）在处理如下拒发执照和纪律处分的有关事宜时,本卷第 190 章（有关纪律处分指南）应当适用于受本章监管的针灸师：

（A）不符合公众健康和福利的执业行为。

（B）违反职业道德或者不光彩的行为。

（C）州委员会和同业组织的纪律处分性措施。

（D）重复和反复遭到医疗责任索赔。

（E）加重和减轻因素。

（F）刑事定罪。

（2）如果第 190 章的规定与本章的法案或者条例出现矛盾,则应当以本章的法案和规则为准。

（e）根据《得克萨斯州针灸法》第 205.352 条、本卷第 187.9 条(有关委员会措施)以及本卷第 187.13 条(有关获取执照资格的非正式委员会程序),委员会可以实施非纪律处分性的补救措施,以解决对申诉的调查或者作为颁发执照的条件。

第 183.7 条　执业范围

（a）针对在针灸治疗前十二个月内对经过医师或者牙医评估的人,针灸师可以酌情开展针灸治疗。

（b）对于得克萨斯州脊椎按摩师考试委员会颁发执照的执业医生转诊的患者,持证人可以在转诊日之后的三十日内实施针灸。

以针灸二十次或者两个月之中最先发生为判别标准,如果实施针灸后患者没有实质性改善,持证人应将患者转诊给另一名医生。

（c）尽管本条(a)和(b)款另有规定,持有当前有效执照的针灸师可以在没有医师、牙医和脊医的评估和转诊的情形下,对吸烟成瘾、体重减轻、酗酒、慢性疼痛和药物滥用的人进行针灸治疗。

（d）以针灸二十次或者两个月之中最先发生为判别标准,如果患者的慢性疼痛没有实质性改善,执业针灸师应当由得克萨斯州执业医师和牙医进行建议和评估。

（e）以针灸二十次或者两个月之中最先发生为判别标准,如果患者的酗酒或者药物滥用情况没有实质性改善,执业针灸师应当由得克萨斯州执业医师和牙医视情况进行建议和评估。

第 183.8 条　调查

（a）保密性。

委员会拥有、接受和收集的所有涉及申诉、不良申报、调查档案、其他调查报告和其他调查信息,均属于保密性信息。任何员工、代理或者委员会成员均不应当透露这些材料中包含的信息。但是,以下情形除外:

（1）向针灸师持有的执照所属的其他州、哥伦比亚特区或者地区或者国家的执照管理当局提供信息。

（2）如果调查信息表明可能已经犯下罪行,则应当向有关执法机构披露。

（3）根据书面请求后,向医疗机构提供。

委员会向医疗单位披露的信息,应当仅限于委员会纪律处分或者协议和解调查后得到解决的有关针灸师的投诉信息,以及正在积极调查的任何投诉的基本事实和当下进展。

（4）如果在调查进行期间确有需要,可以向其他人披露。

（b）要求提供信息和记录。

（1）患者记录。

根据委员会或者委员会代表的要求,持证人应当在提出要求之日起的十四日内,向委员会提供患者的英文记录副本或者原记录。

（2）执照续期。

如果针灸委员会或者医疗委员会提出要求,持证人应当以书面形式解释其对执照续期申请的问题。

此解释应当包括医学委员会或者针灸委员会可能要求的所有内容,并且应当在医学委员会或者针灸委员会提出要求后的十四日内提供。

（c）职业责任险诉讼和索赔。

持证人在收到针灸委员会针对持证人的索赔通知书和投诉之后,应当在收到医学委员会或者针灸委员会具体的提供材料要求之日起十四日内,向医学委员会或者针灸委员会提供以下材料:

（1）完成调查问卷,以提供诉讼或者索赔的概要信息。

（2）完成调查问卷,以提供评估持证人能力的信息。

（3）持证人的办公室病历记录和医院记录（如适用）的准确、清晰、完整的副本,涉及要求赔偿损失的患者。

（4）有关先前向任一委员会申报的任何诉讼或者索赔状态的最新信息。

（d）调查专业审查措施。

由同行评审委员会或者医疗保健实体向针灸委员会提供的专业评审措施的书面申报,应当包含专业审查措施的结果和情况。

这些结果和情况应当包括:

（1）专业审查的具体措施,无论该行动是否与个体患者的直接治疗有关。

（2）对针灸师的临床特权、专业组织或者协会的成员资格的具体限制,以及此类限制的持续时间。

（e）其他申报。

（1）如果一名针灸师的针灸实践对公众福利构成持续威胁,则应当向针灸委员会报告相关信息,其中应当包括一份叙述声明,声明申报所依据的行为或者不作为的时间、日期和地点。

（2）在同行评审委员会、执业针灸师或者相关针灸学员得出结论并且收集相关信息后,应当尽快向针灸委员会上报针灸师的针灸实践对公众福利构成持续威胁。

（f）申报职业责任险索赔。

（1）申报责任。

对于每位被提起职业责任索赔或投诉的被告针灸师,必须填写申报责任表并将其提交给针灸委员会。

该信息应当由保险公司或者为针灸师提供保险的其他组织进行报告。

如果未经认可的保险公司不予申报,或者针灸师没有保险公司,则责任申报应当由针灸师自行负责。

（2）核实信息的单独报告。

每位投保的被告针灸师应当单独发送一份报告。

在申报第二部分时,应当附随所填写的第一部分或者本条(4)(A)所述的其他识别信息。

(3)时间范围和附件。

表格第一部分中的信息,应当在收到索赔或者诉讼的三十日以内提供,并且应当附有索赔信或者请愿书的副本。

第二部分中的信息,应当在处理索赔后的一百〇五日以内申报。

已处理的索赔,包括那些为已作出法院命令、已达成和解协议或者已撤销或者驳回投诉的索赔。

(4)备用申报格式。

信息可以按照所提供的表格或者以任何其他至少载有所需资料的易读格式申报。

(A)如果申报人选择使用针灸委员会以外的申报格式作为第二部分要求的数据,则应当有充足的识别信息供委员会工作人员使用,以便将结案报告与原始文件相互匹配。

完成此操作所需要的信息包括:

(i)被告针灸师的姓名和执照号码。

(ii)原告姓名。

(B)法院命令或者和解协议是第二部分可接受的替代性的呈递材料。

命令或者和解协议应当包含必要的信息,以便将结案报告与原始文件相互匹配。

如果命令或者协议缺少某些必要的信息,则应当在命令或者协议写明附加信息。

(5)罚款。

合法保险公司未根据本条规定进行申报的,应交由州保险委员会处理。

根据《保险法典》第1.10章第7条的规定,未申报者可能会受到处罚。

(6)定义。

为本款之目的,职业责任索赔或者投诉应当定义为针灸师的诉讼事由,即针灸师在治疗、缺乏治疗或者其他违背公认的医疗保健或者健康标准而直接导致患者受伤或者死亡的理由,无论患者在侵权或者合同的索赔或者诉因是否有效。

(7)无须申报的索赔。

根据本章规定,无须申报但是可以申报的索赔,包括但不限于下列情形:

(A)产品责任索赔(例如,针灸师发明了一种可能伤害患者的设备,但是针灸师与声称被该设备伤害的特定患者之间,不存在针灸师-患者关系)。

(B)反垄断指控。

(C)涉及不当同行评审活动的指控。

(D)侵犯公民权利;或者

(E)对针灸师财产上发生的损害责任的指控,但是不涉及对患者的违约责任(例如,滑倒和跌倒事故)。

(8)但是,根据本章规定不需要申报的索赔可以自愿申报。

(9)申报表格应当如下:

此处设置的表格或者图形材料是不可以显示的。

第Ⅱ部分。在处理完《得克萨斯州行政法典》第 22 卷第 183.8(f)条所界定的包括解雇或者和解在内的索赔申请后填写。在一百○五日内向美国国安局备案索赔处理。法院命令或和解书的副本协议可按《得克萨斯州行政法典》第 22 卷第 183.8(f)条的规定使用。

8. 处理日期：

9. 性格类型：

_____(1) 结算

_____(2) 审判后判决

_____(3) 其他(请注明)

10. 代表被告约定或者下令的赔偿金额：

$_____注：如果在有多个被告的情况下,法院或者保险公司没有确定过错的百分比,保险公司可以报告索赔的总金额,后面加上斜杠和投保的被告人数。(示例：$100 000/3)

11. 上诉,如果已知：_____是_____否。如果是,则是哪一方：

_____

_____

填写本报告的人员_____　　　　　　　　电话号码_____

第 183.9 条　存在身体缺陷的针灸师

(a) 精神或者体格检查。

(1) 如果有理由认为持证人或者申请人具有缺陷,委员会可以要求持证人或者申请人接受委员会指定的一名或者多名医师的精神以及/或者身体检查。

如果由于年龄、疾病、醉酒、过量使用药物、麻醉剂、化学品或者任何其他类型的材料,或者由于精神或者身体状况原因,以致无法以合理的技能和安全的方式对患者进行服务的,则确定其存在身体缺陷。

(2) 合理根据可以包括但不限于以下任何一种：

(A) 在针灸委员会或者州行政听证会办公室作证的两个人宣誓证词,证明某一持证人或者申请人有身体缺陷。

(B) 得克萨斯州针灸协会或者得克萨斯州针灸和东方医学协会官方代表的宣誓证词,证实该代表愿意在委员会为持证人或者申请人存在身体缺陷作证。

(C) 持证人或者申请人在完成酒精或者化学药物依赖治疗项目之前离开该项目的证据。

(D) 持证人或者申请人滥用药物或者酒精的证据。

(E) 持证人或者申请人因为醉酒而一再被捕的证据。

(F) 持证人或者申请人经常在精神病院临时住院的证据;或者

(G) 表明持证人或者申请人患有疾病或者不良状态,导致其无法正常工作的医治记录。

(H) 持证人或者申请人在委员会举行的听证会上采取的行动和陈述,使委员会有理由相信持证人或者申请人具有身体缺陷。

(3) 在行政主管提出可能的原因之后,委员会授权行政主管致函持证人/申请人,要求持证人/申请人在收到行政主管信函后的三十日内,接受身体或者精神检查。

该信函说明要求进行身体或者精神检查的理由、行政主管核准进行此种检查的医学专家以及委员会收到检查结果的日期。

（4）收到要求身体或者精神检查信函的持证人/申请人拒绝接受检查,委员会应当通过行政主管发出的命令,要求持证人/申请人说明不接受检查的原因,并且应当安排至迟于发出通知日期之后三十日就该命令对于持证人举办听证会。

持证人/申请人应当以个人送达或者挂号信作为收件回执。

（5）在（4）规定的听证会上,委员会代表们应当确定持证人/申请人是否应当接受评估,或者是否应当在不应当进行检查的情况下结束该事件。

（A）在听证会中,持证人/申请人以及持证人/申请人的律师（若有）有权出示证词或者其他证据,证明持证人/申请人不应当被要求接受检查。

（B）如果在考虑了在听证会上提出的证据后,合议庭确定持证人/申请人应当接受检查,则委员会代表应当通过其行政主管,在提交要求检查命令之日起六十日内发出命令,要求当事人进行检查。

持证人有权对在听证会提供证词的鉴定人做交叉询问。

（C）如果合议庭确定不需要进行此检查,合议庭将会撤回检查请求。

（D）委员会下令进行的任何精神或者身体检查结果均为保密信息,应当密封交与委员会,以便委员会根据检查结果采取任何必要和适当的行动。

持证人应当提供检查结果,并且有机会在委员会采取行动前三十日做出答复。

（6）在履行《得克萨斯州针灸法》第205.3523条规定的义务时,委员会应当将持证人/申请人转诊给最合适的医学专家进行评估。

除非医学上另有说明,否则委员会不得要求持证人/申请人接受委员会指定专科的医生的检查。

委员会不得要求持证人/申请人在距离此人的家或者营业地不适宜距离的情况下接受检查,除非在持证人/申请人居住和工作的地区能够进行适当检查的医生数量有限。

（7）根据本款通过的指导方针,并不损害或者取代委员会作出的独立许可或者纪律处分性决定的权力,除非程序临时中止。

（b）本卷第180章（有关得克萨斯州医师健康计划和康复令）应当适用于被认为功能缺损并有资格参加得克萨斯州医师健康计划的针灸师。

在2010年1月1日或者之前签订的康复令应当受该日期之前存续法律的约束。

第183.10条 患者病历

（a）根据该《得克萨斯州针灸法》获得执照的针灸师,应当保存并且保留所有患者就诊或者咨询的适当病历记录。这些记录至少应当以英文书写,并且包括以下内容:

（1）患者姓名和居住地址。

（2）生命体征,包括患者初次就诊的体温、脉搏或者心跳、呼吸频率、血压,以及医生认为适用后续治疗的生命体征。

（3）患者主诉。

（4）患病史。

（5）每次患者就诊或者咨询的治疗计划。

（6）任何草药的注释，包括剂量和形式，以及在治疗过程中使用的其他方式，并注明相应的治疗日期。

（7）准确反映患者姓名、提供的服务、提供服务的日期以及每次提供服务的收费或者收费的账单记录的系统。

（8）根据本卷第 183.7(a) 条（有关服务范围），在进行针灸服务之前的十二个月内，是否由医师或者牙医（视情况而定）对患者做过病情评估的书面记录。

（9）根据本卷第 183.7(b) 条（有关服务范围）得克萨斯州脊医审查委员会许可的脊医转诊患者的治疗制度，制作的一份书面记录，说明针灸师在针灸二十次或者两个月后（以最先发生者为判断标准），是否将患者转诊给医生。

（10）如果由得克萨斯州脊医审查委员会颁发的脊医服务执照的医生，将患者转诊给针灸师，针灸师应当记录转诊日期和针灸服务前最近的推拿治疗日期。

（11）根据本卷第 183.7 条（有关服务范围）规定实施评估的文件，或者，在持证人无法确定是否进行评估的情形下，需要一份由患者签署的书面声明，证实其已由医生根据以下表格的复印件上规定的时间实施了评估。

（b）根据《得克萨斯州针灸法》第 205.302 条，针灸师在因吸烟成瘾、药物滥用、酗酒、慢性疼痛或者减肥而对患者进行针灸时，不应当被要求保存和保留(a)(11)规定的文件。

（c）保留病历和账单记录。

（1）执业针灸师应当自针灸师最后一次服务之日起的五年内，保留患者病历和账单记录。

（2）如果患者最后一次接受服务时未满十八周岁，则针灸师应当保留患者的医疗病历和账单记录，直到患者年满二十一周岁或者自上次治疗起满五年，以前两段时间中的较长者为准。

（3）针灸师保留医疗病历和账单记录，应当比其他联邦或者州法规规定的时间更长。

（4）只有在针灸师知道有关的民事、刑事或者行政诉讼已经最终解决，并且至少在前述（1）至（3）规定的时间内保存相关记录的情形下，针灸师才可以销毁与任何民事、刑事或者行政诉讼有关的医疗和账单记录。

（d）披露保密信息应当以书面形式征得患者的同意。如果患者是未成年人，则由其父母或者法定监护人签署意见。如果患者被裁定没有能力管理其个人事务，则由其法定监护人签署意见，或者为患者指定诉讼律师。其法律依据如下：《得克萨斯州精神健康法典》第 7 卷 C 编；《健康与安全法典》；《智障人士法案》第 7 卷第 D 编；《健康与安全法典》第 452 章；《健康和安全法典》关于化学品依赖者治疗的制度；《得克萨斯州遗嘱认证法典》第 5 章；《家庭法典》第 11 章。如患者已去世，则应当委任个人代表，但书面同意应当明确以下事项：

（1）拟披露的信息和记录的范围。

（2）披露的原因和目的。

（3）作为拟披露信息的对象的个人。

（e）患者或者其他被授权同意的人，有权撤回其对发布任何信息的同意。

撤回同意不会影响在书面撤回通知之前披露的任何信息。

（f）任何收到通过本法案所称保密信息的人，只有在获得同意发布信息授权目的一致的范围内，才可以向他人披露信息。

（g）针灸师应当根据（d）所规定的信息发布的书面同意，提供所要求的患者记录的易读副本，或者记录的英文概要或者陈述。除非针灸师确定获取信息，将对患者的身体、精神或者情绪健康有害。

针灸师可以删除另一个没有同意披露的人的保密信息。

针灸师应当在收到要求之日起三十日内提供有关资料。

提供信息的合理费用应当由患者或者代表患者的人支付。

如果针灸师拒绝全部或者部分的请求，针灸师应当向患者提供一份书面声明，签名并注明日期，说明拒绝的理由。

拒绝该请求的声明副本应当保存在患者病历记录中。

本款中的"患者病历记录"，系指与患者的病史、诊断、治疗或者预防有关的任何记录。

第183.11条 投诉程序通知书

根据《得克萨斯州针灸法》第205.152条和本卷第178章（关于申诉）的规定，应当规范针灸师向机构申诉的通知方法。

如果本卷第178章与得克萨斯州针灸法或者本章规定存在冲突，应当本州针灸法和本章规定为准。

第183.12条 医学委员会审查和批准

（a）根据法案第205.202条的规定，针灸委员会应当向符合法案以及根据法案通过的规则的人员颁发该州的针灸执业执照，无须医学委员会批准。

（b）根据法案第205.352条的规定，针灸委员会应当在未经医学委员会批准的情况下对持证人实施纪律处分措施。

（c）根据法案第205.101(b)条的规定，针灸委员会通过的规则应当经医学委员会批准，该批准应当在医学委员会的会议记录、医学委员会的委员会会议记录或者由医学委员会审裁官、秘书，或者授权委员会审裁官在考虑针灸委员会的建议后签署的书面文件中加以说明。

第183.13条 解释

本章的解释应当与得克萨斯州针灸法相一致。

如果本章与其相冲突，应当以该针灸法为准；但是，本章的解释应当使本章与针灸法不冲突的规定继续有效。

第183.14条 针灸戒毒专家

（a）在本章中，"针灸戒毒专家"应当被定义为有资格从事耳穴针灸治疗的人，其目的仅限于治疗酒精中毒、药物滥用和化学药物依赖。

（b）不具有得克萨斯州针灸执照的人，或者未根据《得克萨斯州职业法典》第3卷第C编第205章被授权进行针灸实践的人，均只有在符合本款(1)至(4)所列的条件，取得针灸戒毒专家证书的情况下，才能够作为针灸戒毒专家为治疗酗酒、药物滥用或者药物依赖提供服务：

（1）在医学委员会颁发证书后，支付规定的费用，并收到医学委员会发出证书的书面确认书。

（2）完成为治疗酒精中毒、药物滥用或者化学药物依赖开设的针灸实践培训课程。该培训课程已获医学委员会批准,并征求了针灸委员会的意见。

耳穴针灸类课程应当长达七十学时,并应当包括经医学委员会批准的洁针技术课程或者同等的通用感染控制预防程序课程。

（3）如果个人持有得克萨斯州相关监管机构颁发的不受限制的现行执照、注册或者证书,授权作为社会工作者、持证专业咨询师、持证心理学家、持证药物依赖咨询师、持证职业护士或者持证注册护士执业;而并不禁止监管机构将这种戒毒疗法,授权给社会工作者、专业咨询师、心理学家、化学药物依赖咨询师、持证职业护士或者注册护士实施。

（4）根据书面协议,在执业医师或执业针灸师监督下开展服务。监督者是在可以通过电话或者其他通讯方式随时联系,且目前处于积极执业的得克萨斯州执业医生或者执业针灸师。

此类协议应当经得克萨斯州执照监督者和针灸戒毒专家同意并签署,每年至少审查和签署一次,并在现场保存。

针灸戒毒专家应当在变更或者增加日期之后的三十日内提交作为监督医生的人员或者作为针灸戒毒专家的针灸师的各项变更或者增加的通知。

（c）在本章中,耳穴针灸的定义是指仅限于将针头插入耳内五个穴位的针灸实践。

这些穴位是肝、肾、肺、交感神经和神门穴。

（d）针灸戒毒专家的认证,应当根据与《得克萨斯州针灸法》第205.351条的规定基本相似的各种理由,或者因违反本章规定从事针灸实践,被吊销、撤销或者终止。

（e）被认证为针灸戒毒专家的从业人员应当保留患者的治疗记录,至少应当包括治疗日期、治疗目的、患者姓名、使用的穴位以及被认证者的姓名、签名和职称。

（f）用于治疗酒精中毒、药物滥用或者药物依赖的针灸戒毒专家的认证费,其数额应当足以支付管理和执行本节规定的合理费用,不得动用医学委员会或者针灸委员会所产生的各项其他资金。

本卷第175.1条和第175.2条(关于申请和管理费以及注册和续期费)对申请和续期费进行了定义。

（g）本章规定的证书持有人应当在医学委员会备案一个最新的邮寄和执业地址,并应当在地址变更后的十日内以书面形式通知医学委员会。

（h）根据本章规定作为针灸戒毒专家执业的个人,应当确保以书面形式通知各位接受针灸服务的患者有关提供针灸服务的个人的资格和向医学委员会提出投诉的程序,并应当确保在患者的记录中保留该通知的副本。

（i）作为针灸戒毒专家的认证申请,应当以经医学委员会批准的表格以书面形式提交,表格中应当载有本条(b)规定的材料,以及证实该材料所需的各份证明文件。

（j）每位经认证为针灸戒毒专家的人员,可以每年通过填写和向医学委员会提交经批准的续期表格以及本款(1)至(3)所列的下列文件续期认证:

（1）证明本条(b)(3)所要求的证书或者执照仍然有效的文件。

（2）根据本卷第183.21条(关于针灸戒毒专家的针灸继续教育)的规定,获得的各项针灸继续教育（CAAE）证明。

（3）支付本卷第175.2条规定的证书续期费。

（k）每位根据本条规定获得针灸戒毒专家认证的人员，只能使用"针灸戒毒认证专家"或者"C.A.S."的称谓，以证明其专业训练。

第183.15条　专业头衔的使用

（a）除本条（b）规定外，持证人应当在与有关针灸执业的广告或者其他公众可见的材料上，在其姓名后紧跟使用"执业针灸师""Lic.Ac."或者"L.Ac."等头衔。

只有获得针灸执照的人才可以使用这些头衔。

在得克萨斯州同时获得医师、牙医、脊椎指压治疗师、验光师、足科医生和/或兽医执照的持证人不需要在其姓名后紧接其针灸头衔。

（b）如果持证人使用各种额外的头衔或者名称，则持证人应对遵守《治疗技术鉴定法案》，即《得克萨斯州执业法典》注释版第104章的规定，应当标记使用该头衔的权威机构，或者授予使用该头衔的学院或者荣誉学位。

持证人可以在本条（a）所述的材料中，在"执业针灸师""Lic.Ac."或者"L.Ac."等头衔之前或者之后，使用附加的头衔或者名称。

第183.16条　得克萨斯州针灸学校

（a）在得克萨斯州经营针灸学校的合法得克萨斯州针灸师，如尚未获得美国针灸及东方医学审核委员会（ACAOM）的认证或者获得ACAOM认证的候选资格，或者在该学校享有各项所有权的得克萨斯州执业针灸师，或者在该学校任教或者经营该学校的得克萨斯州执业针灸师，均应当确保该学校的学生及该学校的申请人知悉《医疗服务法案》有关针灸服务的条文，以及得克萨斯州针灸审查委员会所采纳的规则和条例，以及获得得克萨斯州针灸执照的教育要求，包括本条（b）所述的为获得得克萨斯州针灸审查委员会为针灸执照目的而设立的经批准的针灸学校的标准的规则和条例。

（b）为遵守本条（a）的规定，应当向学生和申请人提供得克萨斯州针灸法第H节的副本、《得克萨斯州医学委员会规则》所载的本法第183节（针灸）的副本以及以下打印说明。

（c）得克萨斯州执业针灸师在完全或者部分经营、任教或者拥有未经ACAOM认证或者未申请ACAOM认证的得克萨斯州针灸学校时，不得直接或者间接、明确或者暗示地说明，不得以口头或者书面形式，亲自或者通过针灸师或者学校的代理人为达到各种目的，说明该学校是得克萨斯州针灸审查委员会认可、注册、附属或者以其他方式批准的。

（d）不遵守本条的规定或者禁令，得克萨斯州执业针灸师在得克萨斯州经营、任教或者全部或者部分享有未经ACAOM认证或者未申请ACAOM认证的得克萨斯州针灸学校的所有权，将构成对该针灸师实施纪律处分的理由。

这种纪律处分措施应当以违反基于法案第205.351（a）（6）条规定的《得克萨斯州针灸审查委员会规则》为依据。

（e）为了对在得克萨斯州执业的针灸师进行许可和管理，ACAOM批准得克萨斯州的针灸学校符合本卷第183.2条（关于定义）所列的标准，可以以符合得克萨斯州法律的方式颁发东方医学硕士学位。

得克萨斯州针灸审查委员会应当承认各个基于此合法颁发的学位。

为了对在得克萨斯州执业的针灸师进行许可和管理，得克萨斯州的针灸学校如果是 ACAOM 针灸和东方医学硕士水平项目的候选学校，并且在候选期间已经颁发了文凭或者学位，则在获得 ACAOM 完全认证后，可以将其学位升级为硕士学位。

得克萨斯州针灸审查委员会应当承认各个基于此合法升级的学位。

第 183.17 条　遵守规定

本卷第 189 章（关于遵守规定）应当适用于接受委员会命令的针灸师。如果第 189 章的规定与得克萨斯州针灸法或者本章的规则相冲突，则应当以该针灸法和本章规定为准。

第 183.18 条　行政罚款

（a）根据《得克萨斯州针灸法》第 205.352 条和《医疗服务法案》第 165 章的规定，委员会可以根据《行政程序法案》的规定，通过命令对违反法案或者依据法案通过的规则或者命令的获发执照的人员或者受法案约束的人员收缴行政罚款。

该罚款的收缴应当符合得克萨斯州针灸法和《行政程序法案》的规定。

（b）对违法行为的罚款金额不得超过五千美元。

就处罚而言，违法行为持续或者发生的每一日都是一个单独的违法行为。

（c）在委员会命令收缴行政罚款之前，应当通知当事人，并使当事人有机会在合规的程序中就每个问题提出行政罚款的依据作出回应，提出证据和论点。

（d）罚款金额应当根据本卷第 190 节（关于纪律处分规则）规定的因素确定。

（e）如果委员会通过命令确定发生了违规行为，并对持证人或者受监管的人进行行政处罚，则委员会应当将委员会的命令通知该人，其中应当包括该人有权对该命令寻求司法审查的声明。

（f）可以根据本条规定，针对下列情形收缴罚款：

（1）未能及时遵守委员会发出的传票，应当对每项违规行为处以不低于一百美元不超过五千美元的行政罚款。

（2）未能及时遵守委员会命令的条款、条件或者要求，应当对每项违规行为处以不低于一百美元不超过五千美元的行政罚款。

（3）未能及时向委员会报告地址的变更，应当对每项违规行为处以不低于一百美元不超过五千美元的行政罚款。

（4）未能及时回复和患者的沟通，应当对每项违规处以不低于一百美元不超过五千美元的行政罚款。

（5）不遵守本章第 183.11 条（关于投诉程序通知）所规定的投诉程序通知要求的，应当对每项违规行为处以不低于一百美元不超过五千美元的行政罚款。

（6）未在规定时间内提供合规程序的信息的，应当对每项违规行为处以不低于一百美元不超过五百美元的行政罚款。

（7）除治疗质量问题外，委员会认为适当的各种其他违规行为，应当对每项违规行为处以不少于一百美元不超过五千美元的行政罚款。

（g）根据本条规定提出的各项命令，应当由委员会最后批准。

（h）未能支付通过命令施加的行政罚款,将成为委员会根据得克萨斯州针灸法第205.351(a)(10)条对可能欺骗或者伤害公众的违反职业道德或者不光彩的行为实施纪律处分措施的理由,也将成为行政主管将该事项提交给总检察长以收取罚款的理由。

（i）在作出行政处罚的命令后,如果一个人在经济上无力支付行政罚款,在该人以书面形式宣誓证明其有充分理由的情况下,委员会的纪律处分和道德委员会可以酌情批准给予从行政罚款到期之日起不超过一年的延期或者推迟。

在这样的延期或者推迟结束后,如果没有按照规定的方式和金额进行支付,将实施有关命令或者本条(h)的措施。

第183.19条　针灸广告

针灸师不得授权或者使用虚假的、误导性的或者欺骗性的广告。此外,不得有下列各种行为:

（1）将自己标榜为医生或者外科医生,或者使用上述术语的任何组合或者衍生词,除非根据《得克萨斯州医疗服务法案》,即《得克萨斯州职业法典》第151.002(a)(13)条(关于定义)的规定获得医学委员会颁发的医生或者外科医生执照。

（2）使用"经委员会认证"字样,除非该广告还披露授予该认证的委员会的完整名称;或者

（3）在刊登、广播或者以其他方式公布有关广告时,所刊登的委员会认证已到期且未续期时,使用"经委员会认证"或者各种可能具有相同含义的类似词汇或者短语。

第183.20条　针灸继续教育

（a）目的。

本条旨在通过为持有针灸执照的得克萨斯州针灸师制定针灸继续教育（Continuing Acupuncture Education,CAE）的最低要求,以进一步提高他们的专业技能和知识,从而促进得克萨斯州人民的健康、安全和福利。

（b）针灸继续教育最低要求。

作为两年一次的针灸执照注册的先决条件,针灸师应当每二十四个月完成三十四学时的CAE。

（1）所规定的学时应当是从修读时符合下列其中一项标准的课程获得:

（A）由得克萨斯州针灸师考试委员会根据本条(n)所述的教育委员会对课程内容的审查和建议,指定或者以其他方式批准学分。

（B）由得克萨斯州针灸师考试委员会批准的提供者提供。

（C）已被另一个州的针灸委员会批准为CAE学分至少三年,并首先通过了该州的正式批准程序。

（D）被NCCAOM批准为专业发展活动学分;或者

（E）在美国境外由委员会认可的针灸继续教育机构提供。

（2）要求的CAE学时应当包括以下核心学时:

（A）至少有八学时一般的针灸疗法。

（B）至少有两学时道德和安全方面的课程。

（C）至少有六学时草药学课程。

（D）至少有四学时生物医学课程。

（3）剩余的 CAE 学时可以来自本款(1)所批准的其他课程,但要符合本款(5)至(7)的限制。

（4）课程可以通过现场讲授、远程学习或者互联网进行教学。

（5）每个注册期所需的总学时中,与商业惯例或者办公室管理有关的课程不得超过四学时。

（6）根据(1)(D)或者(1)(E)完成的总学时数,不得多于十六学时,适用于每段注册期所规定的总时数。

（7）根据(1)(A)至(1)(C)批准每段登记期所规定的总学时数应当最少为十八学时。

（8）所需的 CAE 应当包括完成得克萨斯州卫生与公共服务委员会执行委员批准的人口贩卖预防课程。

该课程可以被视为根据(1)(A)至(1)(C)批准的最少十八学时的一部分。

（c）报告针灸继续教育。

针灸师应当在持证人的注册表格上报告该持证人在过去两年内是否完成了所要求的针灸继续教育。

（d）豁免接受针灸继续教育的理由。

针灸师可以以书面形式提出要求,并可能因为以下一个或者多个原因而免除两年一次的针灸继续教育最低要求:

（1）持证人患有严重疾病的。

（2）服兵役满一年的。

（3）持证人在美国境外的针灸实践和居住时间超过一年。

（4）持证人在书面申请中表明正当理由并向委员会提供符合要求的证明,证明其无法遵守针灸继续教育的规定。

（e）豁免请求。

豁免申请应当经委员会行政主管批准,并应当在执照有效期届满前至少三十日以书面形式提出。

（f）豁免期限和续期。

根据(d)和(e)的规定授予的豁免不得超过一年,但可以在当前豁免的有效期届满前至少三十日提交书面请求后,每两年延长一次。

（g）学分的核实。

委员会可以要求各持证人提供针灸继续教育学时的书面证明,持证人应当在要求之日起三十日内提供所要求的证明。如果不及时提供所要求的证明,委员会可能会实施纪律处分。

（h）因针灸继续教育不足而不予续期。

除非根据本条规定获得豁免,否则针灸师没有按照本节的要求和规定获得并及时报告三十四学时的继续教育学时,将导致执照无法续期,直到该针灸师获得并报告所需学时为止;但是,委员会行政主管可以向该针灸师颁发临时执照,其编号与未续期的执照相对应。

根据本款规定颁发的临时执照,可以允许委员会核实与针灸师继续教育学时有关信息的准确性,并允许未获得或者未及时报告所需学时的针灸师有机会纠正各个不足之处,以避免终止正在进行的患者保健服务。

(i) 颁发临时执照的费用。

根据本条规定颁发临时执照的费用应当符合本卷第 175.1 条(关于申请费)规定的金额;该费用不需要在颁发临时执照之前支付,但是应当在续期永久执照之前支付。

(j) 额外学时的申请。

为满足前一注册期的要求而获得的针灸继续教育学时,作为执照续期的先决条件,应当首先计入该前一注册期要求的学时数。一旦满足上一注册期的要求,则各额外获得的学时应当计入当前注册期针灸继续教育要求的学时数。持证人可以将两年期注册报告前获得的超过两年期三十四学时要求的 CAE 学时结转,这些超额学时可以用于下一注册期要求的学时数,但本条(b)(8)规定的课程除外。超出的总学时数最多可以结转三十四学时。超过该学时的注册日期后的两年,超出的 CAE 学时不得结转或者应用于两年一次的 CAE 报告。

(k) 虚假报告/陈述。

如果持证人就针灸继续教育学时向委员会故意作出虚假报告或者陈述,委员会将根据得克萨斯州针灸法第 205.351(a)(2)条和第 205.351(a)(6)条的规定对其实施纪律处分。

(1) 罚款。

未能获得并及时报告针灸继续教育学时数以续期执照的持证人将因逾期注册而被罚款,罚款金额见本卷第 175.2 节条和第 175.3 条(关于注册和续期费用以及罚款)的规定。

(m) 纪律处分措施、附条件执照和解释。

本条应当解释为允许委员会为纪律处分措施及附条件的执照而规定完成额外的针灸继续教育学时。

(n) 针灸继续教育课程要求的内容。

针灸继续教育课程应当满足下列要求:

(1) 该课程、项目或活动的内容与针灸或者东方医学服务有关,并且应当:

(A) 与针灸实践所需的知识和/或技术技能有关;或者

(B) 与直接和/或间接的患者治疗有关。

(2) 教学方法足以教授该课程、项目或者活动的内容。

(3) 教员的证书表明其有能力和足够的培训、教育和经验来教授特定的课程、项目或者活动。

(4) 教育提供者对完成课程、项目或者活动的个人保持准确的出席/参与记录。

(5) 课程、项目或者活动的一学分等于至少五十分钟的实际指导或者培训。

(6) 课程、方案或者活动是由知识渊博的卫生保健提供者或者声誉良好的学校、州或者专业组织提供的。

(7) 课程说明提供充分的信息,以便每个参与者了解项目的基础以及要实现的目标和目的。

(8) 教育提供者在每个项目结束时获得书面评估,将评估整理成统计小结,并根据要求向委员会提供小结。

（o）针灸继续教育批准申请。

所有为满足 CAE 学分要求而提出的课程、项目或者活动的批准申请,均应当以书面形式提交给委员会的教育理事会,并附上各项所需的费用,准确描述课程、项目或者活动的信息、文件和材料,以便核实是否符合本条(n)的要求。

委员会或者教育理事会可以根据需要要求补充信息、文件和材料,以获得对课程、项目或者活动的充分描述,并核实是否符合本条(n)的要求。

根据委员会或者教育理事会的决定,在决定批准申请时可能需要检查原始证明文件。

针灸委员会有权对课程、项目或者活动进行随机和定期检查,以确保教育提供者已经满足并将继续满足本条(n)的教育审批标准。

在要求对课程、项目或者活动进行批准时,教育提供者应当同意针灸委员会或者其指定人进行此类检查,并进一步同意提供针灸委员会酌情决定的课程、项目或者活动的批准或者继续批准可能需要的补充信息、文件和材料,以描述课程、项目或者活动。

如果教育提供者未能提供必要的信息、文件和材料,以证明其符合本条(n)的标准,则可以作为拒绝 CAE 批准或者取消有关课程、项目或者活动的事先批准的理由。

（p）有关拒绝批准请求的复议。

针对拒绝批准 CAE 课程、项目或者活动的决定,可以由教育理事会或者委员会根据有关课程、项目或者活动的补充信息,或者在表明有正当理由复议的情况下复议。

拒绝裁定的复议决定,应当是基于考虑补充资料或者所表明的正当理由而作出的酌情处理决定。

复议请求应当由教育机构以书面形式提出,委员会工作人员或者委员会的理事会可以口头或者书面形式提出。

（q）有关批准的复议。

教育理事会或者委员会可以根据有关课程、项目或者活动的补充信息,或者在有充分理由的情况下,针对批准 CAE 课程、项目或者活动的决定进行复议。复议批准裁定的决定,应当是基于对补充信息或者正当理由的考虑而作出的酌情决定。复议请求可以由公众成员以书面形式提出,也可以由委员会工作人员或者委员会的理事会以口头或者书面形式提出。

（r）提供者的准入标准。

（1）要成为获得批准的医疗服务提供者,则其应当以委员会核准的表格向委员会提交医疗服务提供者申请表,并连同所需费用一同提交。所有提交给委员会的提供者申请表和文件都应当使用英文。

（2）要成为一位获得批准的提供者,则该提供者应当向委员会提交证据证明其连续三年在得克萨斯州至少提供一门不同的 CAE 课程的经验,并且其中的每一年都得到了委员会的批准。此外,该提供者应当没有向委员会投诉或者训诫的历史。

（3）获得批准的提供者在委员会批准后三年内到期,并可以在提交规定的申请和各项规定的费用后续期。

（4）根据本卷第 183.2(2)条(关于定义)的规定,已经获得委员会批准的针灸学校和学院,如果想成为获得批准的提供者,则应当向委员会提交一份获批提供者编号申请。

(s)提供者获得批准的要求。

(1)就本节而言,除非另有规定,否则只有个人或者组织提交申请表提供者并获得提供者编号时,才能使用"经批准的提供者"的称谓。

(2)一个人或者组织只能获得一个提供者编号。

当两个或者两个以上经批准的提供者共同主办一门课程时,该课程应当仅由一个提供者编号进行标识,该提供者应当负责记录保存、广告宣传、颁发证书和教员资格证书。

(3)获得批准的提供者应当提供由符合本条(t)规定的最低标准要求的人员讲授或者指导的 CAE 课程。

(4)获得批准的提供者应当在一个确定的地点保存以下记录,为期四年:

(A)每门课程的课程大纲。

(B)每门课程的时间和地点的记录。

(C)课程教员的履历表或者简历。

(D)每门课程的出勤记录。

(E)每门课程的学员评价表。

(5)获得批准的提供者应当在委员会要求的十日内向委员会提交以下资料:

(A)显示参加课程的各位执业针灸师的姓名、签名和执照号码的出席记录副本。

(B)该课程的学员评估表。

(6)获得批准的提供者应当在课程结束后六十日内,向每个完成课程的学员颁发包含以下信息的结业证书:

(A)提供者的名称和编号。

(B)课程名称。

(C)参加者的姓名(如果适用)和针灸执照号码。

(D)课程的日期和地点。

(E)完成的继续教育学时数。

(F)学时描述,说明所完成的学时是一般针灸学、伦理学、中药学、生物医学,还是服务管理。

(G)指导针灸师在完成课程后保留至少四年证书的声明。

(7)获得批准的提供者应当在三十日内通知委员会有关提供者和/或负责提供者的继续教育课程的组成部分的各种变化,包括姓名、地址或者电话号码的变化。

(8)提供者的批准不得转让。

(9)委员会可以在合理的工作时间内对获得批准的提供者的记录、课程、教师和相关活动进行审核。

(t)讲师。

(1)针灸师讲师的最低资格。

讲师应当:

(A)在得克萨斯州或者其他州持有有效的针灸执照,并且没有受到州执照颁发机构的各种纪律处分令或被列入察看状态。

（B）在课程主旨方面具有知识渊博、与时俱进和熟练的技能，可以通过以下任何一项证明：

（i）在官方认可的学院或者大学或者中等以上教育机构至少获得硕士学位，主修与所提交课程内容直接相关的学科。

（ii）在过去两年内，在其所任教的专业领域有教授类似学科内容的经验。

（iii）在过去两年内有至少一年在其任教的专业领域的经验；或者

（iv）已毕业于本卷第183.2(2)条规定的可接受的针灸学校，并已完成三年的针灸执业专业经验。

（2）非针灸师讲师的最低资格。

讲师应当：

（A）在适当的情况下，目前在其专业领域获得执照或者认证。

（B）提供专门培训或者经验的书面证明，可以包括但不限于某一学科领域的培训证书或者高级学位证书。

（C）在过去两年内，在其所任教的专业领域有至少一年的教学经验。

（u）CAE 课程教学学分。

经委员会批准的 CAE 课程或由经批准的提供 CAE 学分的机构提供的课程的讲师可以从每学时的授课中获得三学时的 CAE 学分，每年不超过六学时的继续教育学分，无论授课多少学时。

作为被批准课程的小组演示的成员，参与者不能获得作为讲师的 CAE 学分。

学校教职员工在完成常规教学任务时不得获得 CAE 学分。

（v）批准的到期、拒绝和撤回。

（1）CAE 课程的批准自批准之日起三年后终止。

（2）如果提供者被判定犯有与提供者的活动密切相关的罪行，则委员会可以撤销对提供者的批准或者拒绝批准申请。

（3）服务提供者或者申请人在需要提交给委员会的各项信息中对事实的任何重大误述，都是撤回批准或者拒绝申请的理由。

（4）委员会可以在向提供者发出书面通知，说明撤回理由，并给其一个合理的机会向委员会或者委员会指定的人作出陈述后，撤回对提供者的批准。

（5）如果委员会拒绝批准提供者，则该提供者可以通过向委员会提交说明理由的信件，对这一行动提出上诉。

上诉信应当在邮寄给申请人关于委员会拒绝的通知后的十日内提交给委员会。

委员会应当考虑该上诉。

（w）针灸师，如果是军人，则可以要求延长时间，但不得超过两年，以完成各项 CAE 要求。

第 183.21 条　针灸戒毒专家的针灸继续教育

（a）目的。

本条的目的是通过规定经过认证的针灸戒毒专家进行耳穴继续针灸教育（Continuing

Auricular Acupuncture Education,CAAE)的最低要求,进一步提高他们的专业技能和知识,从而促进得克萨斯州人民的健康、安全和福利。

（b）耳穴继续针灸教育的最低要求。

作为重新获得针灸戒毒专家认证书的先决条件,针灸戒毒专家应当向医学委员会提供文件,证明该人已成功达到医学委员会规定的继续教育要求,其中包括本款（1）至（2）所列的要求：

（1）每年至少有六学时的 CAAE 是关于耳穴针灸的实践。

（2）所要求的学时应当来自学习课程时医学委员会指定或者以其他方式批准的学分课程。

（c）报告耳穴针灸继续教育。

针灸戒毒专家应当在证书持有人的再认证表格上报告上一年完成的耳穴针灸继续教育的学时数和类型。

（d）豁免耳穴针灸继续教育的理由。

针灸师可以以书面形式提出申请,并可以根据本款（1）和（2）所列的一个或者多个原因免于遵守每年最低耳穴针灸继续教育的要求：

（1）灾难性的疾病。

（2）服役时间超过一年的军人。

（e）豁免请求。

豁免申请应当经医学委员会行政主管批准,并应当在证书到期前至少三十日以书面形式提交。

（f）豁免期限和延期。

根据本条（d）和（e）给予的豁免期不得超过一年,但是如果在本次豁免到期前至少三十日提交书面申请,则可以每年续期。

（g）学分的核实。

委员会可以要求各位经认证的针灸戒毒专家提供耳穴针灸继续教育学时的书面证明,证书持有人应当在要求之日起三十日内提供所要求的证明。如果不及时提供所要求的证明,可能会导致委员会的纪律处分措施。

（h）批准耳穴针灸继续教育。

耳穴针灸继续教育（CAAE）学分学时数应当由医学委员会批准,并应当包括由 ACAOM 认证的学校或者其他国家认证的机构、组织或者医学委员会批准的培训项目提供的教育。课程应当于 1999 年 1 月 1 日或者之前获得批准。2000 年续期认证时,应当要求 CAE 首次报告。

批准应当基于教育提供者证明：

（1）该课程、项目或者活动的内容与针灸实践有关,而不是关于加强服务、业务或者办公室管理的课程。

（2）教学方法足以教授该课程、项目或者活动的内容。

（3）教员的资格证明其有能力和足够的培训、教育和经验来教授特定的课程、项目或者活动。

（4）教育提供者对完成该课程、项目或者活动的个人保持准确的出勤/参与记录。

（5）该课程、项目或者活动的每一学分等于至少五十分钟的实践教学或者培训。

（i）虚假报告/陈述。

如果证书持有人在报告获得的针灸继续教育学时方面故意作虚假报告或者陈述，则将构成委员会根据《得克萨斯州针灸法》第205.351（a）（2）条和第205.351（a）（6）条实施纪律处分措施的依据。

（j）罚款。

如果未能获得并及时报告用于证书续期的耳穴针灸继续教育学时，则证书持有人应当受到本卷第175.2条（关于注册和续期费用）和本卷第175.3条（关于处罚）规定的逾期注册罚款。

（k）纪律处分措施、附条件执照和解释。

本条应当解释为允许委员会为纪律处分措施及附条件的执照而规定完成额外的耳穴针灸继续教育学时。

第183.22条　语言要求

（a）所有病历和处方均应当用英文书写，但针灸术语（包括草药）除外，这些术语在适当情况下更常用中文或者拼音翻译。

（b）给患者的所有书面指示应当用英文书写。

如果患者不会说英语，则针灸师应当做出合理的努力将其翻译成患者的母语。

第183.23条　语言要求

根据《得克萨斯州针灸法》第205.3522条的规定，委员会可以接受自愿放弃针灸执照。

本卷第196章（关于自愿交出医疗执照）应当以类似于该节适用于医疗执照的方式管理自愿放弃的针灸执照。本卷第183.4条（关于执照）的规定应当管辖自愿放弃后的重新申请。

第183.24条　程序

本卷第187章（关于程序规则）的规定应当在适用的情况下管辖与针灸师有关的程序。

如果第187章的规定与《得克萨斯州针灸法》或者本章的规则相冲突，则应当以该针灸法和本章规定为准。

第183.25条　非执业状态的执照

（a）持证人可以通过向委员会申请将其执照置于非执业状态。

处于非执业状态的持证人不得在得克萨斯州从事针灸师工作。

（b）为了使持证人处于非执业状态，持证人应当具有一个当前的注册许可以及一个信誉良好的执照。

（c）持证人在非执业状态下在得克萨斯州作为针灸师执业，被视为无证执业。

（d）持证人可以通过向委员会申请，支付与针灸执照申请费相同的申请费，遵守法案对执照续期的要求，提供该针灸师在其他各州持有针灸执照的有效证明，并遵守本条（e）的规定，恢复执业状态。

（e）非执业状态的持证人申请恢复执业状态，应当向委员会提供足够的文件，证明申请人在收到恢复执照申请之前的两年内,按照本卷第183.4(a)(9)(B)条的定义,全职积极从事针灸工作,或者在可以接受的经批准的针灸学校中担任教职员工。不符合这一要求的申请人,在符合本款(1)至(4)规定的一个或者多个条件或者限制的情况下,可以由委员会决定是否恢复执照。

(1)完成本卷第183.20条(关于针灸继续教育)规定的针灸继续教育学时资格。

(2)将申请人的执业活动限制和/或排除在特定的执业活动之外。

(3)辅导教育。

(4)其他补救性或者限制性的条件或者要求,这些条件或者要求是由委员会决定的,以确保保护公众和确保申请人作为针灸师安全执业的最低能力。

(f)在非执业状态五年后,持证人的执照应当按照要求被取消。该针灸师可以通过遵守获得初始执照的要求和程序来获得新的执照。在执照取消后,针灸师可以申请新的执照。针灸师应当遵守获得执照的标准要求和程序。

第183.26条 停用执照

(a)注册续期费不适用于停用执照的持证人。

下列持证人将被置于停用状态:

(1)持证人应当没有受到委员会的调查或者正在执行的命令,或者拥有限制性的执照。

(2)持证人应当以书面形式向委员会申请将其执照置于正式停用状态。

(b)对于执照处于正式停用状态的持证人,应当适用以下限制性规定:

(1)持证人不得在各个州从事针灸实践。

(2)持证人的执照不得背书到各个其他州。

(c)持证人可以按照以下方式申请恢复积极执业:

(1)处于停用状态的持证人,如果处于停用状态不到两年,则可以通过向委员会申请,支付与针灸执照申请费相同的申请费,遵守法案对执照续期的要求,并遵守本款(2)(A)至(2)(D)的规定(如果适用),来申请恢复执业状态。

(2)处于停用状态的持证人,如果其执照已被置于正式停用状态两年或者更长时间,则其寻求恢复执业状态的请求应当提交给委员会的执照委员会审议,并向全体委员会提出批准或者拒绝该请求的建议。

在审议了该请求和执照委员会的建议后,委员会应当批准或者拒绝该请求。如果该项请求被批准,则可以无条件获得批准,或受制于委员会为充分保护公众而制定的条件,包括但不限于:

(A)完成了本卷第183.20条(关于针灸继续教育)规定的针灸继续教育学时。

(B)将申请人的执业活动限制和/或排除在特定的执业活动之外。

(C)补救教育。

(D)委员会为确保保护公众和确保申请人安全执业的最低能力所要求的,其他补救性或者限制性的条件。

(3)如果持证人的执照被置于正式停用状态不足两年,则其寻求恢复执业状态的请求可以由委员会的行政主管批准,或者由行政主管提交委员会审议,并向全体委员会提出批准或者拒绝请求的建议。在行政主管将申请提交给委员会执照委员会的情况下,执照委员会应当向全体委员会提出批准或者拒绝的建议。在对申请和执照委员会的建议进行审议后,委员会应当批准或者拒绝该申请,但是应当符合委员会确定的充分保护公众所需的条件,包括但不限于本款(2)(A)至(2)(D)规定的选项。

(4)在评估恢复执业状态的申请时,执照委员会或者委员会全体成员可以要求申请的持证人出席委员会办公室,并可以要求由一名或者多名医生经行政主管、财务长秘书、执照委员会或者委员会多数票决定的人事先书面批准的其他医疗保健提供者对其进行身体或者精神检查。

第 183.27 条　豁免某些军人配偶的执照

(a)得克萨斯州医学委员会行政主管应当根据《得克萨斯州职业法典》第 55.0041(a)条的规定,在无须获得执照的情形下,授权合格的军人配偶在得克萨斯州从事针灸实践。

这种执业授权对于该军人在得克萨斯州军队就职期间有效,但不得超过三年。

(b)为获得执业授权,军人配偶应当:

(1)在其他州、准州、加拿大省或者国家具有有效的针灸执照,并且:

(A)其执照要求经委员会认定与得克萨斯州的执照要求基本相同。

(B)没有受到任何限制、纪律处分措施、察看或者调查。

(2)以委员会规定的表格通知委员会该军人配偶计划在得克萨斯州执业。

(3)根据得克萨斯州《政府法典》第 437.001(1)条(关于定义)的规定,提交军人配偶在本州的居住证明、配偶的军人身份证复印件,以及该军人作为现役军人的身份证明。

(c)当军人配偶被授权在得克萨斯州进行针灸实践时,应当遵守适用于得克萨斯州针灸实践的所有其他法律法规。

(d)一旦委员会收到有关军人配偶拟在得克萨斯州执业的通知表格,委员会将核实该军人配偶持有的另一个州、准州、加拿大省或者国家颁发的执照是否有效并且信誉良好。

此外,委员会还将确定该司法管辖区的执照要求是否与得克萨斯州的执照要求基本相同。

夏 威 夷 州

夏威夷州针灸法[①]

第 436E‑1 条　规制必要性声明

立法机关特此声明,针灸是治疗疾病和残疾以及稳固和强身健体的理论和方法,它影响着公众健康、安全和福利,因此有必要对于从事针灸实践的个人进行规制。

第 436E‑2 条　定义

在本章所用术语如下:

"针灸医师"系指从事针灸实践的个人。

"委员会"系指针灸委员会。

"部门"系指商业和消费者事业部。

"主管"系指商业和消费者事业部主管。

"已获学位"系指学术或者临床获得的学位(非荣誉学位)。

"针灸实践"系指刺激人体上某个针灸穴位,以控制和调节人体内能量的流动与平衡。

该实践包括通过针刺穿人体皮肤技术,以及通过使用指压、电气、机械、热或者其他传统治疗手段进行点刺激的技术。

第 436E‑3 条　执照要求

除法律另有规定外,任何人不得在本州从事无偿或者有偿的针灸实践,或者不得主动提出从事针灸实践,也不得在没有本州颁发的有效且未被撤销的执照或者实习许可的情况下,公开或者私下宣布其准备或者有资格进行针灸实践。但是,在委员会根据本法第 436E‑3.6 条初步通过规定之前,不得执行获得许可的相关要求。

第 436E‑3.5 条　医师和骨科医师不可豁免

根据《夏威夷州议会法》修订版第 453 章获得执照的人员,如希望从事针灸实践,应当按照本章规定获得执照。

---

① 　根据《夏威夷州议会法》修订版第 2 卷第 25 编第 436E 章"针灸执业者"译出。

第 436E - 3.6 条　针灸实习生许可证相关规定

（a）除法律另有规定之外，任何人在未事先获得委员会许可证的情况下，不得在本州无偿或者有偿作为针灸实习生从事针灸实践。该许可证允许申请人在根据本章获得正式执照的执业针灸师的直接监督下从事为期四年的针灸实践。

（b）针灸实习生许可证可以补发一次，期限不超过一年，但应当向委员会提出书面要求并缴纳所需费用。

（c）委员会应当根据《夏威夷州议会法》修订版第 91 章通过的规则，界定针灸实习生的职能，确定针灸实习生许可证的申请人应当满足的要求，并指定由执业针灸师直接监督针灸实习生的程序。

第 436E - 4 条　豁免

另一州或者国家的执业针灸师在针灸或者医学会会议或者针灸学校进行演示或者讲座时，应当豁免本章规定的许可程序。

第 436E - 5 条　考试的资格

（a）除非本人已通过考试，并且被认定具有委员会根据《夏威夷州议会法》修订版第 91 章通过规则中规定的必要资格，否则任何人不得获得针灸执照。

（b）在 2000 年 9 月 1 日之前，除本条（c）另有规定外，任何申请人在有资格参加考试之前，应当向委员会提供足够材料，证明其已经接受不少于一千五百学时的教育和培训，其中包括：

（1）在委员会批准的研究所或者学校进行的针灸学（传统中医）的正式课程：

（A）应当不少于两学年（不少于六百学时）。

（B）应当获得证书或者文凭。

（2）在执业针灸师的监督下，在临床实习计划中进行一年临床实习（不少于十二个月以及不少于九百学时）；前提是临床实习的九百学时可以从颁发证书或者文凭的学院或者学校中获得，也可以在不隶属于学院或者学校的执业针灸师的监督下获得。

（c）在 1984 年 12 月 31 日之前开始在委员会批准的学校接受培训，以及在 1989 年 12 月 31 日之前完成培训并在 2000 年 9 月 1 日之前向委员会提交申请的学生应当：

（1）不丧失继续教育的权利，以及所获得和累计得学分。

（2）为本章之目的，应当符合第 436D 章规定的考试和执照要求，以及 1984 年 12 月 31 日委员会执行的规则；前提是学校没有为了降低完成课程的标准而更改课程。

此类学生如能提交下列课程的证明，便有资格参加考试：

（A）至少十八个月（至少五百七十六学时）的专业培训。

（B）在执业针灸师的监督下，接受至少六个月（至少四百八十学时）的人体针灸临床培训。

（d）尽管第（b）款和第（c）款另有规定，自 2000 年 9 月 1 日起，在任何申请人有资格参加执照考试之前，申请人应当向委员会提供充分证据，证明申请人已经完成正式针灸课程，并且总计接受了至少两千一百七十五学时的学术和临床培训，其中包括至少一千五百一十五学时的针灸学课程（传统东方医学）和至少六百六十学时的临床培训，并获得证书或者文凭。

对于毕业于美国或者其管辖区的机构、学校或者学院的申请人,该机构、学校或者学院应当获得美国教育部认可的美国针灸或者东方医学认证机构的认证或认证候选人。

对于拥有针灸学正式课程的外国机构、学校或者学院毕业的申请人,申请人应当自费由委员会批准和指定的专业评估员评估申请人的成绩单和课程,该评估员应当确定成绩单和课程是否至少与美国认可的针灸课程具有同等效力,并且该外国机构应当由适当的政府机构或者相应国家的司法管辖区政府机构认可的机构许可、批准或者认可,且应当被委员会批准。

第 436E‑6 条　针灸委员会

(a)应当设立一个针灸委员会,其成员应当由州长指定。

委员会应当由五人组成,其中两人为普通公民,其中三人为根据本章拥有执照的针灸师。

(b)自 1992 年 7 月 1 日起,此后,被任命为委员会成员的每位成员任期四年,连续任期不得超过两届。自 1992 年 7 月 1 日之前被任命为委员会成员的,应当允许继续在委员会任职,直到自首次任命之日起最多连续任职满八年为止。

第 436E‑7 条　委员会的权利和职责

除法律授权的任何权利和义务外,委员会应当:

(1)根据《夏威夷州议会法》修订版第 91 章通过规定,执行本章的宗旨,特别强调公众健康与安全。

(2)制定执照标准。

(3)准备,管理和评定考试成绩,前提是委员会可以与测试机构签订提供这些服务的合同。

(4)颁发、续期、吊销和撤销执照。

(5)对执照申请人和持证人进行注册登记。

(6)调查并就任何违反本章和委员会任何规定的行为举行听证会。

(7)保存其诉讼记录。

(8)履行本章规定的职能、权利和义务所需的一切事项。

第 436E‑8 条　根据 1992 年法案第 202 章第 181 条废除

第 436E‑9 条　两年一次的续期

每位根据本章获得执照的人,应当在每个奇数年的 6 月 30 日或者之前向委员会登记并且缴纳两年的费用。未缴纳两年续期费,将自到期之日没收执照。执照被没收后,可以在提交申请并且缴纳执照恢复费的一年之内予以恢复。

第 436E‑10 条　撤销或者吊销执照

除法律授权的任何其他行动外,本章规定的针灸执照均可以被针灸委员会以任何法律授权的原因撤销或者吊销,包括但不限于以下原因:

(1)以保证可以永久治愈明显无法治愈的疾病为由获取酬金。

(2)使用虚假、欺诈或者欺骗性广告,并且做出不真实或者不可能的陈述。

(3)习惯使用任何易上瘾的管制药物,例如鸦片或者其任何衍生物、吗啡、海洛因或者可卡因。

（4）通过欺诈、谎报或者欺骗获得执照。

（5）职业不端行为或者严重粗心或者在针灸实践中明显无实践能力。

（6）违反本章通过的任何规定。

第436E‑11条　根据1992年法案第202章第182条废除

第436E‑12条　罚款

（a）除根据本章获发执照的人员外，任何人如果在没有委员会颁发的执照或者许可证的情况下，在针灸实践的任何阶段提供实践、治疗或者指导，或者使用任何文字或者头衔诱使他人相信其正在从事某种类型的针灸实践，均属轻罪，并且应当因每次违规行为处以不少于五十美元或者不超过一千美元的罚款。

（b）除了执业针灸师以外，任何人不能：

（1）从事或者试图从事针灸实践。

（2）购买、出售或者欺诈性地获得任何文凭或者针灸执照，无论是否记录在案。

（3）不遵守本章规定，使用"针灸师""D.Ac"或者"D.O.M."头衔或者任何单词或者头衔误导人们相信该人正在从事针灸实践。

（4）违反本章规定。

应当按（a）的规定进行处罚，该部门亦可寻求所有可获得的法律及公平补救，包括寻求禁令救济。

第436E‑13条　头衔的使用

（a）持证人如获得本州委员会颁发的针灸执照，可以在针灸广告中使用"执业针灸师"或者"L.Ac"头衔，并且注明持证人姓名，或者在持证人的姓名后标明或者附加标注。

（b）如果持证人已获得博士学位，并且其学位是由美国教育部认可的地区或者国家认证机构认可的学校或者学院授予，则该持证人可以在针灸广告中使用"Ph.D"头衔，或者在其姓名后标明或者附加标注该头衔。

委员会根据本款承认的博士持证人应当使用非执业医师头衔，而非（c）款所指出的"针灸师"或"针灸医师"。

（c）经委员会批准使用针灸医师称号的持证人，可以使用"针灸医师"或者"D.Ac"头衔，或者在持证人姓名前添加"医师"或者"Dr."前缀，但是如果"医师"或者"Dr."前缀单独使用，则"针灸师"一词应当紧接在持证人姓名后。

（d）在任何持证人有资格使用针灸医师头衔之前，持证人应当向委员会提供符合委员会要求的证据，证明持证人已经获得针灸（传统中医）博士学位。

对于毕业于美国或者美国管辖的任何准州的研究机构、学院或者学校的持证人，该研究机构、学院或者针灸和中医专业的研究生与博士课程的认证或者预认证（候选）应当由美国教育部认可的地区或者国家机构认证或者确定为认证候选人。

对于毕业于外国的研究机构、学校或者学院的持证人，持证人应当自费将成绩单和课程安排由经委员会批准和指定的专业评估人员评估，该评估人员应当确定成绩单和课程是否至少与美国认可的针灸和中医博士课程具有同等效力，以及该外国研究机构是否获得许可、批准或者由适当的政府在该外国管辖的政府当局承认的机构认可，其课程应当经委员会批准。

（e）除本条另有规定外,不得使用其他头衔、前缀或者名称。

第436E-14条　外国学校课程和标准

如果外国学校或者学院的课程和标准,并不等同于或者低于委员会认可和批准的、从事针灸研究或者实践的美国机构,针灸委员会将不承认和不认可其获得的博士学位。

夏威夷州针灸行政法①

第1节　总　　则

第16-72-1条　废止

第16-72-2条　目的

本章旨在澄清和实施《夏威夷州议会法》修订版（HRS）第436E章,以使该章的规定得到最好的执行,并最有效地满足公众利益。

第2节　定　　义

第16-72-3条　定义

《夏威夷州议会法》修订版第436E章中出现的术语定义应当作为参考。

此外,在本章中使用时,应当包括以下定义:

"针灸针"系指由针灸医师将不同长度和直径的笔直细长的针杆,尖端用于刺入皮肤,另一端用于操纵或者保持针的位置,并插入人体的穴位。

订书针不是针灸针。

"针灸医师"系指持有本州针灸委员会颁发的有效执照的人。

"获批的高等教育学校"或者"高等教育学校"系指:

（1）经美国教育部认可的认证机构认证或者被认可为候选认证的学院、学校或者大学。

（2）在申请人完成针灸课程时,已经被美国教育部认可的认证机构或者作为候选认证机构的学院、学校或者大学;或者

（3）其课程被委员会认可,但由于针灸或者其他医学研究领域的认证尚不存在,而未被认证或者被确认为认证候选者的学院、学校或者大学。

如果是外国学校,"获批的高等教育学校"系指由适当的政府当局或者该国政府当局认可的机构许可、批准或者认证的学院、学校或者大学,其课程由委员会核准。

"获批的学校""委员会批准的学校",或者类似的词语或者短语,在提到针灸或者传统东方医学的研究所、学校、学院或者包括针灸的课程时,系指:

（1）对于在2000年9月1日之前向委员会提交申请的人来说,指的是在申请人毕业时,由适当的政府当局或者该司法管辖区、州或者国家的政府当局认可的机构许可、核准、候

---

① 根据《夏威夷州行政法典》第16卷第72章"针灸执业者"译出。

选认证或者认可的针灸或者传统东方医学的研究所、学校、学院或者项目,并且其课程由委员会核准;或者

(2)对于在 2000 年 9 月 1 日或者之后向委员会提交申请的人来说,指的是在申请人毕业时被美国教育部认可的针灸或者传统东方医学认证机构认证或者被认可为候选认证的针灸或者传统东方医学研究所、学校、学院或者项目。

但"获批的学校"就外国学校而言,系指具有针灸或者传统东方医学科学的正式课程的研究所、学校、学院或者项目,该项目由该国适当的政府当局或者政府当局认可的机构许可、核准或者认可,且其课程由委员会核准。

"委员会"系指针灸委员会。

"面授学时"或者"学时"系指至少五十分钟的有组织的课堂教学或者临床实践培训。

"部长"系指商业和消费者事务部部长。

"功能障碍"系指人体的一种状况而不是器质性障碍,其症状不能指任何器质性病变或者结构的改变。

"办公场所"系指用于针灸实践的实体设施。

"传统东方医学"系指治疗技术系统,主要强调人体能量的流动和平衡,是在健康和疾病中保持身体健康的最重要因素,包括针灸和草药的实践。

第 3 节　授权实践;执业范围;执照

第 16－72－4 条　经授权的针灸实践

针灸师被授权通过刺激某个或者某些穴位对人体进行治疗,以达到控制和调节体内能量流动和平衡的目的。

这种实践包括通过插针刺入皮肤的技术,以及通过使用穴位按摩、电、机械、热疗、艾灸、拔罐或者传统治疗手段进行穴位刺激。

第 16－72－5 条　针灸的执业范围

针灸被广泛地应用于治疗。

然而,委员会认识到应当对针灸医师的执业范围进行指导,并规定了以下允许的授权治疗做法,其中包括止痛和镇痛;功能性和肌肉骨骼疾病,包括疾病的功能性组成部分,以及维持健康,促进健康和生理平衡。

第 16－72－6 条　病历

持证人应当保持其治疗的每名患者的准确病历记录。病历应当包括患者的姓名、治疗的指征和性质,以及持证人认为重要的任何其他相关数据。病历应当至少留存七年,并应当在任何时候开放给委员会或者经其正式授权的代表检查。

第 16－72－7 条　废止

第 16－72－8 条　执照的展示

执照证书应当在提供针灸的办公场所的醒目位置展示。

第 16－72－9 条　地址的变更

持证人应当在地址变更后的 30 日内通知委员会。

第 16‐72‐10 条　废止

第 16‐72‐11 条　针灸实习生临床培训中的监督和职能

（a）持证人不得允许针灸实习生在没有持证人的直接监督下从事针灸实践。

直接监督系指在实习生对患者进行治疗之前、期间和之后，持证人都要亲自在场，指导和积极引导实习生对患者进行诊断和治疗。

此外，持证人应当确保：

（1）所有患者应当被告知并同意接受针灸实习生的治疗。

（2）在持证人监督下的每名针灸实习生都应当佩戴醒目的名牌，上面写有该人的姓名和"针灸实习生"字样。

"针灸实习生"的字样应当至少有 1.27 厘米高。

（b）针灸实习生提供的针灸实践可以包括本法第 16‐72‐5 条规定的针灸执业范围中所确定的项目。

（c）任何违反本条规定的行为都将构成渎职。

第 4 节　教育和培训要求

第 16‐72‐14 条　正规教育和培训要求

（a）对于 2000 年 9 月 1 日前申请的申请人：

（1）申请人应当提交从获批的学校毕业的证明，以及完成不少于一千五百学时正规教育和临床培训课程的证明。

（2）为满足正规教育的要求，申请人应当完成一门学习课程，并获得证书或者文凭，其中包括不少于两个学年（不少于六百学时）的针灸或者传统东方医学课程学习。

学习课程应当包括，但不限于以下科目：

（A）传统东方医学的历史和哲学（《内经》、道家、气功、阴阳等）。

（B）传统的人体解剖学，包括穴位的位置。

（C）传统生理学，包括五行脏腑理论。

（D）传统的临床诊断，包括脉诊。

（E）病理学，包括六淫和七情。

（F）针灸的规律（母子、夫妻、五行）。

（G）穴位的分类和功能。

（H）针刺技术。

（I）并发症。

（J）禁忌穴位。

（K）抢救。

（L）安全和预防措施。

（M）使用电气设备进行诊断和治疗。

（N）公众健康和福利。

（O）卫生和环境卫生。

（P）东方草药研究。

（Q）临床针灸实践。

（3）为满足临床培训的要求，申请人应当在一名执业针灸师的直接监督下，完成不少于十二个月（不少于九百学时）的临床实习培训课程。

临床实习培训的要求可以从获批的学校或者其他临床机构、私人诊所的执业针灸师处获得，或者从以上任何组合中获得。

提供直接监督的执业针灸师应当：

（A）在申请人的临床实习培训开始前，已经获得执照并积极服务不少于五年。

（B）在监督过程中拥有现行的、有效的、未受限制的执照。

（b）尽管有本条（a）的要求，在 1984 年 12 月 31 日之前在委员会核准的学校开始培训，并在 1989 年 12 月 31 日之前完成所需培训的申请人，在 2000 年 9 月 1 日之前向委员会提交申请，有资格获得执照，但申请人应当符合《夏威夷州议会法》修订版第 436D 章规定的考试和执照的要求。只要学校没有改变其课程以降低完成该课程的标准，且申请人应当提交毕业证明，以及完成正规教育和临床培训课程的证明，包括至少一千〇五十六学时。

（1）为满足正规教育的要求，申请人应当完成至少为期十八个月（至少五百七十六学时）的针灸或者传统东方医学学习课程。

该学习课程应当包括但不限于（a）（2）所列的科目。

（2）为满足临床培训要求，申请人应当已经完成至少为期六个月（至少四百八十学时）的培训课程，在执业针灸师的直接监督下对人体提供针灸服务。

临床培训的要求可以是在获批的学校，或者其他临床环境，从私人诊所的执业针灸师或者从任何组合中获得。

（c）在 2000 年 9 月 1 日或者之后提出申请的申请人，应当提交获批的学校毕业的证明，以及完成至少两千一百七十五学时的正规教育和临床培训课程的证明。

（1）为满足正规教育的要求，申请人应当完成不少于一千五百一十五学时的针灸和传统东方医学课程的学习。该学习课程应当包括但不限于（a）（2）所列的科目。

（2）为满足临床培训要求，申请人应当在执业针灸师的监督下完成不少于六百六十学时的培训课程。临床培训要求应当在获批的学校获得，不得从私人诊所或者其他临床机构的执业针灸师处获得，除非它是获批的学校的临床培训课程的一部分。

第 16-72-15 条　废止

第 16-72-16 条　废止

第 16-72-17 条　头衔使用的学术标准

（a）在遵守本规定的前提下，如果持证人已经在核准的学校完成教育，包括与学位有关的针灸课程，则可以使用已获得的学位头衔。

（b）以前被委员会授权使用博士头衔的持证人可以继续使用该头衔，直到 2000 年 9 月 1 日。

（c）从 2000 年 9 月 1 日起，任何持证人不得使用"针灸学博士""D.Ac."或者类似的博士头衔，除非该持证人已经向委员会申请并获得核准使用该头衔。

为使持证人获得委员会的核准,持证人应当证明其具有以下条件:

(1)从获批的学校获得针灸或者传统东方医学博士学位,或者已经完成委员会核准的针灸或者传统东方医学研究或者实践的课程,其中包括至少五百学时的高级学术教育和培训,超过了L.Ac.入门水平的要求。

这五百学时可以包括2000年4月6日题为"博士课程"的"附录A"中所列第一类和第二类课题的任何组合,以确定证书评估。

(2)至少一千五百学时的针灸、传统东方草药或者传统东方理疗的临床培训和实践,其中可包括实验室工作和学术指导,且该培训和实践是在其开始攻读博士学位后获得的。

(d)在确定持证人是否符合使用博士头衔的要求时,委员会可以要求提供额外的信息,包括但不限于持证人的学校目录课程说明和针灸临床培训和实践的文件。

(e)已经获得博士头衔的持证人,如果希望在2000年9月1日之后使用博士头衔,应当遵守本条(c)的规定。

(f)已经获得针灸或者传统东方医学"博士学位"的持证人,应当被视为非执业医师,并允许其按照《夏威夷州议会法》修订版第436E-13(b)条的规定使用"博士学位"的头衔。

第5节 执照的申请

第16-72-20条 申请

(a)每位申请针灸执照的人,或者希望在本州使用涉及针灸的头衔的人,应当使用委员会提供的表格提交申请。

所有申请应当以英文填写,并附上以下资料:

(1)根据《夏威夷州议会法》修订版第91章,由主管通过的规则中规定的申请费,并以个人支票、本票或者邮政汇票的形式支付。

(2)所需教育和培训的证明,如适用。

(3)由申请人签署的宣誓书,声明申请人已经阅读并将遵守委员会关于针灸实践的法律和规则(《夏威夷州议会法》修订版第436E章和本章)。

(4)委员会认为必要的其他文件。

(b)已经参加并通过第16-72-33条规定的考试的申请人,可以在任何时候提出执照申请,并应当附上本条(a)规定的项目。

申请人应当责成考试承办机构直接向委员会核实第16-72-36条规定的考试合格分数。

第16-72-20.1条 针灸实习生许可证的申请

(a)申请人可以在任何时候向委员会提出申请,要求在执业针灸师的直接监督下从事为期四年的针灸实习工作,并应当附上所需费用。

委员会可以授权其执行官员向合格的申请人颁发针灸实习生许可证。

(b)申请人应当向委员会提供以下证明。

(1)证明申请人已经在获批的学校完成了至少三个学期的教学,并且目前正在获批的学校就读或者已经毕业的证明文件。

(2)申请人的毕业证书或者获批的学校的正式成绩单的复印件,显示申请人的毕业日期,或者获批的学校的院长或者注册官的信件,说明申请人已经完成至少三个学期的学习,应当与申请一起提交。

(3)负责监督的针灸医师的姓名和执照编号;但从 2000 年 9 月 1 日起,申请人还应当提供获得临床培训的获批的学校的名称。

(c)在向委员会提出书面申请并支付所需费用后,可以重新颁发针灸实习生许可证,期限不超过一年。

第 16－72－21 条　废止

第 16－72－22 条　废止

第 16－72－23 条　教育和培训的证明

(a)对于在 2000 年 9 月 1 日之前申请的申请人,只要符合第 16－72－14(a)条或者第 16－72－14(b)条的要求,就应当提交以下文件作为申请人的教育和培训证明,如适用:

(1)在获批的学校进行的学术或者教育研究和培训的证明,包括:

(A)委员会直接从获批的学校收到的经认证的成绩单,以及获批的学校的文凭、证书或者其他经认证的文件的复印件,并盖有学校的公章,证明完成了包括针灸在内的针灸或者传统东方医学的课程,以及证明在获批的学校学习的课程的复印件;或者

(B)如果学校不再存续,或者学校的记录由于某种合理的原因而被销毁,申请人可以提交一份宣誓书,说明学校的名称、地址、入学日期和完成的课程,委员会可以酌情要求申请人提供适当的政府当局或者政府当局认可的机构关于学校关闭或者学校记录不可用的证明,以及委员会可能认为必要的其他信息和文件。

(C)认证机构或者适当的政府主管部门的声明,说明该学校已经被美国教育部认可的针灸认证机构认证或者正在申请认证,或者该学校已被该司法管辖区、州或者国家的适当政府主管部门或者政府主管部门认可的机构许可、批准或者认证。

(2)临床培训的证明,包括:

(A)申请人接受临床培训的执业针灸师的姓名、医师执照号码、医师执照日期的证明、营业的街道地址、申请人完成培训的学时数、日期和时间,以及对申请人接受培训的描述。

(B)由针灸医师宣誓签署的证明,证明申请人按照第 16－72－14(a)(3)条或者第 16－72－14(b)(2)条的要求,在该针灸医师的指导下完成了临床培训课程,如适用;或者

(C)如果针灸医师已经去世或者下落不明,申请人应当如此说明,并应当提交一份宣誓书,证明申请人已经完成临床培训,以及委员会认为必要的其他文件。

(b)对于 2000 年 9 月 1 日或者之后申请的申请人,应当提交以下文件作为申请人在核准的学校接受教育和临床培训的证明,但这些文件应当符合第 16－72－14(c)条的要求:

(1)直接从获批的学校收到的经认证的成绩单,以及由获批的学校提供的、盖有学校公章的文凭、证书或者其他经认证的文件的复印件,证明其完成了针灸或者传统东方医学的课程,其中包括针灸,还包括证明在获批的学校学习的领域的课程的复印件;或者

(2)如果学校不再存续,或者学校的记录由于某种合理的原因而被销毁,申请人可以提交一份宣誓书,说明学校的名称、地址、入学日期和完成的课程,还应当提供美国教育部承认的针灸认证机构的证明。如果是外国学校,则应当提供适当的政府当局或者政府当局认可

的机构对学校关闭或者无法获得学校记录的证明,以及委员会认为必要的其他信息和文件。

(3)认证机构或者适当的政府机构的声明,说明该学校已经被美国教育部认可的针灸认证机构认证或者正在申请认证。如果该学校为外国学校,则应当说明该学校已经被该国适当的政府部门或者其认可的机构许可、批准或者认证。

第 16 - 72 - 24 条　废止

第 16 - 72 - 25 条　外语文件

所有以外语提交的文件应当附有准确的英文翻译。

每份译文都应当附有翻译者的宣誓书,证明翻译者在文件语言和英语方面都具有胜任力,且译文是外语原文的真实和完整的翻译,并经公证处宣誓。

与个人申请有关的任何文件的翻译费用应当由申请人承担。

第 16 - 72 - 26 条　文件的充分性

在任何情况下,委员会对文件材料是否充分具有最终决定力。

委员会可以要求申请人提供进一步的资格证明,也可以要求与申请人进行个人面谈以确定申请人的资格。

第 16 - 72 - 27 条　提交执照申请的截止日期

应当在考试日前七十五日提交执照申请及其附件。

第 16 - 72 - 28 条　听证请求

任何因委员会拒绝授予、续期、恢复或者重新颁发执照,或者因委员会不允许使用学术头衔而感到不满的人,应当自拒绝日起的六十日内根据《夏威夷州议会法》修订版第 91 章和《夏威夷行政法典》第 16 - 201 章的服务和程序规则,提交争议案件听证的请求。

根据《夏威夷州议会法》修订版第 91 - 14 章或者其他规则,只能根据委员会的最终命令向巡回法院提出上诉。

第 16 - 72 - 29 条　废止

第 6 节　考　　试

第 16 - 72 - 33 条　考试

(a)每名申请针灸执照的人都应当通过国家针灸与东方医学认证委员会(NCCAOM)的书面综合考试或者委员会确定的其他书面考试。

(b)考试应当符合《夏威夷州议会法》修订版第 436E 章和本章规定的针灸实践的操作和理论要求。

考试应当以其自身的价值为依据。

申请人应当通过考试,才能获得提供针灸实践的资格。

(c)委员会可以与独立的考试承办机构签订合同,为委员会提供考试。

(d)残疾的申请人可以得到特殊的考试安排和便利,但应当在委员会提供的表格上提出适当的申请,且符合委员会或者其指定人员所确定的资格。

第 16 - 72 - 34 条　考试频次

考试应当至少每年进行一次。

第 16－72－35 条　考试语言

考试应当以英语进行;但委员会可以根据申请人的要求并在私立考试承办机构提供这种考试的情况下以另一种语言进行笔试。

第 16－72－36 条　合格分数

书面综合笔试的合格分数应当由委员会的考试承办机构根据标准心理测量程序和推荐的入门水平能力的最低分数确定。委员会要求的其他书面考试的合格分数应当由委员会决定。

第 16－72－37 条　废止

第 16－72－38 条　废止

第 16－72－39 条　废止

第 16－72－40 条　废止

第 16－72－41 条　废止

第 16－72－42 条　废止

第 7 节　执 照 续 期

第 16－72－46 条　续期

无论执照何时颁发,都应当在每个奇数年的 6 月 30 日或者之前采用委员会提供的表格提出续期申请,并附上主管根据《夏威夷州议会法》修订版第 91 章通过的规则所规定的适当续期费用。

第 16－72－47 条　续期到期日

如果信封上有每个奇数年的 6 月 30 日或者之前的邮戳,则通过邮寄方式发送的费用应当被视为到期时提交。

续期费用应当以个人支票、银行本票或者邮政汇票的形式支付。

第 16－72－48 条　未续期;丧失;恢复

如果没有支付到期的续期费用,执照将自动失效。

因未支付续期费用而失效的执照,在符合法律规定的执照续期要求,并由申请人提出书面申请和支付适当的执照恢复费用后,可以自失效日期起一年内恢复效力。该规则由主管根据《夏威夷州议会法修订版》第 91 章通过。

自失效之日起一年后,执照将无法被恢复。当事人应当被视为新申请人,并应当满足新申请人的所有要求。

第 8 节　公共卫生和环境卫生设施

第 16－72－52 条　办公场所

在住宅建筑物内进行针灸实践时,应设置一个或者多个房间分开作为针灸诊所的办公场所,并应当只用于此目的。

办公场所内应当配备盥洗室和厕所设施。

在正常营业时间内,委员会或者商业和消费者事务部的任何授权雇员可以随时对针灸办公场所进行检查。

第 16‒72‒53 条　卫生设施操作标准

操作服务应当包括以下标准：

（1）应当为每位患者的检查台上使用干净的一次性纸或者新的床单。

（2）在处理针头之前和在治疗不同患者之间，应当以肥皂和水洗手。

（3）穿刺针应当事先未使用过并经过消毒。

（4）穿刺针每次治疗不得使用超过一次，使用后应当立即按下文（8）规定的方式处理。

（5）在使用针头之前，针灸手术区域的皮肤应当用杀菌液彻底拭擦。

（6）如果未使用的针或者器械的无菌性受到影响，在使用前应当在最低温度 121℃下以每平方英寸十五磅的压力进行不少于三十分钟的消毒。

（7）可以重复使用的器械或者不穿刺的针灸针在用于患者之前，应当在最低温度 121℃下以每平方英寸十五磅的压力进行不少于三十分钟的消毒。

（8）所有待处置的针头应当放在符合卫生部门规定标准的危险废物容器中。

对该容器的所有操作，包括但不限于处理、运输和处置该容器，应当符合卫生部门的规章和规则。

（9）应当遵循政府机构或者制造商推荐的其他合理的卫生程序和操作，以保护患者和公众的健康和安全。

第 16‒72‒57 条　头衔的使用

（a）针灸师不得在广告中虚报自己的学术头衔、专业头衔、资格和隶属关系。

（b）获批的大专院校、中专学校、获批的学校或者委员会批准的学校授予的博士学位，并符合第 16‒72‒17 条规定的学术标准的持证人，可以使用"Doctor""Dr.""Doctor of Acupuncture""D.Ac."等头衔，但应当在持证人的名字后面紧跟"针灸师"一词。

（c）在本章通过之前已经被委员会核准使用博士头衔的持证人可以继续使用该头衔，直至 2000 年 9 月 1 日。

为了在 2000 年 9 月 1 日之后继续使用博士头衔，持证人应当申请使用学术头衔，并应当向委员会提供符合第 16‒72‒17 条学术标准的证明。

如果持证人未能在 2000 年 9 月 1 日前提出申请并达到第 16‒72‒17 条的学术标准，将导致其丧失继续使用博士头衔的所有权利，持证人应当立即停止使用该头衔。

第 16‒72‒58 条　废止

第 16‒72‒59 条　废止

第 16‒72‒63 条　行政执行和程序

本法的执行和程序的规则应按照《夏威夷州议会法行政规则》第 16‒201 章的规定，即商业和消费者事务部的执行和程序规则，该规则通过引用而纳入本章并成为其一部分。

第 16‒72‒67 条　口头证词

（a）委员会应当接受关于委员会议程上的任何项目的口头证词，但该证词应当符合下列条件：

（1）希望提供口头证词的每个人都应当在会议前四十八小时内通知委员会，届时应当说明要提供的证词的项目。

(2)委员会可要求任何提供口头证词的证人,以书面形式将其言论或者摘要提交委员会。

(3)委员会可以重新安排列入议程的项目,以便提供最有效和方便地提供口头证词。

(4)提供口头证词的证人在开始作证时,应当表明自己的身份和所代表的组织(若有)。

(5)委员会可以将口头证词限制在一个特定的时间内,但在任何情况下都不得少于五分钟,而且在开始作证之前,应当告知证人将被限制的时间。

(6)委员会可以拒绝听取任何与所提交的议程项目无关、不重要或者不适当地重复的证词。

(b)本章不得要求委员会听取或者接受某人有关如下议题的口头或者书面证据,即该事项是与《夏威夷州议会法行政规则》第16-201章的听证救济、宣告性救济或者规则救济规则相关的待决事项。

(c)本章的任何内容都不妨碍委员会请出席会议的人员发表口头意见,或者邀请人员就委员会议程上的任何特定事项向委员会报告。

第16-72条 附录A-博士项目

2000年4月6日

第I类:东方医学科学

A. 东方医学哲学和年代学研究

传统哲学文学和文化视角下的东方医学研究,包括与针灸与东方医学的发展有关的古典历史。

B. 诊断与症状学进阶

诊断技术的研究,包括必要数据的相关性和统计分析来评估结果。

进一步研究器官系统和特定的针灸程序,以发展更精准的诊断技能,包括比较古典和现代技术。

C. 经络系统进阶

有关人体系统如何与针灸经络系统的内部和不同途径整合的研究。

D. 穴位及其功能进阶

基于形态反应的穴位科学分析,包括经典和现代穴位测定方法的系统。

进一步研究新的穴位,并对禁忌证进行科学回顾。

E. 中药学进阶

传统东方中药配方的成分和药理分析研究。

对基于传统东方医学的新配方和药典进行进一步的研究回顾。

F. 传统病理学和病因学

传统东西方病理和病因学方面的先进研究。

研究"脏腑"的形态结构和外部、内部、非外部/非内部因素的影响以及与中国生物钟机制的病理关系。

研究针灸应用对体液过滤的生物系统功能。

研究针灸对器官的病理进展、转化和分子代谢的影响。

第Ⅱ类：应用于普通医学的针灸科学

A. 免疫学

针灸与东方医学对过敏反应和自身免疫性疾病的人体免疫生理机制和活性生理物质变化的调节研究。

B. 妇科和泌尿科

针灸与东方医学在妇科、产科问题和女性内分泌系统的研究。

研究肾脏和泌尿生殖系统，确定针灸与东方医学应用的临床意义。

C. 神经病学

针灸对内源性和血管舒缩控制的影响研究。

对中枢和周围神经系统进行神经解剖学和组织学研究，以确定针灸应用的意义。

D. 矫正手术

针灸对骨科疾病的起源和影响的研究。

骨学研究和 X 线分析。

E. 老年病学/康复学/慢性病

针灸与东方医学在衰老相关疾病中的应用的研究。

研究可扩展到康复、慢性疾病和疼痛管理。

F. 儿科学

回顾婴儿和儿童相关疾病，与围产期护理相关的针灸与东方医学治疗的临床应用。

小儿针灸治疗器械的研究与实践。

第Ⅲ类：相关先进临床针灸与东方医学

针灸的临床培训实践，以及东方理疗。

临床学分可能包括实验室工作和学术指导。

新墨西哥州

新墨西哥州针灸法①

第 61 - 14A - 1 条　简称

《新墨西哥州议会法》注释版（NMSA）第 61 卷第 14A 章可以被引用为"针灸和东方医学实践法"。

第 61 - 14A - 2 条　目的

为了公众健康、安全和福利，并保护公众免受针灸和东方医学的违反职业道德、不适当、不称职和非法实践的侵害，有必要提供法律和法规来管理针灸和东方医学的实践；针灸和东方医学委员会的主要责任和义务是保护公众。

第 61 - 14A - 3 条　定义

在《针灸和东方医学实践法》中使用的定义如下：

A."针灸"系指通过控制和调节能量和功能的流动和平衡，在身体的特定位置使用针灸针插入和拔出，以及使用其他装置、方式和程序来预防、治疗或者纠正疾病、伤害、疼痛或者其他病症，以恢复和保持健康。

B."委员会"系指针灸和东方医学委员会。

C."东方医学医生"系指持证人，可以从事针灸和东方医学实践，有能力独立执业，作为初级保健提供者，必要时与其他卫生保健提供者合作。

D."艾灸"系指在身体特定部位或者针灸针上使用热力，以此预防、治疗或者纠正任何疾病、伤害、疼痛或者其他病症。

E."东方医学"系指利用东方医学所有的传统和现代技术，通过控制和调节能量、形态和功能的流动和平衡，诊断、治疗和开出处方，以预防、治疗或者纠正疾病、伤害、疼痛或者其他身体或者精神状况的独特的初级卫生保健系统。

F."初级卫生保健提供者"系指在卫生保健执照范围内执业的卫生保健从业者，为个人的健康需求提供第一级的基本或者一般卫生保健，包括诊断和治疗服务，向其他卫生保健从

---

① 根据《新墨西哥州议会法》注释版第 61 卷第 14a 章"针灸与东方医学服务"译出。

业者的转诊,并在适当时保持连续护理。

G."东方医学技术"系指:

(1)东方医学中使用的诊断和治疗技术,包括诊断程序、针灸、艾灸、手法疗法,也称为推拿;其他物理医学模式和治疗程序;呼吸和功法;以及饮食、营养和生活方式咨询。

(2)开具、分配、制作和提供草药、顺势疗法药物、维生素、矿物质、酶、腺体产品、天然物质、天然药物、原生质、活细胞产品、玻尿酸原液、氨基酸、膳食和营养补充剂、新墨西哥州药品、设备和化妆品法中定义的化妆品以及药房法中定义的非处方药。

(3)开具、分配和提供新墨西哥州药品、设备和化妆品法中定义的设备、限制性设备和处方设备,前提是委员会通过规则确定这些设备在东方医学服务中是必要的,并且开具处方的东方医学医生已经按照委员会颁布的规则满足了对本段所列设备的处方权要求。

H."导师"系指具有至少十年临床经验的东方医学医生,是针灸和东方医学的教师。

第61-14A-4条 执照要求

除非根据《针灸和东方医学实践法》获得东方医学医生执照,否则任何人不得:

A.从事针灸或者东方医学实践。

B.使用该头衔或者代表自己为东方医学的合法医生,或者使用任何其他头衔、缩写、字母、数字、标志或者设备,表明该人作为合法的东方医学医生进行实践;或者

C.广告、向公众宣传或者以任何方式,代表他被授权从事针灸和东方医学实践。

第61-14A-4.1条 经认证的耳穴戒毒专家、监督员和培训项目;费用

A.非东方医学医生或者未根据《针灸和东方医学实践法》获得耳穴戒毒专家认证的人,不得:

(1)采用耳穴针灸治疗酗酒、药物滥用或者化学药物依赖。

(2)使用或者代表作为经认证的耳穴戒毒专家的头衔,或者使用任何其他表明该人作为耳穴戒毒专家执业的头衔、缩写、字母、数字、标志或者设备;或者

(3)宣传、向公众展示或者以任何方式表示该人被授权从事耳穴戒毒疗法。

B.委员会应当向已支付申请费并已满足委员会要求的人颁发耳穴戒毒专家证书;委员会应当通过规则,要求申请人符合以下条件:

(1)完成国家针灸戒毒协会培训或者经委员会批准的同等培训,包括洁针技术培训。

(2)证明在治疗、预防疾病、减少伤害和咨询酗酒、药物滥用或者化学药物依赖患者方面的经验,或者受雇于一个药物滥用治疗计划。

(3)完成委员会批准的培训计划,其中包括洁针技术、法学和委员会要求的其他技能的考试。

(4)在向委员会申请证明之前,证明至少连续两年没有因毒品或者酒精相关罪行而被定罪的记录。

C.经认证的耳穴戒毒专家,有权进行耳穴针灸和在耳部使用委员会批准的不穿透皮肤的简单设备,以治疗和预防酗酒、药物滥用或者化学药物依赖;专家应当使用五耳穴国家针灸戒毒程序或者委员会规则批准或者建立的耳穴程序,并且只能在委员会批准的方案中治疗或者预防酗酒、药物滥用或者化学药物依赖,该方案应证明在疾病预防、减少伤害或者治

疗或者预防酗酒、药物滥用或者化学药物依赖方面有经验。

D. 根据本条认证的人应当使用"认证的耳穴戒毒专家"或者"C.A.D.S."头衔，以此向公众宣传耳穴针灸服务。

E. 经认证的耳穴戒毒专家，应当向委员会申请续期该认证；如申请人支付续期费并达到了委员会规则的要求，委员会应当为其续期一年；申请人在认证有效期的截止日期前没有申请续期，可以根据委员会的规则缴付滞纳金；委员会应当认定在该日期后的六十日内未申请续期的证书为到期，而寻求有效认证的申请人应当向委员会申请新的证书；委员会应当根据规则，要求申请续期证明的申请人在向委员会申请续期前，证明至少一年无因毒品或者酒精有关的罪行而被定罪的记录。

F. 经认证的耳穴戒毒专家应当在委员会注册的东方医学注册医生的监督下实践；东方医学指导医生应当直接或者通过电话向执业耳穴戒毒专家咨询，并且监督对象不得超过委员会允许的人数限制；监督要求应当由委员会的规则来规定。

G. 东方医学医生如果监督经认证的耳穴戒毒专家，应当向委员会申请注册；委员会应当向符合其要求者发布确认注册的信息；委员会应当根据规则要求注册申请人列出将受到监督的认证耳穴戒毒专家，支付注册申请费，并展示治疗或者咨询酗酒、药物滥用或者化学药物依赖患者的临床经验。

H. 培养耳穴戒毒专家认证的培训计划应当向委员会申请批准；委员会应当批准符合委员会规定的要求并支付申请费的培训计划；该批准的有效期至首次批准后的 7 月 31 日。

I. 经委员会批准的提供耳穴戒毒专家认证培训的培训方案，应当向委员会申请重新获得批准；委员会应当批准对符合其要求的计划续期，有效期为一年；申请人在续期批准有效的最后一个日期前未续期的，应当缴纳滞纳金；委员会应当将在该日期后六十日内未续期的计划确定为到期计划；拟提请委员会批准的计划，应当向委员会重新申请。

J. 委员会应当征收下列费用：

（1）不超过一百五十美元的耳穴戒毒专家认证申请费。

（2）不超过七十五美元的耳穴戒毒专家证书续期费。

（3）不超过二百美元的耳穴戒毒专家认证督导的注册申请费。

（4）不超过二百美元的耳穴戒毒专家培训计划的批准申请费。

（5）不超过一百五十美元的耳穴戒毒培训专家培训计划的批准续期费。

（6）在根据本节颁发的注册、认证、批准或者续期的最后有效日期之后提出的续期申请，收取不超过五十美元的滞纳金。

K. 按照程序规定的统一执照法案，委员会发现某人违反了其建立的规则，可以拒绝、撤销或者吊销所有的认证，注册、批准或者续期请求。

第 61－14A－5 条　头衔

任何根据《针灸和东方医学实践法》的规定获得执照的人，在向公众宣传其服务时，应当使用"东方医学医生"的头衔或者"D.O.M."。"东方医学医生"或者"D.O.M."应当取代包括"医生"或者首字母"医生""M.D."在内的所有其他头衔，除非该人是根据《医疗执业法》的规定获得执照的医生。

第 61－14A－6 条　豁免

A.《针灸和东方医学实践法》中的任何内容,都并非旨在限制、干扰或者阻止任何其他类别的持证医疗专业人员在其执照范围内执业,但他们不得通过使用任何包含针灸、针灸师或者东方医学一词的头衔或者服务描述,向公众或者任何私人团体或者企业展示自己,除非他们根据《针灸和东方医学实践法》获得执照。

B. 如果当事人不自称为东方医学医生或者从事针灸或者东方医学实践,则《针灸和东方医学实践法》不适用于或者干涉下列做法:

（1）在紧急情况下提供无偿服务。

（2）家庭救济的家庭管理。

（3）关于呼吸、运动技巧的咨询或者教学和演示。

（4）膳食、营养方面的咨询、教学。

（5）某人或者精神团体的精神或者生活方式咨询,或者服务教会的宗教教义。

（6）提供关于草药、顺势疗法药物、维生素、矿物质、酶或者腺体或者营养补充剂的一般用途的信息;或者

（7）为诊断之目的而使用针灸针,以及由有执照的卫生保健专业人员为使用诊断药物或者治疗药物而使用针灸针。

第 61－14A－7 条　委员会成立;任命;官员;薪酬

A. "针灸和东方医学委员会"业已成立。

B. 该委员会在行政上隶属于政府监管和行政许可部门。

C. 委员会由州长任命的七名成员组成,每届任期为三年;委员会的四名成员应当是东方医学医生,他们在被任命前至少有五年在新墨西哥州居住并从事针灸和东方医学实践;三名成员应被任命为公众代表,不得在本州或者任何其他地区从事针灸和东方医学实践,也不得在所监管的行业中有任何经济利益;委员会成员不得担任提供针灸和东方医学教育计划的机构的所有者、负责人或者委员;来自以下每个类别的委员会成员不得超过一人:

（1）提供针灸和东方医学教育课程的机构的教职员工。

（2）针灸和东方医学的导师;或者

（3）针灸和东方医学专业协会的官员或者负责人。

D. 委员会成员应当由州长任命,任期为三年,委员会成员的任期应当于 7 月 1 日届满;委员会成员应当任职至其继任者被任命并合格为止;在未届满的剩余期限内,应按照与原任命相同的方式填补空缺。

E. 委员会成员不得连续担任超过两个完整的任期,如果委员会成员在收到通知后,连续三次没有出席会议,除非有委员会规定的理由,否则应当被建议解除委员会成员资格。

F. 委员会应每年从其成员中选出一名主席和其他高级管理人员,以履行其职责。

G. 委员会应每年至少召开一次会议,并在认为必要的其他时间召开;其他会议可由主席、多数委员会成员或者州长召集;在任的委员会成员超过半数即构成委员会的法定人数。

H. 委员会成员应当按照《每日津贴和里程法》的规定进行报销,不得领取其他补偿、津贴或者补贴。

第 61－14A－8 条　委员会；权力

委员会有权：

A. 执行《针灸和东方医学实践法》的规定。

B. 根据《州规则法案》，颁布实施和执行《针灸和东方医学实践法》规定所需的所有规则。

C. 采用道德准则。

D. 采用并使用印章。

E. 检查经批准的教育计划、外部项目和持证人办公室的设备。

F. 颁布实施继续教育要求的规则，以保护该州公民的健康和福祉，并保持和持续了解专业知识和意识。

G. 根据《统一执照法》：

（1）在发出预期行动的通知之前，发出调查传票，以调查针对持证人的投诉。

（2）就委员会管辖范围内的任何事项主持宣誓和收集证言。

（3）对与持证人的纪律处分有关的指控进行听证，包括拒绝、吊销或者撤销执照。

（4）根据《针灸和东方医学实践法》或者委员会的规定，颁发、拒绝颁发、续期、吊销或者撤销针灸和东方医学执业证书，或者颁发、拒绝颁发、续期、吊销或者撤销教育计划和外部项目的批准。

第 61－14A－8.1 条　扩大实践和处方权；认证

A. 委员会应当根据委员会的规则，向提交了委员会提供的完整表格、支付了认证申请费并提交了顺利完成委员会规则要求的额外培训证明的东方医学医生颁发证书，该证书只能用于 C 款第（1）和（2）项段中列举的内容的扩大实践和处方权限；委员会应当采用药学委员会确定的规则，对咖啡因、普鲁卡因、氧气、肾上腺素和生物相同激素的处方、给药、配制或者分发进行额外培训；委员会和药学委员会应当根据情况进行协商。

B. 委员会应当颁发基本注射疗法、注射疗法、静脉注射疗法和生物同质性激素疗法这四种扩大实践的证书。

C. 扩大实践和处方权应当包括：

（1）草药、顺势疗法药物、维生素、矿物质、氨基酸、蛋白质、酶、碳水化合物、脂质、腺体产品、天然物质、天然药物、原生质、活细胞产品、玻尿酸原液、膳食和营养补充剂、新墨西哥州药品、设备和化妆品法中定义的化妆品以及药房法中定义的非处方药的开具、分配、配制和分发。

（2）下列危险药品或者《新墨西哥州药品、设备和化妆品法》《管制药物法》或者《药房法》中规定的管制药物的处方、分配、配置和分发，条件是开具处方的东方医学医生已按照委员会颁布的关于本段所列药物的规则满足扩大实践和处方权的要求：

（a）无菌水。

（b）无菌盐水。

（c）沙拉平①或者其仿制品。

---

① 沙拉平：即 sarapin，是从猪笼草蒸馏得到的一种悬浮液，同糖皮质激素一样可以减轻炎症，用于慢性疼痛的治疗［《实用疼痛学杂志》，2010,6（6）］。

（d）咖啡因。

（e）普鲁卡因。

（f）氧气。

（g）肾上腺素。

（h）蒸汽冷却喷雾剂。

（i）生物同质性激素。

（j）生物制品,包括治疗性血清。

（k）本款(1)列举的任何药物或者物质,如果这些药物或者物质在任何时候都被归类为危险药物或者管制药物。

D. 当为患者配制药物时,获得扩大实践和处方权认证的东方医学医生应当遵守《美国药典》和《国家处方集》中对持证卫生保健专业人员的配制要求。

第 61－14A－9 条　委员会;职责

委员会应当:

A. 确定费用。

B. 根据《针灸和东方医学实践法》的规定,对申请成为东方医学执业医师的申请人进行考试。

C. 记录所有所举行的考试,以及所有参加考试的人的姓名、地址和考试结果。

D. 在考试结果向委员会公布后二十一日内,以书面形式通知各申请人。

E. 保存持证人的记录,其中应当记录所有持证人的姓名、地址和执照号码,以及所有执照续期、吊销和撤销的记录。

F. 规定颁发和续期执照和批准教育计划。

G. 准确记录其所有的会议、收支情况。

第 61－14A－10 条　颁发执照的要求

委员会应向符合以下条件的人颁发针灸和东方医学执照。

A. 向委员会提交的材料包括:

（1）在委员会提供的表格上填写完整的执照申请。

（2）由委员会确定的所需文件。

（3）所需的费用。

（4）一份宣誓书,说明申请人没有被发现有违反职业道德的行为或者不称职的情况。

（5）委员会确定的证据,证明申请人已经完成了《针灸和东方医学执业法》和委员会规则中规定的经委员会批准的针灸和东方医学教育课程。

（6）证明已通过委员会批准的考试。

B. 符合委员会的各项其他要求。

第 61－14A－11 条　考试

A. 委员会应当制定程序以确保每年至少提供一次执照考试。

B. 委员会应当制定受理考试申请的期限以及有关许可考试、重新参加考试的规定。

C. 委员会应当制定其批准的考试的合格线。

D. 委员会可以批准用于国家认证或者其他考试的考试,并将其作为颁发执照的依据。

E. 委员会应当要求每个合格的申请人通过一个有效的、客观的书面考试,考试内容不包括在委员会批准的其他考试中,至少包括以下科目:

（1）解剖学和生理学。

（2）病理学。

（3）诊断。

（4）药理学。

（5）针灸和东方医学的原理、实践和治疗技术。

F. 委员会可以要求每个合格的申请人通过一个有效的、客观的实践考试,考试内容不包括在委员会批准的其他考试中,证明他在应用针灸和东方医学的诊断和治疗技术方面的知识和技能。

G. 委员会应要求每个合格的申请人通过以下科目的书面考试或者实践考试,或者同时通过:

（1）个人卫生、环境卫生和洁针技术。

（2）针灸针和器械的消毒技术。

H. 委员会可以要求每个合格的申请人通过与针灸和东方医学有关的州法律和规则的书面考试。

I. 如果英语不是申请人的主要语言,委员会可以要求申请人通过委员会规定的英语水平考试。

第 61－14A－12 条　颁发临时执照的要求

A. 委员会应当制定向州外的东方医学医生颁发临时执照的标准。

B. 委员会可以向符合以下条件的人颁发临时执照:

（1）在另一州或者国外被合法认可从事针灸和东方医学实践,或者在另一州或者国外被合法认可从事另一种卫生保健职业,并拥有东方医学医生执业范围内的知识和技能。

（2）由新墨西哥州执业东方医学医生或者新墨西哥州提供经委员会批准的教育课程的机构的赞助,或与其存在合作关系。

（3）在委员会提供的表格上提交完整的临时执照申请。

（4）提交所需的文件,包括由委员会确定的充分教育和培训证明。

（5）提交所需的临时执照申请费。

（6）提交一份宣誓书,说明申请人没有被发现有违反职业道德的行为或者不称职的情况。

（7）提交由新墨西哥州东方医学医生或者新墨西哥州研究所的赞助和联系机构出具的宣誓书,证明申请人的资格和申请人将开展的活动。

C. 委员会可以授予临时执照,允许临时持证人从事以下工作:

（1）教授针灸和东方医学。

（2）与赞助的东方医学医生一起,为赞助医生的患者提供咨询。

（3）与主办医生合作,对主办医生的患者进行专门的诊断或者治疗技术。

（4）协助开展针灸和东方医学的研究。

（5）协助实施与针灸和东方医学有关的新技术。

D. 临时持证人只能从事临时执照授权的活动。

E. 临时执照应当注明赞助和合作的新墨西哥州东方医学医生或者研究所。

F. 临时执照的颁发期限由规则确定；但临时执照的发放期限不得超过十八个月，包括续期。

G. 在提交以下材料后，临时执照可以续期：

（1）用委员会提供的表格填写的临时执照续期申请。

（2）所需的临时执照续期费用。

H. 在委员会定期会议之间，只要合格的申请人提交了申请并遵守了本条的所有其他要求，委员会主席或者委员会授权的代表就可以颁发临时执照，直到委员会下次定期会议为止。

第 61－14A－13 条　颁发加急执照的要求

A. 如果申请人已经在另一个执照管辖区，按照《新墨西哥州议会法》注释版第 61－1－31 条规定获得了针灸和东方医学的执照、认证、注册或者法律认可，委员会应当在无须考试的情形下授予其执照：

（1）在委员会提供的表格上提交完整的加急执照申请。

（2）提交由委员会确定的所需文件。

（3）提交所需的快速颁发执照申请费。

（4）通过与针灸和东方医学有关的州法律和规则的书面考试，如果委员会要求正常的执照申请人通过这种考试。

B. 委员会应当在可行的情况下尽快颁发加急执照，并且不得迟于该人提交申请和所需费用的三十日内；该申请人应当提交证明，证实其持有有效的、不受限制的执照，且在其他执照管辖区的执照委员会中信誉良好，并在申请前至少在新墨西哥州执业了两年；如果委员会向某人颁发加急执照，而该人以前的执照管辖区不需要考试，委员会可以要求该人在执照续期前通过考试。

C. 委员会应当规定美国各州和准州以及哥伦比亚特区不接受加急执照申请，并且确定接受加急执照申请的其他国家的范围；委员会应当在其网站上公布上述不同的执照管辖区的名单；不被批准的执照管辖区的名单中还应当包括不被批准的具体原因；这些名单应当每年审查一次，以确定是否需要做出修正。

第 61－14A－14 条　教育计划的批准

A. 委员会应当根据规则确定委员会批准针灸和东方医学教育计划的标准；对于获得委员会批准的教育计划，应当向委员会提交证明，证明该教育计划至少：

（1）期限不少于四年。

（2）包括至少九百小时的受监督的临床服务。

（3）由合格的教师或者导师授课。

（4）作为毕业时所有班级和诊所的个人出席的先决条件，并至少完成以下科目：

（a）解剖学和生理学。

（b）病理学。

（c）诊断。

（d）药理学。

（e）东方的生命治疗原理，包括膳食、营养和咨询。

（f）东方医学的理论和技术。

（g）针灸治疗的注意事项和禁忌证。

（h）经络脉象评估和经络穴位的理论和应用。

（i）传统和现代的气或者生命能量评估方法。

（j）中药的处方和使用的注意事项和禁忌。

（k）个人卫生、环境卫生和洁针技术。

（l）针灸针设备的护理和管理。

（m）针灸针和器械的消毒技术。

（5）在完成所有教育计划要求后，颁发证书或者文凭。

B. 所有州内的针灸和东方医学的教育计划，其目的是让学生毕业后有资格成为委员会执照考试的申请人，每年由委员会批准；申请人应当提交以下材料：

（1）已完成的教育计划审批申请。

（2）由委员会确定的所需文件。

（3）证明由委员会确定，符合本条 A 款规定的教育要求。

（4）申请批准教育计划所需的费用。

C. 州外的针灸和东方医学教育计划，如果打算让学生毕业后有资格成为委员会执照考试的申请人，可以向委员会申请批准；申请人应当提交以下材料：

（1）已完成的教育计划审批申请。

（2）由委员会确定的所需文件。

（3）证明由委员会确定，符合本条 A 款规定的教育要求。

（4）申请批准教育计划所需的费用。

D. 每个州内批准的教育计划应每年续期，并在委员会规定的日期前提交：

（1）按照委员会提供的表格填写教育计划续期申请。

（2）证明由委员会确定，符合本条 A 款规定的教育要求。

（3）申请批准教育计划所需的费用。

E. 每个州外批准的教育计划可以每年续期，在委员会规定的日期之前提交：

（1）按照委员会提供的表格填写教育计划续期申请。

（2）证明由委员会确定，符合本条 A 规定的教育要求。

（3）申请批准教育计划所需的费用。

F. 在批准期结束后，应允许每个教育计划有六十日的宽限期，在此期间，可以通过提交以下材料续期批准：

（1）按照委员会提供的表格填写教育计划续期申请。

（2）证明由委员会确定，符合本条 A 款规定的教育要求。

（3）申请续期教育计划所需的费用。

（4）延期续期所需的费用。

G. 宽限期结束前未续期的,视为到期,教育计划应当另行申请。

第 61－14A－14.1 条　学生和校外实习生;指导实践

A. 参加经过批准的教育计划的学生,可以在教师或者导师的直接指导下开展针灸和东方医学实践,作为该教育计划的一部分。

B. 委员会可以颁布规则管理实习生从事的针灸和东方医学实践;该规则应当包括实习生和东方医学导师或者其他卫生保健专业导师的资格,以及允许的执业范围;委员会可能会对批准和续期已经批准的实习计划收取一笔费用;作为实习生参与计划是选择性的,并不作为获得执照的条件。

第 61－14A－15 条　执照续期

A. 每名持证人应当每年在委员会确定的日期之前提交以下材料:

（1）按照委员会提供的表格填写完整的执照续期申请。

（2）每年的执照续期所需的费用。

B. 委员会可要求继续教育证明或者其他能力证明作为续期的要求。

C. 在执照有效期之前,应当允许每个持证人有六十日的宽限期,通过提交下列材料续期执照:

（1）按照委员会提供的表格填写的续期申请。

（2）每年的执照续期所需的费用。

（3）所需缴纳的滞纳金。

D. 宽限期结束后未续期的执照视为到期,持证人将没有资格在州内执业。

对于在续期日期的一年内恢复已到期的执照,委员会应当制定除每年执照续期费用外的各项要求或者费用,并可以要求前持证人作为新的申请人重新申请。

第 61－14A－16 条　费用

除了《新墨西哥州议会法》注释版第 61－1－34 条规定外,委员会应当制定一个合理的不可退还的费用表,不超过以下金额:

A. 申请执照八百美元。

B. 加急执照申请七百五十美元。

C. 申请临时执照五百美元。

D. 考试,不包括任何国家认可的考试费用七百美元。

E. 年度执照更新四百美元。

F. 逾期执照续期二百美元。

G. 到期执照续期四百美元。

H. 临时执照续期一百美元。

I. 申请批准或者延长批准的教育计划六百美元。

J. 逾期续期的教育计划批准两百美元。

K. 年度继续教育机构注册两百美元。

L. 拓展或者扩大处方权的申请五百美元。

M. 外聘导师注册申请五百美元。

N. 申请外部人员认证五百美元。

O. 支付合理和必要的行政开支。

第 61‑14A‑17 条　纪律处分程序;司法审查;《统一执照法》的适用

A. 根据《统一执照法》,如果委员会发现持证人或者申请人存在以下情形,可以拒绝、撤销或者吊销任何根据《针灸和东方医学实践法》持有或者申请的永久或者临时执照:

（1）在获取或者试图获取执照时犯有欺诈或者欺骗行为。

（2）已被判定犯有重罪;定罪记录的核证副本应是这种定罪的确凿证据。

（3）犯有委员会规则所定义的不称职的行为。

（4）习惯性酗酒,沉迷于使用成瘾药物,或者沉迷于任何恶习,以至于不适合作为一名东方医学医生实践。

（5）犯有委员会规定的违反职业道德的行为。

（6）犯有任何违反《管制药物法》的行为。

（7）违反了《针灸和东方医学实践法》的规定或者委员会颁布的规则。

（8）未能向委员会、其调查员或者代表提供委员会所要求的信息。

（9）故意或者因疏忽而超出《针灸和东方医学实践法》规定的针灸和东方医学的范围进行实践。

（10）存在未能充分监督被赞助的临时执照持证人的行为。

（11）存在协助或者教唆未经委员会批准的人从事针灸和东方医学实践的行为。

（12）存在以假名行医或者企图行医的行为。

（13）以明知虚假陈述的手段做广告。

（14）以《针灸和东方医学实践法》或者委员会规则所禁止的不道德的方式进行宣传或者试图吸引顾客。

（15）被正规机构宣布为精神不健全的。

（16）在美国或者外国的任何司法管辖区,曾因类似于本款所述的行为而被撤销、吊销或者拒绝颁发东方医学医生的执照、证书或者注册;采取这种纪律处分的司法管辖区的记录的核证副本将是确凿的证据;或者

（17）在诊断或者治疗患者时,没有掌握或者应用在类似情况下合理胜任的东方医学医生通常使用的知识或者技能和护理,并适当考虑到所涉地区。

B. 纪律处分程序可以由任何人提起,应当通过宣誓控诉,并应当符合《统一执照法》的规定;听证会的任何一方都可以获得听证会记录的副本,但要支付副本的费用。

C. 任何提出宣誓控诉的人,如果是善意的,没有实际的恶意,应当免于承担因民事诉讼而产生的责任。

D. 除非被免除责任,否则持证人应当承担纪律处分程序的费用。

第 61‑14A‑18 条　基金创建

A. 在本州财政部设立"针灸和东方医药基金委员会"。

B. 委员会根据《针灸和东方医学实践法》收到的所有款项,应当存放于州财政部,记入

针灸和东方医学基金委员会名下。

州财政部应当按照其他州资金的投资方式一样进行投资。

基金内的所有余额应留在基金内,不得归还给普通基金。

C. 针灸和东方医学委员会的资金是拨给委员会的,只能用于支付执行《针灸和东方医学实践法》规定的必要费用。

第61－14A－19条　处罚

A. 违反《针灸和东方医学实践法》规定的,即属轻罪,经定罪后,将按照《新墨西哥州议会法》注释版第31－19－1条的规定进行处罚。

B. 除了刑事处罚以外,无证从事针灸或者东方医学实践的人也会受到委员会的纪律处分程序。

尽管第61－1－3.2条另有规定,委员会仍可以对该人判处不超过两千美元的民事罚款,并向该人收缴行政费用,包括调查费用和进行听证的费用。

罚款应当存入现有学校基金的名下。

第61－14A－20条　刑事罪犯就业法

《刑事罪犯就业法案》的规定应当适用于《针灸和东方医学实践法》所要求或者允许的任何对犯罪记录的考虑。

第61－14A－21条　执业针灸师;执照根据新法有效

根据本州先前法律获得有效针灸执照的人,应当被视为根据《针灸和东方医学实践法》的规定获得执照。

第61－14A－22条　机构存续的终止;延迟废止

根据《日落法案》,针灸和东方医学委员会将于2023年7月1日终止。

该委员会将继续按照《针灸和东方医学实践法》运作至2024年7月1日。

届时,《新墨西哥州议会法》注释版第61卷第14A章被废止。

新墨西哥州针灸行政法①

第1节　总　　则

第16－2－1－1条　发证机构

新墨西哥州针灸和东方医学委员会。

第16－2－1－2条　适用范围

适用于所有东方医学执照医生、申请人、临时执照持证人、临时执照申请人、获得扩大实践资格认证的东方医学医生、认证、教育课程、实习生、耳穴戒毒专家、教育计划和获得教育计划批准的申请人。

---

① 根据《新墨西哥州行政规则法典》第16卷第2章"针灸和东方医学执业者"译出。

第 16－2－1－3 条　法定权限

本部分是根据 1978 年《针灸和东方医学实践法案》,即《新墨西哥州议会法》注释版(NMSA,下同)第 61－14A－1 条、第 61－14A－2 条、第 61－14A－3 条、第 61－14A－7 条、第 61－14A－8 条、第 61－14A－8－1 条、第 61－14A－14－1 条和第 61－14A－9 条颁布的。

第 16－2－1－4 条　有效期

永久生效。

第 16－2－1－5 条　生效日期

2022 年 2 月 11 日,除非某一条款的末尾引用了一个更晚的日期。

第 16－2－1－6 条　目的

本部分除了提供了法案中的定义外,还提供了规则中使用的术语的定义,列出委员会的职责,澄清非公开记录的内容,规定委员会公共记录的检查制度,并提供电话会议。

第 16－2－1－7 条　定义

以下定义适用于本规则和法案:

A. 首字母"A"术语的定义:

(1)"A4M"系指美国抗衰老医学科学院。

(2)"ACAM"系指美国替代医学院。

(3)"ACAOM"系指针灸及东方医学教育审核委员会。

(4)"法案"系指《针灸和东方医学实践法案》,NMSA 第 61－14A－1 条至第 61－14A－22 条。

(5)"AMA"系指美国医学会。

(6)"动物针灸"系指对除人类以外的任何动物进行的针灸。

动物针灸是在新墨西哥州注册的兽医医生的监督下授权的,只有在《新墨西哥州兽医执业法案》,即 NMSA 第 61－14－1 条至第 61－14－20 条和新墨西哥州兽医委员会规则,即《新墨西哥州行政法典》(即 NMAC,下同)第 16－25－9－15 条的指导下才可以实施。

(7)"申请人"系指已向委员会提交东方医学医生执照申请的人。

(8)"临时执照申请人"系指已向委员会提交作为东方医学医生的临时执照申请的人。

(9)"耳穴针灸戒毒"系指一种与针灸相关的技术,仅用于治疗和预防酗酒、药物滥用和化学药物依赖。

耳穴针灸戒毒可以被描述或者称为"耳穴戒毒""针灸戒毒""耳穴针灸戒毒"或者"穴位戒毒"。

(10)"耳穴戒毒专家督导"系指根据 NMAC 第 16－2－16－18 条的规定,在委员会注册的东方医学医生。

(11)"耳穴戒毒专家培训计划"系指由委员会根据 NMAC 第 16－2－16－26 条的规定批准的一个培训计划,旨在培训经认证的耳穴戒毒专家和耳穴戒毒督导。

(12)"耳穴戒毒专家培训计划培训师"系指耳穴戒毒专家培训计划的工作人员,虽然不一定获得国家执照或者认证,但是在耳穴戒毒专家培训计划的目的和培训期间,才应被视为一名经认证的耳穴戒毒专家。

（13）"授权药物"系指 NMAC 第 16－2－20 条 4 项认证中定义的特定药物,根据 NMSA 第 61－14A－8(1)条的授权,由 NMAC 第 16－2－19 条定义的特定扩大实践类别的东方医学医生进行开具、管理、配制和分发。

B. 首字母"B"术语的定义：

（1）"生物同质性激素"系指这些化合物或者这些化合物的盐形式,它们与人体产生的激素具有完全相同的化学和分子结构。

（2）"生物医学诊断"系指根据最新版本或者国际疾病分类、第九修订、临床修订(ICD－9－CM)中公认的《传统生物医学指南》对一个人的医疗状况的诊断。

（3）"生物医学"系指将自然科学原理应用于临床医学的方法。

C. 首字母"C"术语的定义：

（1）"认证耳穴戒毒专家"系指一个人通过委员会 NMAC 第 16－2－16－10 条规定的认证后,从事仅针对耳朵的戒毒服务,只有在一个既定的治疗程序,在一名在该委员会注册的耳穴戒毒监督员的监督下实践。

根据 1978 年 NMSA 第 61－14A－4 条 B 款(1)项获得认证的人应当使用"经认证的耳穴戒毒专家"或者"C.A.D.S."的头衔。

（2）"总干事"系指委员会主席或者其指定人员,负责管理纪律处分程序的审前程序事项。

（3）"临床经验"系指该法案中定义的针灸和东方医学的实践,在任何司法管辖区获得初步许可、认证、注册或者法律认可后,才能进行针灸和东方医学实践。

一年的临床经验应包括在一个日历年内不少于五百患者小时的针灸和东方医学实践,在该年内至少接诊二十五名不同的患者。

一患者小时系指与患者在东方医学实践中花费的一小时。

（4）"临床技能考试"系指一种委员会批准的、经过验证的、客观的执业考试,证明申请人在针灸、东方医学和生物医学的诊断和治疗技术应用方面具有入门级知识、能力和技能。

（5）"申诉人"系指投诉方。

（6）"投诉委员会"系指由投诉委员会主席和投诉管理人组成的委员会。

（7）"投诉委员会主席"系指由委员会主席任命的委员会成员。

（8）"投诉管理人"系指委员会的管理人员或者由委员会主席任命的任何委员会成员。

D. 首字母"D"术语的定义：

（1）"部门"系指新墨西哥州的监管和许可部门。

（2）"戒毒"系指整合医学中的一个概念,其原理是有毒物质(毒素)在体内积聚可引起疾病。

消除这些毒素的治疗支持是戒毒。

（3）"东方医学医生"系指根据该法案获得针灸和东方医学执照的医生,因此作为初级保健医生或者独立专科护理医生对其患者负有责任。

E. 首字母"E"术语的定义：

（1）"教育课程"系指委员会批准的全面学习基础,以证明在特定知识方面的入门级能力以及在扩大实践中获得四种认证所需的技能。

教育课程不等于教育计划,因为这个术语在法案和规则中使用,其定义参见 NMAC 第 16－2－1 节。

(2)"教育计划"系指一个由委员会批准的、完整的正式计划,其目标是培养符合该法案 NMSA 第 61－14A－14 条和 NMAC 第 16－2－7 节要求的个人,以便其获得新墨西哥州的东方医学医生执照,培训时间至少四学年。

(3)"扩大实践"系指由 NMSA 第 61－14－8.1 条授权,并授予已经满足了 NMAC 第 16－2－19 节规定的许可要求的,经委员会认证的东方医学医生。

扩大实践是对根据 NMSA 第 61－14A－3 条 G 款(2)项确定的所有东方医学执业医生规定权利的补充。

(4)"实习生"系指正在接受外聘导师监督临床培训的申请人,其已满足外部认证的申请要求,并已获得了委员会根据 NMAC 第 16－2－14 节颁发的实习认证。

(5)"实习期"系指根据 NMAC 第 16－2－14 节,在新墨西哥州由外聘导师监督下从事的有限制的东方医学实践活动。

(6)"外聘导师"系指具有至少五段临床经历、运营一个临床设施并保持适当的专业和设施保险、满足委员会对外聘导师的申请要求,并获得委员会根据 NMAC 第 16－2－14 条颁发的外聘导师注册证书的东方医学医生。

F. 首字母"F"术语的定义：[保留]

G. 首字母"G"术语的定义："正当理由"系指由于严重事故、伤害或者疾病而无法遵守,或者由于存在无法预见的、超出主张正当理由的人的控制的、会造成过度困难的特殊情况而无法遵守。

主张正当理由的人应当有责任证明正当理由的存在。

H. 首字母"H"术语的定义：[保留]

I. 首字母"I"术语的定义：

(1)"非执业执照"系指信誉良好的持证人,其执照被委员会置于非执业状态,因此被视为符合 NMAC 第 16－2－15 节规定的非执业执照。

(2)"ICE"系指卓越认证研究所。

(3)"IFM"系指功能医学研究所。

J. 首字母"J"术语的定义：[保留]

K. 首字母"K"术语的定义：[保留]

L. 首字母"L"术语的定义：

(1)"持证人"系指根据本法案获得执照的东方医学医生。

(2)"执照"与 NMSA 第 61－1－34F(1)条定义的含义相同。

(3)"执照候选人"系指首次申请东方医学医生的执照申请已获委员会批准的申请人。

(4)"执照费用"与 NMSA 第 61－1－34(2)条中定义的含义相同。

(5)"执照背书"是在建立现行教育标准之前完成针灸和东方医学初始教育的经验丰富医生的执照程序以及通过结合 NMAC 第 16－2－17 节定义的教育、考试、授权的合法实践和临床经历来证明其能力的人。

通过背书程序获得的执照,可以获得作为东方医学医生的完全执照。

(6)"受限临时执照"系指根据 16.2.5.12 NMAC 的规定颁发的专门用于教授针灸和东方医学单一完整课程及协助实施针灸和东方医学新技术的执照,包括由除新墨西哥州之外的司法管辖区获得执照、注册、认证或法律认可的卫生保健从业者学习该等技术。

如果不是持证人或者临时执照持证人,对于在教学或者协助实施新技术时对他人演示、实践或者实施诊断和治疗技术的人,须持有受限临时执照。

受限临时执照不应当发给教授全学期课程的教师,这些课程是经批准的教育计划的一部分。

(7)"活细胞产品"是来自腺体组织和其他组织的活细胞。

M. 首字母"M"术语的定义:"现役军人"的含义与 NMSA 第 61-1-34 条 F 款(3)项的定义相同。

N. 首字母"N"术语的定义:

(1)"天然物质"系指存在于自然界中或者由自然界产生的,在性质或者用途上没有发生实质性改变的物质。

(2)"NCA"系指一种预期行动的通知。

(3)"NCCAOM"系指国家针灸及东方医学认证委员会。

O. 首字母"O"术语的定义:

(1)"办公室"系指用于针灸、东方医学和耳穴戒毒实践的物理设施。

(2)"氧化医学"系指理解和评价人体的氧化和还原生化功能,以及物质的处方或者管理,以及使用设备和疗法来改善身体的氧化和还原功能和健康。

P. 首字母"P"术语的定义:"原形态体"是腺体组织的提取物。

Q. 首字母"Q"术语的定义:〔保留〕

R. 首字母"R"术语的定义:

(1)"答辩人"系指投诉的对象。

(2)"规则"系指根据本法案颁布的、管理 NMAC 第 16-2 章中所述的有关法案实施和管理的规则。

S. 首字母"S"术语的定义:

(1)"基本同等"系指委员会认为,另一司法管辖区的议会法和规则中所载的教育、考试和经验要求,等同或者超过《针灸和东方医学实践法案》(即 NMSA 第 61-14A-1 条及以下内容)的相关要求。

(2)"受监督的临床观察"系指处于适当监管之下,对针灸和东方医疗实践的观察。

(3)"受监督的临床实践"系指处于适当监管之下,对针灸和东方医疗实践的应用。

(4)"监督"系指由 NMAC 第 16-2-7 节规定的合格教师或者导师提供的,学生在培训或者从事临床实践中的直接协调、指导和持续评估。

受监督临的床实践学生不超过四人,随时由合格的教师监督临床观察。

T. 首字母"T"术语的定义:

(1)"临时执照持有人"系指根据 NMSA 第 61-14-12 条和 NMAC 第 16-2-5 节持

有临时执照的东方医学医生。

（2）"治疗性血清"系指一种从血液中获得的产品,能去除凝块或者凝块成分和血细胞。

（3）"治疗方案"系指根据 NMAC 第 16-2-16-28 条的规定在经委员会批准的固定场所或者不固定单位提供的一项综合方案,可能包括预防疾病、减少伤害或者治疗或者预防酗酒、药物滥用或者化学药物依赖的医疗和咨询服务。

U. 首字母"U"术语的定义:"USP 797"是《美国药典》第 797 章的药物复合物。

V. 首字母"V"术语的定义:"退伍军人"的含义与 NMSA 第 61-1-34F（4）条的定义相同。

W. 首字母"W"术语的定义:〔保留〕

X. 首字母"X"术语的定义:〔保留〕

Y. 首字母"Y"术语的定义:〔保留〕

Z. 首字母"Z"术语的定义:〔保留〕

第 16-2-1-8 条　委员会职责

除该法案中所述的职责外,委员会还应当:

A. 保存所有经批准的教育计划的档案。

B. 颁发教育计划的批准证书。

C. 如果符合要求,就授权其部长职责。

D. 如有委员会成员连续三次缺席会议,通知州长。

E. 在每年 1 月 1 日之后的第一次委员会会议上选出一名主席和一名副主席。

F. 委员会应当履行其他职责,并应当行使依法授予的其他权力,或者行使从该等法定权力和职责中合理暗示的权力,以及在履行其本法案规定的职责时合理必要的权力。

第 16-2-1-9 条　公共记录

除另有规定外,根据《新墨西哥公共记录审查法》（即 NMSA 第 14-2-1 条以下的规定）,委员会保存的所有记录均可供公众查阅。

A. 在处理和调查投诉的过程中,以及在委员会就是否驳回投诉或者发布统一许可法（即 NMSA 第 61-1-1 条及以下）规定的预期措施通知进行投票之前,为了保持对投诉、披露机密来源、方法、信息或者持证人的调查的完整性,应当保密,不得接受公众审查。

该等记录应当包含通过投诉或代表任何调查代理机构的委员会的持证人收到或汇编的任何形式的证据。

B. 在对投诉的处理和调查完成后,在委员会决定驳回投诉或者发出预期行动的通知时,NMAC 第 16-2-1-9 条 A 所赋予的保密特权将解除,与投诉和投诉调查有关的记录、文件或者其他证据,应当供公众查阅。

C. 申请人接受的所有测试和测试问题不得供公众查阅,因为有一项相悖的公共政策,要求这些记录保密,以确保执照考试的诚信,旨在保护公众健康、安全和福利不受不称职人员的伤害。

D. 委员会或者其管理人可对 11 英寸×17 英寸或者更小的文件收取每页不超过一美元的费用。

第 16－2－1－10 条　电话会议

根据经修订的《公开会议法案》(即 NMSA 第 10－15－1.C 条),委员会成员难以或者不可能出席会议时,该成员可以通过会议电话或者类似的通信设备参加委员会会议,前提是在发言时可以确定通过电话参加会议的每个委员会成员。所有与会者都能够同时相互发表意见,出席会议的公众应当能够听到委员会成员在会议期间发言的声音。

委员会成员通过这种方式参与,即构成出席会议。

第 16－2－1－11 条　灾害或者紧急情况的规定

获得执照、信誉良好或者其他方面符合新墨西哥州执照要求的东方医学医生、教育计划和耳穴戒毒专家,当其所在州宣布发生联邦灾害后的四个月内,可以根据 NMAC 第 16－2－1－11 条在新墨西哥州申请执照。

应当向委员会申请紧急临时执照,并提供以下资料:

A. 根据本规定向委员会提出的申请,应采用委员会提供的完整的英文表格,其中应包括申请人的姓名、地址、出生日期和社会保障号码,并附上身份证明,其中可能包括政府签发的驾驶证、护照或者其他有照片的身份证明复印件;申请人在申请表上的签名。

B. 一份宣誓书证明申请人因联邦灾难所遭受的后果。

C. 符合 NMAC 第 16－2－3 节、第 16－2－4 节、第 16－2－7 节、第 16－2－10 节和第 16－2－16 节规定条件的证据。如果申请人无法从联邦申报的灾区获得文件,或者受阻于宣称的联邦灾难,委员会可以接受其他文件,以代替 NMAC 第 16－2－3 节、第 16－2－4 节、第 16－2－7 节、第 16－2－10 节和第 16－2－16 节所要求的表格。委员会保留在批准执照之前要求补充文件的权利,包括但不限于推荐表格和工作经验的验证表格。

D. 有正当理由可以例外。

E. 一份证明书,证明与申请一并提交的所有文件都是真实和准确的,或者是原始文件的副本。

F. 本节所有内容,均不构成对 NMAC 第 16－2－3 节、第 16－2－4 节、第 16－2－7 节、第 16－2－10 节和第 16－2－16 节的颁发执照要求的豁免。

G. 申请人有责任阅读、理解和遵守新墨西哥州关于本次申请以及针灸和东方医学实践相关的法规。

第2节　执业范围

第 16－2－2－1 条　发证机构

新墨西哥州针灸和东方医学委员会。

第 16－2－2－2 条　适用范围

本节规定适用于所有根据 NMAC 第 16－2－19 节的定义的执业东方医学医生,所有获得扩大实践的执业东方医学医生,只从事所授权的活动临时执照持证人,只从事实习期规定活动的实习生,以及参与委员会批准的针灸和东方医学教育计划的学生,此类学生由在该计划中的教师直接监督下工作。

第 16－2－2－3 条　法定权限

本节是根据《针灸和东方医学实践法案》,NMSA 第 61－14A－3 条、第 61－14A－4 条、第 61－14A－6 条、第 61－14A－8 条和第 61－14A－8.1 条颁布的。

第 16－2－2－4 条　有效期

永久生效。

第 16－2－2－5 条　有效期

除非某一条款的末尾引用了一个更晚的日期。

第 16－2－2－6 条　目的

本节阐明了东方医学医生、临时执照持证人、实习生、学生和获得扩大实践认证的东方医学医生的执业范围。

第 16－2－2－7 条　定义

参考 NMAC 第 16－2－1－7 条(第 1 节第 7 条)中的定义。

第 16－2－2－8 条　执业范围

根据 NMSA 第 61－14A－3 条的规定,东方医学实践在新墨西哥州是一个独特的初级卫生保健系统,其目标是预防,治疗,或者纠正任何疾病、伤害、疼痛或者其他身体或者精神病症,通过控制和调节能量的流动和平衡,形式和功能来恢复和维持健康。

东方医学包括针灸和东方医学医生所使用的所有传统和现代的诊断、处方和治疗方法。

东方医学医生的执业范围应包括但不限于:

A. 评估、管理和治疗服务。

B. 诊断性检查、检测和程序。

C. 安排诊断成像程序和实验室或其他诊断试验。

D. 针灸外科手术等相关程序。

E. 利用气、针、热、冷、色、光、红外线、紫外线、激光、声音、振动、压力、磁性、电力、电磁能、放血、吸力等装置或者手段对穴位、身体部位或者体内物质的刺激。

F. 物理医学的治疗方式、治疗程序和治疗设备。

G. 治疗性运动、气功法、呼吸技巧、冥想,以及使用生物反馈装置等设备,利用热、冷、色、光、红外线、紫外线、激光、声音、振动、压力、磁性、电力、电磁能等治疗手段。

H. 膳食和营养咨询,以及食品、饮料和膳食补充剂的处方或者管理。

I. 关于生活方式中的身体、情感和精神平衡的咨询和教育。

J. 开具、管理、配置、提供、合成、分发任何非注射草药、顺势疗法药物、维生素、矿物质、酶、腺产品、天然物质、原生质、活细胞产品、氨基酸、膳食和营养补充剂;《新墨西哥药品、器械和化妆品法案》中定义的化妆品以及《药房法案》中定义的非处方药。

K. 由符合 NMAC 第 16－2－2－9 条要求的东方医学医生在《新墨西哥药品、器械和化妆品法案》(第 26－1－1 条)中定义的器械、限制设备和处方设备的处方或者管理。

第 16－2－2－9 条　设备;受限设备和处方设备

该委员会确定,《新墨西哥药品、器械和化妆品法案》(NMSA 第 26－1－1 条)中定义的设备、限制性设备和处方设备在东方医学实践中是必要的。

接受过该设备制造商推荐过的培训的东方医学医生应当被授权开具处方、管理或者分发该设备。

第 16－2－2－10 条　扩大实践的执业范围

A. 除了新墨西哥州东方医学执业医生的执业范围外,在扩大实践中获得认证的执业范围应当包括以下任何或者所有模块的认证:基础注射治疗、注射治疗、静脉注射治疗和生物同质性激素治疗。

先前认证为 Rx1 扩大处方授权的从业人员,将获得基本注射治疗认证,而先前认证为 Rx2 扩大处方授权的从业人员,将获得注射治疗、静脉治疗和生物同质性激素治疗认证。

B. 扩大实践的范围应当包括:

(1) 草药、顺势疗法药物、维生素、矿物质、氨基酸、蛋白质、酶、碳水化合物、脂质、腺体产品、天然物质、天然药物、原生质、活细胞产品、玻尿酸原液、膳食和营养补充剂的处方、管理、配药和分发,在《新墨西哥药品、器械和化妆品法案》(1978 年 NMSA 第 26－1－1 条)中定义的化妆品,以及《药房法案》(NMSA 第 61－11－1 条)中定义的非处方药。

(2) 根据《新墨西哥药物、器械和化妆品法案》《管制药物法案》(1978 年 NMSA 第 30－31－1 条)或者《药房法案》中定义的下列危险药物或者受控物质的处方、管理、配制和分发:

(a) 无菌水。

(b) 无菌盐水。

(c) 沙拉平或者其仿制药。

(d) 咖啡因。

(e) 普鲁卡因。

(f) 氧气。

(g) 肾上腺素。

(h) 蒸汽冷却喷雾剂。

(i) 生物同质性激素。

(j) 生物制品,包括治疗性血清。

C. 在为患者配制药物时,经扩大实践和处方权限认证的东方医学医生应当遵守《美国药典》和国家处方中执业卫生保健专业人员的配制要求。

第 16－2－2－11 条　[保留]

第 16－2－2－12 条　处方笺

东方医学医生在开具处方时,应使用印有其姓名、地址、电话号码、执照号的处方笺。

东方医学医生使用印有多个东方医学医生姓名的处方笺的,每位东方医学医生应设有单独的签名行,注明名称和执照号。

每份特定处方应注明该处方的东方医学医生的姓名。

第 16－2－2－13 条　[保留]

第 16－2－2－14 条　[保留]

第 3 节　执 照 申 请

第 16－2－3－1 条　发证机构

新墨西哥州针灸和东方医学委员会。

第 16－2－3－2 条　适用范围

所有申请东方医学医生执照的申请人。

第 16－2－3－3 条　法定权限

本节是根据《针灸和东方医学实践法案》,NMSA 第 61－14A－4 条、第 61－14A－6 条、第 61－14A－8 条、第 61－14A－9 条和第 61－14A－10 条的规定颁布的。

第 16－2－3－4 条　有效期

永久生效。

第 16－2－3－5 条　生效日期

2022 年 2 月 11 日,除非某一条款的末尾引用了一个更晚的日期。

第 16－2－3－6 条　目的

本节列出了申请者应当满足的要求,以便其申请东方医学医生的执照。

第 16－2－3－7 条　定义

参考 NMAC 第 16－2－1－7 条中的定义。

第 16－2－3－8 条　一般要求

A. 受到 NMAC 第 16－2－3－8 条第 A 款所包含的行动或者程序影响的申请人,将会受到纪律处分,包括根据 NMSA 第 61－14A－17 条,《统一执照法案》(即 NMSA 第 61－1－1 条及以下规定)以及《刑事罪犯就业法案》(即 NMSA 第 28－2－1 条及以下规定)实施的拒绝、吊销或者撤销执照。

B. 向委员会提供虚假信息或者作出虚假陈述的申请人,可能会受到纪律处分,包括根据 NMSA 第 61－14A－17 条的规定和《统一执照法》(即 NMSA 第 61－1－1 条及以下规定)拒绝颁发、吊销或者撤销执照。

第 16－2－3－9 条　教育计划要求

申请人应当提供充分的证据,证明他完成了 NMSA 第 61－14A－14 条和 NMAC 第 16－2－7 节中定义的委员会批准的教育计划。

如果该教育计划已不存在,或者如果申请人因正当理由而无法提供相关记录,申请人应当提交一份宣誓书,对该教育课程进行说明,并应当提供地址、入学日期和完成的课程,以及委员会认为必要的其他信息和文件。

委员会可以自行决定是否接受或者拒绝此类充分的证据,以代替所需的记录。

第 16－2－3－10 条　刑事定罪

A. 凡有以下罪行,或者在其他司法管辖区有同等的犯罪记录,都可能导致申请人被取消其获得或者持有的执照,包括临时执照和耳穴戒毒专家证书的资格。这些犯罪包括:

(1) 杀人。

(2) 严重袭击、严重殴打、绑架、非法监禁、贩卖人口,或者其他针对个人的暴力犯罪。

(3) 抢劫、盗窃、入室盗窃、敲诈勒索、接收赃物、拥有盗窃工具、非法占有机动车,或者其他涉及盗窃或者侵占个人财产或者资金的犯罪。

(4) 强奸、性侵入、性接触、乱伦、猥亵、引诱儿童,或者其他构成性犯罪的罪行。

(5) 在申请日期之前的五年内,在醉酒或者毒品的影响下驾驶。

（6）在申请日期之前的五年内贩运管制药物,具体不包括大麻或者大麻衍生产品。

（7）涉及虐待或者忽视儿童的罪行。

（8）欺诈、伪造、洗钱、挪用公款、信用卡欺诈、造假、金融剥削,或者其他改变影响他人权利或者义务的文书的罪行。

（9）在宣誓中或者在任何官方文件中做出虚假陈述。

（10）企图、教唆或者共谋本款中涉及的任何重罪。

第 16－2－3－11 条　初次申请执照

符合下列要求的执照申请一经批准,委员会将颁发执照,其有效期至初次颁发执照后的 7 月 31 日,但 5 月 1 日之后首次颁发的执照将在 NMAC 第 16－2－8－9 条规定的下一个续期的 7 月 31 日之前到期;执照的申请要求是委员会收到下列材料:

A. NMAC 第 16－2－10 节规定的执照申请费。

B. 在委员会提供的表格上用英文填写的执照申请,其中应当包括申请人的姓名、地址、出生日期和社会保险号码(若有)。

C. 两张申请人的护照类型的照片,拍摄时间不超过提交申请前的六个月。

D. 在"初次执照申请"中提供的宣誓书,说明申请人是否:

（1）在任何司法管辖区受到过与针灸和东方医学有关的纪律处分,或者与任何其他职业(包括申请人有执照、证书、注册或者法律认可的其他卫生保健专业)有关的纪律处分,包括在纪律处分程序或者潜在纪律处分程序调查期间辞职、撤回或者放弃执照、证书或者注册。

（2）曾是任何司法管辖区内与申请人的针灸和东方医学实践或与任何其他职业(包括申请人被许可、认证、注册或法律认可从事的其他卫生保健专业)相关的诉讼的一方当事人。

（3）拖欠法院判决的儿童抚养费。

（4）违反了该法案或者规则的任何规定。

E. 正式执照历史记录。申请人根据《新墨西哥州针灸和东方医学实践法》以外的任何部门在任何司法辖区获得执照、认证、注册或法律认可以从事任何专业实践(包括卫生保健专业)的,由该司法管辖区出具的一份证明,说明申请人的纪律处分记录。

F. "初次执照申请"中提供的宣誓书,声明申请人理解:

（1）根据 NMSA 第 61－14A－17 条的规定,已经受到 NMAC 第 16－2－3－10 条第 D 款包含的任何诉讼或者程序的申请人,可能受到包括拒绝、吊销或者撤销执照在内的纪律处分。法律依据包括《统一执照法案》(即 NMSA 第 61－1－1 条)、《刑事罪犯就业法案》(即 NMSA 第 28－2－1 条)。

（2）根据法案 NMSA 第 61－14A－17 条和《统一执照法案》(NMSA 第 61－1－1 条)的规定,向委员会提供虚假信息或者向委员会作出虚假陈述的申请人,可能会受到包括拒绝、吊销或者撤销执照在内的纪律处分。

G. "初次执照申请"中提供的宣誓书,声明申请人理解:

（1）申请人负责阅读、理解和遵守新墨西哥州有关此次申请以及针灸和东方医学服务的法律和规则。

（2）执照应当在每年 7 月 31 日前续期。

（3）如果申请人的地址发生变化,申请人应当在十日内通知委员会。

H. 申请人的教育计划证书或者文凭的副本,证明完成了要求的计划;该副本应当包括一份宣誓书,证明其为原件的真实副本。

I. 申请人成绩单的正式副本,应当由申请人获得证书或者文凭的教育机构,使用密封信封直接发送给委员会,并应当证明申请人顺利完成了要求的学术和临床教育,标明完成的科目和每个科目的学习时间;或者,该副本应当保留在密封信封中并加盖教育机构公章,并应当由申请人将其连同申请文件,一并发送给委员会。

J. 提交的所有外文文件的准确英文翻译;每份翻译文件应当附有翻译者的宣誓书,证明其能够胜任文件的语言和英语,且该翻译是外文原件的真实的翻译;每份翻译文件还应当附有申请人的宣誓书,证明该翻译是对原件的真实的翻译;每份宣誓书应当在公证人面前签署;与申请有关的任何文件的翻译费用应当由申请人承担。

第 16 - 2 - 3 - 12 条　考试要求

NMAC 第 16 - 2 - 4 节中规定的考试要求应当在委员会办公室收到首次申请后十二个月内提交给委员会办公室,但国家针灸与东方医学认证委员会(NCCAOM)的分数要求除外,该分数要求需要在首次申请后二十四个月内提交给委员会办公室。

第 16 - 2 - 3 - 13 条　外文文件

所有提交的外文文件应当附有准确的英文翻译。

每份翻译文件应当附有翻译者的宣誓书,证明他或者她能够胜任文件的语言和英语,且该翻译是外文原件真实可信的翻译。

每份翻译文件还应当附有申请人的宣誓书,证明该翻译是对原件的真实可信的翻译。

每份宣誓书应当在公证人面前签署。

申请人应当承担与其申请有关的任何文件的翻译费用。

第 16 - 2 - 3 - 14 条　文件的充分性

委员会应当确定执照申请支持文件的充分性。

委员会可以酌情要求提供进一步的资格证明,或者要求与申请人进行面谈,以确定其资格。

如果委员会要求,所有进一步的资格证明应当在临床技能考试日期前至少四十五日寄至委员会办公室。

委员会将决定所需面试的时间。

第 16 - 2 - 3 - 15 条　完成所有执照要求的截止日期

委员会办公室应当在收到首次申请后的十二个月内收到颁发执照所需的文件。NCCAOM 的分数要求除外,该要求需要在初次申请后的二十四个月内提交给委员会办公室。

第 16 - 2 - 3 - 16 条　颁发执照的通知

在委员会收到所有文件后,应当在不超过二十一日内通过邮寄方式通知申请人,批准或者拒绝其已完成的申请要求(包括考试要求)。

委员会应当向所有符合 NMAC 第 16－2－3 节和第 16－2－4 节要求的申请人颁发执照。

第 16－2－3－17 条　申请到期和放弃

如果在初次申请的二十四个月内没有满足所有的申请要求,申请将到期并被视为放弃。

如果有正当理由,委员会可以酌情给予例外处理。

如果申请被放弃,而申请人想重新申请执照,申请人应当要求提交完整的现行申请表,支付现行的申请费,并满足再次申请时有效条件要求。

第 4 节　考　　试

第 16－2－4－1 条　发证机构

新墨西哥州针灸和东方医学委员会。

第 16－2－4－2 条　适用范围

所有申请东方医学医生执照的申请人。

第 16－2－4－3 条　法定权限

本节是根据《针灸和东方医学实践法案》,NMSA 第 61－14A－8 条、第 61－14A－9 条、第 61－14A－10(F)条和第 61－14A－11 条的规定颁布。

第 16－2－4－4 条　有效期

永久生效。

第 16－2－4－5 条　生效日期

1996 年 7 月 1 日,除非在某条末尾引用了一个较晚的日期。

第 16－2－4－6 条　目的

本节明确了执照考试的内容、语言、数量和类型,颁发执照的要求,考试的频次以及在不合格的情况下的复试要求。

第 16－2－4－7 条　定义

参考 NMAC 第 16－2－1－7 条(第 1 节第 7 条)中的定义。

第 16－2－4－8 条　经批准的考试

委员会批准的考试,应当包括笔试和实践考试。

在参加临床技能考试之前,应当完成所有要求的 NCCAOM 考试。

A. 委员会批准的笔试应当是:

(1) NCCAOM 东方医学基础模块。

(2) NCCAOM 针灸模块。

(3) NCCAOM 中草药学模块。

(4) NCCAOM 生物医学模块。

(5) NCCAOM 批准的洁针技术课程。

(6) 委员会批准并管理的法学考试,涵盖了法案和规则。

B. 委员会批准的实践考试应当是:

(1) NCCAOM 穴位定位模块。

（2）临床技能考试;临床技能考试包括针灸、中草药和生物医学能力的考试。

C. 委员会可以采用其他必要的考试,以评估其批准的考试。

第 16－2－4－9 条　考试用语

委员会要求的所有考试均应当以英语进行。

第 16－2－4－10 条　执照考试要求

以下是执照考试要求。

国家承认的考试的所有费用应当由申请人支付,不包括在委员会收取的费用中。

A. 在参加临床技能考试之前,达到 NCCAOM 确定的以下各项的合格分数。

（1）NCCAOM 东方医学基础模块。

（2）NCCAOM 针灸模块。

（3）NCCAOM 中草药学模块。

（4）NCCAOM 生物医学模块。

（5）NCCAOM 穴位定位模块。

B. 在临床技能考试中达到至少百分之七十五的合格分数。

当申请人由多个考官进行评定时,为了确定合格分数,如果申请人由两个考官进行评定,申请人应当获得至少百分之七十五的平均分数;如果申请人由三个考官进行考试,申请人应当从大多数考官那里获得至少百分之七十五的分数。

C. 顺利完成国家针灸与东方医学认证委员会批准的洁针技术课程。

D. 在委员会批准和管理的涵盖法案和规则的法学考试中,达到不低于百分之九十的合格分数。

E. 在 2004 年 6 月之前完成国家针灸与东方医学认证委员会（NCCAOM）针灸和中草药学考试的申请者,不需要通过 NCCAOM 东方医学基础模块。

第 16－2－4－11 条　临床技能考试频率和截止日期

委员会应当每年至少举行一次临床技能考试,前提是执照申请尚未得到批准。

NMAC 第 16－2－3－11 条规定的初次申请,应当在下一次预定的临床技能考试日期前至少六十日送达委员会办公室。

委员会应当在下一个预定的临床技能考试日期前至少四十五日,向申请人发出书面答复,告知其申请的完整性或者需要的文件。

委员会办公室应当在下一个预定的临床技能考试日期前至少三十五日收到完成初次执照申请所需的所有文件。

如果委员会办公室在截止日期后收到申请要求,申请将被搁置,直到下一次临床技能考试的截止日期安排时才会处理。

对于第 16－2－3－11 条中规定的已完成的初次执照申请,应当在下一次预定的临床技能考试日期前至少二十五日,通过邮件或者电子方式通知申请人获准或者拒绝。

第 16－2－4－12 条　临床技能考试确认

在收到 NMAC 第 16－2－10 节规定的临床技能考试费后十五日内,应当将提供给申请人的委员会批准的确认卡发给申请人。

临床考试通过确认卡的有效期为自首次申请之日起二十四个月。

二十四个月过后,申请人应当重新参加临床考试,并作为新的申请人重新申请,并支付 NMAC 第 16－2－10 节规定的所需费用。

第 16－2－4－13 条　支付临床技能考试费

NMAC 第 16－2－10 节规定的不可退还的临床技能考试费应当以美国基金的支票或者汇票支付,并在下一次预定的临床技能考试前至少三十一个日历日送达委员会办公室。

第 16－2－4－14 条　临床技能考试承诺

申请人收到下一次预定的临床技能考试的临床技能考试费后,应当参加考试,否则费用不予退还。

按照 NMAC 第 16－2－4 节第 15 条的规定,不予退还的临床技能考试费可以用于后续考试。

第 16－2－4－15 条　没收临床技能考试费

一旦委员会办公室收到临床技能考试费,申请人应当参加下一次预定的临床技能考试,否则将没收临床技能考试费。

在特殊情况下,申请人可获准参加后续临床技能考试,而无须支付额外的考试费。

第 16－2－4－16 条　分数不及格

如果申请人未能在临床技能考试中取得及格成绩,可以按照 NMAC 第 16－2－4－17 条的规定提出申请,并必须支付所需费用。

第 16－2－4－17 条　重新考试

未能通过临床技能考试的申请人可以申请参加下一次临床技能考试。

申请人应当在下一次临床技能考试日期前至少六十日,向委员会办公室提交一份书面签名信,告知其参加下一次临床技能考试的承诺。

其后,委员会应当在下一次临床技能考试日期前至少四十五日,通过邮件或者电子方式通知申请人接受其参加下一次临床技能考试。

申请人应当按照 NMAC 第 16－2－4－13 条的规定支付临床技能考试费。

如果申请人没有通过下一次预定的临床技能考试,申请人应当填写委员会现行表格,重新提出申请,支付所有规定的费用,并满足申请时的条件。

如果申请人通过了考试,但没有在二十四个月内完成执照申请,申请人将不得不作为首次申请人重新申请。

第 16－2－4－18 条　考官

委员会应当选取一批东方医学医生作为临床技能考试的考官。

选中的考官,应当具有五年的临床经验。

委员会或者其指定机构应当培训考官,使其有能力判断参加委员会批准的临床技能考试的申请人,在应用针灸和东方医学的诊断和治疗技术方面的水平。

第 16－2－4－19 条　临床技能考试分数审查

申请人可以要求委员会或者其考试委员会对其临床技能考试结果进行复核,以确定是否存在重大的程序或者计算错误。申请人应当在通知其临床技能考试结果的二十五个日历日内，向委员会办公室提出复核请求。

第 5 节　临 时 执 照

第 16－2－5－1 条　发证机构

新墨西哥州针灸和东方医学委员会。

第 16－2－5－2 条　适用范围

所有持证人、申请人、临时执照持证人、临时执照申请人、实习生、教育课程和教育课程审批申请人。

第 16－2－5－3 条　法定权限

本节根据《针灸和东方医学实践法案》，NMSA 第 61－14A－8 条、第 61－14A－9 条和第 61－14A－12 条颁布。

第 16－2－5－4 条　有效期

永久生效。

第 16－2－5－5 条　生效日期

2022 年 2 月 11 日，除非某一条款的末尾引用了一个更晚的日期。

第 16－2－5－6 条　目的

本节规定临时执照和受限临时执照的要求，先前与其他执照有关的纪律处分，先前的诉讼和先前的重罪、临时执照的教育要求、临时执照的续期周期和临时执照的续期要求。

第 16－2－5－7 条　定义

参考 NMAC 第 16－2－1－7 条中的定义。

第 16－2－5－8 条　一般要求

A. 根据《针灸和东方医学实践法案》，NMSA 第 61－14A－17 条、《统一执照法案》，NMSA 第 61－1－1 条、《刑事罪犯就业法案》、NMSA 第 28－2－1 条的规定，受到 NMAC 第 16－2－5－10 条第 E 款和 NMAC 第 16－2－5－12 条第 D 款规定的各项措施或者程序约束的临时执照申请人或者受限临时执照申请人，可能随时受到纪律处分，包括拒绝颁发、吊销或者撤销执照。

B. 根据《针灸和东方医学实践法案》，NMSA 第 61－14A－17 条、《统一执照法案》，NMSA 第 61－1－1 条的规定，向委员会提供虚假信息或者作出虚假陈述的临时执照申请人或者受限临时执照申请人，可能受到包括拒绝、吊销或者撤销执照在内的纪律处分。

第 16－2－5－9 条　临时执照的教育要求

A. 临时执照申请人应当提供符合要求的证明，以证明其已经完成批准的教育计划。

在各州或者其他国家获得法律承认，从事另一种卫生保健专业并拥有东方医学执业范围内的知识和技能的临时执照申请人，应当提供符合要求的证明，以证明其已经完成在该州或者其他国家获得法律承认所需要的教育。

B. 如果委员会有正当理由认为新墨西哥公民的健康和安全不会受到危害，则委员会可以通过召开的正式的委员会会议，经过多数成员的投票，决定无须要求临时执照申请人完成 NMAC 第 16－2－5－9 条第 A 款的要求。

第 16－2－5－10 条　临时执照申请

符合以下要求的临时执照申请一经批准,委员会将颁发临时执照,其有效期为执照上规定的日期,但不得超过六个月。

临时执照应当包括临时执照持证人的姓名、执照的生效日期、赞助的新墨西哥州东方医学医生或者新墨西哥州教育计划的名称,以及一份声明,说明该执照的唯一目的是用于以下一项或者多项:教授针灸和东方医学;与赞助医生一起为赞助医生的患者提供咨询;与赞助医生一起为赞助医生的患者进行专门的诊断或者治疗技术;协助进行针灸和东方医学的研究;或者协助实施与针灸和东方医学有关的新技术和科技。

受限临时执照的申请条件是,委员会应当收到以下材料:

A. NMAC 第 16－2－10 节规定的临时执照申请费。

B. 在委员会提供的表格上用英文填写的临时执照申请书,其中应当包括申请人的姓名、地址、出生日期、社会安全号码(若有),以及赞助和合作的新墨西哥州东方医学医生或者新墨西哥州教育计划的名称。

C. 一张申请人的护照型照片,拍摄时间不超过提交申请前的六个月。

D. 由新墨西哥州东方医学医生或者新墨西哥州教育计划的赞助方和联合方提供的"临时执照申请"上的宣誓书,证明申请人的资格和申请人将要进行的活动。

E. 在"临时执照申请"中提供的宣誓书,证明申请人是否:

(1) 在各司法管辖区受到过与针灸和东方医学有关的纪律处分,或者与各种其他专业(包括申请人有执照、证书、注册或者法律认可的其他卫生保健专业)有关的纪律处分,包括在纪律处分程序或者潜在纪律处分程序调查期间辞职、撤回或者注销申请人的执照、证书或者注册;或者

(2) 曾经在各司法管辖区成为与申请人的针灸和东方医学实践有关的诉讼当事人,或者与各种其他专业有关的诉讼当事人,包括申请人获得执照、认证、注册或者法律承认的其他卫生保健专业;或者

(3) 拖欠法院判决的儿童抚养费。

F. 一份正式的执照记录,即每个司法管辖区出具的证明,说明申请人的纪律处分记录,申请人根据新墨西哥州《针灸和东方医学实践法案》以外的规定在各司法管辖区获得执照、认证、注册或者法律承认从事各种其他职业(包括其他卫生保健专业)的各司法管辖区出具的证书。

G. "临时执照申请"上提供的宣誓书,说明申请人理解:

(1) 根据《针灸和东方医学实践法案》,NMSA 第 61－14A－17 条、《统一执照法案》,NMSA 第 61－1－1 条、《刑事罪犯就业法案》1978 年 NMSA 第 28－2－1 条的规定,受到 NMAC 第 16－2－5－10 条第 E 款规定的各项措施或者程序约束的申请人,可能随时受到包括拒绝颁发、吊销或者撤销执照在内的纪律处分。

(2) 根据《针灸和东方医学实践法案》,NMSA 第 61－14A－17 条、《统一执照法案》,NMSA 第 61－1－1 条的规定,向委员会提供虚假信息或者作出虚假陈述的申请人可能受到包括拒绝、吊销或者撤销执照的纪律处分。

H."临时执照申请"上提供的宣誓书,说明申请人知晓:

(1)申请人有责任阅读、理解并遵守新墨西哥州有关本申请以及针灸和东方医学实践相关的法律和规则。

(2)如果申请人的地址发生变化,或者申请人与赞助和合作的新墨西哥州东方医学医生或者新墨西哥州教育计划的关系情况发生变化,申请人应当在十日内通知委员会。

(3)申请人只能从事临时执照上授权的活动,并且只能在临时执照上规定的有限时间内与赞助和合作的新墨西哥州东方医学医生或者新墨西哥州教育计划进行合作。

I.申请人的执照、证明或者注册文件或者其他文件的副本,证明申请人在另一个州或者国家被合法承认从事针灸和东方医学或者其他卫生保健专业,并且拥有东方医学医生执业范围内的知识和技能。

副本上应当包括申请人的宣誓书,并证明它是原件的真实副本。

对于在美国没有获得法律承认的州行医资格的申请人,只需提供 NCCAOM 颁发的针灸、中草药或者亚洲身体疗法的认证文件(适合他们将要教授或者学习的材料类型为准)的副本即可。

副本上应当包括申请人的宣誓书,并证明它是原件的真实副本。

对于美国以外的申请人,如果在没有具体法律承认文件的国家实践,但从适当的教育计划毕业是实践的法律要求,则本款的上述规定不再适用。

J.申请人从教育计划毕业的学位证书的副本,且该学位证书是在申请人实践的州或者国家获得执照、认证、注册或者受法律认可的要求。

副本上应当包括申请人的宣誓书,并证明它是原件的真实副本。

K.申请人的成绩单的正式副本应当由申请人获得证书或者文凭的教育计划直接装在密封信封里寄给委员会,该成绩单应当证实申请人完成了规定的学术和临床教育并合格,并应当指明完成的科目和每个科目的学习时间。

该成绩单副本应当保存在加盖教育计划公章的密封信封中,并应当由申请人连同申请人的执照申请一起发送给委员会。

L.一份宣誓书,说明申请人已经被委员会正式书面通知已满足以下两项要求之一:

(1)申请人毕业的针灸和东方医学教育计划已被委员会批准为教育计划;或者

(2)委员会在正式召开的会议上以多数成员的投票决定不要求临时执照的申请人从NMAC 第 16-2-5-9 条第 B 款规定获批的教育计划中毕业。

M.所有外文文件的准确英文译本。每份翻译文件都应当附有翻译者的宣誓书,证明其具备使用该文件的语言和英语语言的能力,并且该译文是外文原文的真实可信的翻译。每份翻译文件还应当附有申请人的宣誓书,证明该翻译是对原件的真实可信的翻译。每份宣誓书应当在公证人面前签署。与申请人的申请有关的任何文件的翻译费用应当由申请人承担。

第 16-2-5-11 条　临时执照续期

委员会颁发的临时执照最多可以续期两次,每次续期的时间为六个月。

续期应当按照顺序进行,当前临时执照期限到期时,应当立即开始续期。

满足以下要求的临时执照续期申请一经批准,委员会应当颁发临时执照。

根据临时执照续期的申请要求,委员会应当收到以下材料:

A. NMAC 第 16-2-10 节规定的临时执照续期费。

B. 在委员会提供的表格上用英语填写完整的临时执照续期申请,其中应当包括申请人的姓名、地址、出生日期、社会安全号码(若有),以及赞助和合作的新墨西哥州东方医学医生或者新墨西哥州教育计划名称。

C. 由赞助和合作的新墨西哥州东方医学医生或者新墨西哥州教育计划提供的宣誓书,证明申请人的资格和申请人将进行的活动。

第 16-2-5-12 条　受限临时执照申请

在批准符合下列要求的受限临时执照的申请后,委员会将颁发受限临时执照,且在执照上规定的日期内有效,但从颁发之日起不得超过连续十二个月,且不可续期。

受限临时执照专门用于教授针灸和东方医学单一完整课程及协助实施针灸和东方医学新技术的执照,包括由除新墨西哥州之外的司法管辖区获得执照、注册、认证或法律认可的卫生保健从业者学习该等技术。

如果不是持证人或者临时执照持证人,对于在教学或者协助实施新技术时对他人演示、实践或者实施诊断和治疗技术的人,须持有受限临时执照。

受限临时执照不应当发给教授全学期课程的教师,这些课程是经批准的教育计划的一部分。

受限临时执照应当包括受限临时执照持证人的姓名、执照的生效日期、赞助的新墨西哥州东方医学医生或者新墨西哥州教育计划的名称,以及一份声明,说明该执照的唯一目的是教授针灸和东方医学,并协助实施针灸和东方医学的新技术,包括由除新墨西哥州之外的司法管辖区获得执照、注册、认证或法律认可的卫生保健从业者学习该等技术。

对受限临时执照的要求应当是:

A. NMAC 第 16-2-10 节规定的受限临时执照申请费。

B. 在委员会提供的表格上用英文填写的临时执照申请书,其中应当包括申请人的姓名、地址、出生日期、社会安全号码(若有),以及赞助和合作的新墨西哥州东方医学医生或者新墨西哥州教育计划的名称。

C. 由赞助和合作的新墨西哥州东方医学医生或者新墨西哥州教育计划提供的"临时执照申请"所提供的宣誓书,证明申请人的资格和申请人将进行的活动。

D. 一份关于申请人是否存在以下行为的宣誓书:

(1)在各司法管辖区受到过与针灸和东方医学有关的纪律处分,或者与各种其他专业(包括申请人有执照、证书、注册或者法律认可的其他卫生保健专业)有关的纪律处分,包括在纪律处分程序或者潜在纪律处分程序调查期间辞职、撤回或者注销申请人的执照、证书或者注册;或者

(2)曾经在各司法管辖区成为与申请人的针灸和东方医学实践有关的诉讼当事人,或者与各种其他专业有关的诉讼当事人,包括申请人获得执照、认证、注册或者法律承认的其他卫生保健专业;或者

(3)拖欠法院判决确认的子女抚养费。

E. "临时执照申请"中提供的宣誓书,声明申请人理解:

(1) 根据《针灸和东方医学实践法案》,NMSA 第 61-14A-17 条、《统一执照法案》, NMSA 第 61-1-1 条、《刑事罪犯就业法案》,NMSA 第 28-2-1 条的规定,受到 NMAC 第 16-2-5-12 条第 D 款规定的各项措施或者程序约束的申请人可能随时受到包括拒绝颁发、吊销或者撤销执照在内的纪律处分。

(2) 根据《针灸和东方医学实践法案》,NMSA 第 61-14A-17 条和《统一执照法案》, NMSA 第 61-1-1 条的规定,向委员会提供虚假信息或者作出虚假陈述的申请人,可能受到包括拒绝颁发、吊销或者撤销执照在内的纪律处分。

F. "临时执照申请"中提供的宣誓书,声明申请人理解:

(1) 申请人有责任阅读、理解并遵守新墨西哥州有关本申请以及针灸和东方医学实践的法律和规则。

(2) 如果申请人的地址发生变化,或者申请人与赞助和合作的新墨西哥州东方医学医生或者新墨西哥州教育计划的关系情况发生变化,申请人应当在十日内通知委员会。

(3) 申请人只能从事临时执照上授权的活动,并且只能在临时执照上规定的有限时间内与赞助和联合的新墨西哥州东方医学医生或者新墨西哥州教育计划合作。

G. 申请人的执照、证明或者注册文件或者其他文件的副本,证明申请人在另一个州或者国家被合法地承认从事针灸和东方医学实践或者其他卫生保健专业,并且拥有东方医学医生执业范围内的知识和技能。副本上应当包括申请人的宣誓书,并证明它是原件的真实副本。对于在美国没有获得法律承认的州行医资格的申请人,只需提供 NCCAOM 颁发的针灸、中草药或者亚洲身体疗法的认证文件(以适合他们将要教授或者学习的材料类型为准)的副本即可。该副本应当包括申请人的宣誓书,并证明它是原件的真实副本。对于美国以外的申请人,如果在没有具体法律承认文件的国家实践,但从适当的教育计划毕业是实践的法律要求,则本款的上述规定不再适用。

H. 申请人从教育计划毕业的学位证书的副本,且该学位证书是在申请人实践的州或者国家获得执照、认证、注册或者法律认可的要求。该副本应当包括申请人的宣誓书,并证明它是原件的真实副本。

I. 所有外文文件的准确英文译本。每份翻译文件都应当附有翻译者的宣誓书,证明其具备使用该文件的语言和英语语言的能力,并且该译文是外文原文的真实可信的翻译。每份宣誓书应当在公证员面前签署;与申请有关的各项文件的翻译费用应当由申请人承担。

第6节 互惠许可

第 16-2-6-1 条 发证机构

新墨西哥州针灸和东方医学委员会。

第 16-2-6-2 条 范围

所有持证人和申请人。

第 16-2-6-3 条 法定权力

本节根据《针灸和东方医学实践法》,NMSA 第 61-14A-8 条、第 61-14A-9 条、第

61－14A－13 条的规定颁布。

第 16－2－6－4 条　有效期

永久生效。

第 16－2－6－5 条　生效日期

2001 年 12 月 1 日,除非某一条款的末尾引用了一个更晚的日期。

第 16－2－6－6 条　目的

本节规定,目前委员会与其他州或者国家之间没有互惠许可协议。

第 16－2－6－7 条　定义

参考 NMAC 第 16－2－1－7 条(第 1 节第 7 条)中的定义。

第 16－2－6－8 条　互惠许可

目前委员会与其他州或者国家之间没有互惠许可协议。

第 7 节　教　育　计　划

第 16－2－7－1 条　发证机构

新墨西哥州针灸和东方医学委员会。

第 16－2－7－2 条　范围

所有注册的东方医学医生、临时注册的东方医学医生、经批准的教育计划以及所有申请东方医学医生执照、临时执照和教育计划批准的申请人。

第 16－2－7－3 条　法定权限

本节根据《针灸和东方医学实践法》,NMSA 第 61－14A－8 条、第 61－14A－9 条、第 61－14A－14 条的规定颁布。

第 16－2－7－4 条　有效期

永久生效。

第 16－2－7－5 条　生效日期

2003 年 10 月 22 日,除非某一条款的末尾引用了一个更晚的日期。

第 16－2－7－6 条　目的

本节规定批准教育计划的要求,申请批准教育计划的要求,批准教育计划的续期以及通知变更的要求。

第 16－2－7－7 条　定义

参考 NMAC 第 16－2－1－7 条(第 1 节第 7 条)中的定义。

第 16－2－7－8 条　教育计划要求

所有的教育计划都应当得到委员会的批准。

根据 NMAC 第 16－2－7－8 条和第 16－2－7－9 条(本法第 7 节第 8 条和第 9 条)的要求,委员会将评估教育计划是否应当被批准。

如果有必要进行访问以评估教育计划,则访问的费用,包括各项行政费用,应当由教育计划预先支付。

A. 基础教育计划的要求应当是四学年的东方医学硕士课程,符合 NCCAOM 在本法定义的认证/等同教育政策。

毕业/教育应当从符合美国针灸及东方医学审核委员会(ACAOM)或者同等教育机构标准的正规教育计划中获得。

证明下列情况之一的计划可被确定为已满足本要求：

(1)ACAOM 的认证或者候选资格；或者

(2)由外国政府的教育部、卫生部或者同级外国政府机构批准；每位候选人应当提交他们的文件，以获得 NCCAOM 认可的外国证书同等服务机构的批准；尝试根据这种方法满足资格要求的计划应当同时满足申请时 ACAOM 有效的课程要求；或者

(3)由外国私人认证机构批准，该机构的认证程序和标准与 ACAOM 的认证程序和标准基本相同，并且为此目的被该外国适当的政府单位所承认；每位候选人应当提交他们的文件，以获得 NCCAOM 认可的外国证书等效服务机构的批准；尝试通过这种方法满足资格要求的计划还应当满足申请时 ACAOM 有效的课程要求。

B. 教育计划应当提供至少四年的计划，并应当包括至少两千四百学时的课堂教育，其中包括至少一千一百学时的针灸和东方医学教学教育，以及至少九百学时的针灸和东方医学监督临床实践、指导和观察。

课程应当提供维持针灸和东方医疗保健适当标准所需的知识和技能。

C. 教育计划应当包括一门授课式课程，以教育和并使有能力从事针灸和东方医学实践，且能够准确诊断、开药和治疗的医生毕业，除法案的要求外，还特别包括东方养生治疗原则，包括中药处方、膳食营养、手法治疗/物理疗法和咨询，不得超过 NMAC 第 16－2－7－8 条第 B 款(本法第 7 节第 8 条第 B 款)规定的两千四百学时中的九百学时，其中包括至少四百五十学时的中药教育。

D. 教育计划应当包括临床课程，包括临床指导和直接接触患者。

教育计划的临床部分应当包括至少九百学时在以下领域受监督的临床实践、指导和观察：

(1)观察和协助应用东方医学的原理和技术，包括诊断、针灸、艾灸、手法治疗/物理疗法、膳食和营养、咨询和中药处方。

(2)至少有四百学时的实际治疗，其中要求学生作为初级实习医生进行完整的治疗。

E. 教育计划应当包括一门课程，教育和使毕业的医生有能力展示与临床相关的、互补的和综合的生物医学和生物医学诊断知识，足以在适当的时候治疗和转诊患者。

F. 该教育计划可以从其他教育计划中获得学分。

G. 所有针灸和东方医学的教学导师、驻校教师和客座教师的姓名和教育资格应当提交给委员会，并应当满足以下要求：

(1)在新墨西哥州从事针灸和东方医学实践的教师均应当具有委员会颁发的在新墨西哥州从事针灸和东方医学实践的执照或者临时执照；违反此规定的教育计划均将被吊销或者撤销批准，或者受到纪律处分，包括 NMAC 第 16－2－12 节(本法第 12 节)规定的罚款。

(2)在新墨西哥州以外的教育计划的针灸和东方医学教师均应当在其实践和教学的州或者国家获得执照、认证、注册或者法律认可；违反此规定的教育计划均应当被吊销或者撤

销批准教育计划,或者受到纪律处分,包括 NMAC 第 16－2－12 节(本法第 12 节)规定的罚款。

(3) 如有正当理由,可以由委员会酌情决定做出豁免处理。

H. 教育计划可以雇佣导师或者与导师签订合同来教授教育计划的各组成部分。

教育计划可以从导师那里获得学分。

导师在该法案中被定义为"具有至少十年临床经验的东方医学医生,担任针灸和东方医学的教师"。

I. 教育计划可以接受委员会的检查。

第 16－2－7－9 条　教育计划证书或者文凭和成绩单要求

教育计划应当提供下列内容:

A. 成绩单,作为学生记录的一部分,包括以下内容:

(1) 学生的姓名。

(2) 学生的地址。

(3) 出生日期。

(4) 课程名称。

(5) 每门课程获得的成绩。

(6) 每门课程的学时数。

B. 证明学生在亲自参加所有规定的课程并顺利完成教育课程要求后,顺利完成教育计划的证书或者文凭。

第 16－2－7－10 条　教育计划年度批准申请

新墨西哥州的所有教育计划都需要每年得到委员会的批准。

新墨西哥州以外的各教育计划,只要愿意,都可以申请获得年度批准。

这些教育计划应当在提交委员会后予以批准:

A. 以美元为单位的保付支票或者汇票支付 NMAC 第 16－2－10 节(本法第 10 节)规定的教育计划年度批准的初始申请费。

B. 在委员会规定的表格上用英语填写完整的申请,其中包括教育计划的入学日期和必要的信息,以核实是否符合 NMAC 第 16－2－7－8 条和第 16－2－7－9 条(本法第 7 节第 8 条和第 9 条)要求的专业教育标准,包括课程的正式副本。

委员会应当在收到申请后的六十日内采取行动,并在采取行动后的七日内以邮件形式书面通知教育计划申请的情况。

第 16－2－7－11 条　教育计划单次批准申请书

没有获得委员会年度批准资格的教育计划,应当在已毕业申请人的教育计划提交给委员会后,获得单个申请人使用的教育计划的单次批准:

A. 以美元为单位的保付支票或者汇票支付 NMAC 第 16－2－10 节(本法第 10 节)规定的教育计划单次审批申请费。

B. 在委员会规定的表格上用英语填写完整的申请,其中包括教育计划的入学日期和必要的信息,以核实是否符合 NMAC 第 16－2－7－8 条和第 16－2－7－9 条(本法第 7 节第 8

条和第 9 条)要求的专业教育标准,包括课程的正式副本。

委员会办公室应当在下一次预定的临床技能考试前至少九十日收到申请书和申请费。

委员会应当在下一次预定的临床技能考试日期前至少八十五日,向申请批准教育计划的申请人发出书面答复,告知申请人申请的完整性或者所需的文件。

委员会办公室应当在下一次预定的临床技能考试日期前至少七十日收到为完成申请而要求的所有文件。

申请的批准或者拒绝应当在下一个预定的临床技能考试日期前至少六十日以邮件形式通知申请人。

请注意,上述截止日期与 NMAC 第 16－2－4－11 条(本法第 4 节第 11 条)规定的临床技能考试申请人的截止日期同步。

第 16－2－7－12 条　年度续期;超期续期和到期批准

为保持年度批准资格,教育计划应当在 5 月 1 日之前提交一份由委员会规定的完整的英文年度续期申请,并以美元为单位的保付支票或者汇票支付 NMAC 第 16－2－10 节(本法第 10 节)规定的教育计划续期批准费。

批准期系指当年的 8 月 1 日至下一年的 7 月 31 日,在 7 月 31 日午夜 12：00 到期。

在任一年的 9 月 30 日之后收到的续期申请应当与 NMAC 第 16－2－10 节(本法第 10 节)规定的滞纳金一并提交,并以美元为单位的保付支票或者汇票支付。

如果在到期后六十日内没有收到年度续期申请和费用,在批准期限之后,年度批准就会到期,教育计划应当提交初始申请书和初始申请费用以获得批准。

第 16－2－7－13 条　变更通知

如果教育计划的所有权发生变化或者教育计划发生重大变化,则教育计划应当在十日内通知委员会。之后,该教育计划可能会接受检查。该教育计划应当处于预备批准状态,直到根据变更情况作出最终批准。

亚利桑那州

亚利桑那州针灸法①

第1节 针灸评审委员会

第 32－3901 条 定义

除文意另有所指外,本章中的术语含义如下:

1.“针灸”:

（a）系指一种以传统实践为基础,并受当代科学影响的医学体系。

（b）包括以下内容:

（i）用细而实心的针灸针插入皮肤,达到皮下结构。

（ii）刺激针灸针以产生积极的治疗反应。

（iii）移除针灸针。

（iv）使用和开具辅助疗法。

（v）使用和开具与针灸师的教育和培训相适应的中药疗法。

（vi）使用诊断支持工具,包括体格检查和临床检查。

（vii）安排诊断成像和临床实验室程序,以确定护理的性质,或者形成转诊给其他有执照的卫生保健专业人员的基础,或者两者都是。

2.“针灸助理”系指已完成委员会批准的培训计划的无证人员,在执业针灸师的监督下,协助完成针灸实践中的基本保健职责,并履行与针灸助理的教育和培训相称的委托职责,但不评估、解释、设计或者修改既定的针灸保健治疗方案。

3.“辅助疗法”系指手工、机械、磁、热、电或者电磁刺激穴位和能量通路,耳穴和戒毒疗法,使用离子线装置,电针,营养咨询,治疗性运动,使用非离子激光和穴位按压。

4.“委员会”系指针灸审查委员会。

5.“草药疗法”系指开具处方、给药、注射、配制和分发草药以及植物、动物、矿物和天然

---

① 根据《亚利桑那州议会法》注释版第 32 卷第 39 章“针灸”译出。

药物。

6."监督"系指监督执业针灸师在针灸助理提供服务的机构内,就执业针灸师授权的以及仍对其负责的程序进行咨询。

7."创伤"系指在任何可怕或危及生命的事件之后经历的重大心理困扰。

8."违反职业道德的行为"包括以下内容,无论发生在本州还是其他地方:

(a)故意泄露专业秘密或者故意违反特许通讯,除非法律另有规定。

(b)犯有重罪,并由有管辖权的法院定罪证明。

(c)习惯性地酗酒或者滥用任何药物,影响安全从事针灸实践的能力。

(d)犯有委员会认定的严重渎职、反复渎职或者各种导致患者死亡的渎职行为。

(e)冒充其他针灸师或者任何其他医术技术的从业人员。

(f)伪装成或者假装成委员会的成员、雇员或者授权代理人。

(g)通过欺诈或者谎报获得或者试图获得本章规定的执照。

(h)拒绝回应委员会的要求向其透露治疗患者的针灸方法。

(i)直接或者间接地给予或者接受,或者协助或者教唆给予或者接受回扣的行为。

(j)明知故犯地做出与针灸实践有关的任何书面或者口头的虚假或者欺诈性陈述。

(k)被美国任何其他州、区或者准州或者任何其他国家拒绝授予、撤销或者吊销执照,除非采取该行动的原因与该人安全和熟练地从事针灸实践的能力有关或者与违反职业道德的行为有关。

(l)实施违反针灸行业公认标准或者道德的行为,或者可能对患者或者公众的健康、福利或者安全构成危险的行为。

(m)犯有可能损害或者有条件损害安全和熟练地从事针灸实践能力的行为。

(n)直接或者间接违反或者试图违反,协助或者教唆违反或者串通违反本章或者委员会规则。

(o)以虚假、欺骗性或者误导性的方式进行广告宣传。

(p)未能或者拒绝保存足够的患者健康记录,或者未能或者拒绝将健康记录及时提供给患者,或者未能在收到适当授权的情况下提供给另一个保健医生或者提供者。

(q)从转诊患者处获得直接或者间接赔偿,而不以书面形式向患者披露赔偿的额度。

(r)从针灸师认可或者向患者推荐的产品中获取经济利益,而不以书面形式向患者披露经济利益的范围。

(s)在针灸实践中与患者发生性关系。

(t)未能适当地控制或者监督由从业者雇用或者分配给从业者的针灸学生从事针灸实践。

(u)当委员会依法要求提供这些信息时,未能及时向委员会或者其调查员或者代表提供信息。

(v)在没有得到委员会批准和注册的情况下,监督或者从事针灸临床培训计划的工作。

(w)故意以书面或者口头形式向委员会作出虚假、欺诈性或者误导性陈述。

(x)没有对患者进行适当的护理,放弃或者忽视需要立即护理的患者,没有为继续护理做出合理的安排,或者在必要时没有将患者转介给其他适当的医疗机构。

（y）未能按照委员会批准的洁针技术原则使用经过消毒的针灸针。

（z）未能展示委员会在规则中规定的专业标准治疗方式的护理和培训及教育资格。

（aa）开具或者给予药品或者药物，但根据本章规定允许的除外。

第 32-3902 条　针灸审查委员会;成员;资格;条款;免职;补偿

A. 设立针灸师审查委员会,由以下成员组成,由州长任命：

1. 截至 2022 年 1 月 16 日,四名根据本章规定获得针灸执照,并在本州或者其他任何州从事针灸实践至少一年的成员。这些成员中,不超过两名是同一所针灸学校或者学院的毕业生。州长可以从全州针灸协会提交的名单中任命这些人员。

2. 截至 2022 年 1 月 17 日,三名消费者,他们：

（a）不受雇于健康行业。

（b）在医学院或者保健机构中没有任何金钱利益。

（c）对本州的健康问题表现出兴趣。

3. 截至 2022 年 1 月 17 日,有两名根据本卷第 8、13、14、17 或者 29 章获得执照的成员。这些成员不得根据同一章节获得执照。

4. 自 2022 年 1 月 17 日起,一名根据本章获得从事耳穴针灸实践的证书或者执照的成员。

5. 自 2022 年 1 月 20 日起,三名根据本章规定获得针灸执照,并在本州或者其他州从事针灸实践至少一年的成员。这些成员中,不超过两名是同一所针灸学校或者学院的毕业生。州长可以从全州针灸协会提交的名单中任命这些人员。

6. 自 2022 年 1 月 18 日或者之后作出的任命,两名符合以下所有条件的消费者：

（a）不受雇于健康行业。

（b）在医学院或者保健机构中没有任何金钱利益。

（c）对本州的健康问题表现出兴趣。

7. 自 2022 年 1 月 18 日或者之后的任命,一名根据本卷第 8、13、14、17 或者 29 章获得执照的成员。

B. 在州长任命之前,委员会的潜在成员应当向州长提交一套完整的指纹,以便根据第 41-1750 条和公法第 92-544 条获得州和联邦犯罪记录检查。公共安全部可以与联邦调查局交换这一指纹数据。

C. 委员会成员在被任命前至少有一年是本州的居民。

D. 委员会成员的任期为三年,从 1 月的第三个星期一开始并结束。成员不得连续任职超过两个任期。

E. 委员会应当在每年 1 月举行会议,选举主席和副主席。

F. 委员会应当每季度召开一次会议,并在主席或者多数委员会成员的召集下召开。

G. 委员会成员有资格获得报酬,金额不超过每日五十美元,用于实际服务于委员会的业务,并有资格获得出席委员会会议的必要和适当费用的报销。

H. 如果委员会成员有渎职、不光彩的行为或者对委员会职责的不专业管理,州长可以将其免职。

I. 成员的任期在辞职或者离开本州超过六个月时自动结束。州长应当以与常规任命相同的方式填补任期未满的空缺。

J. 委员会成员和委员会雇员在为促进本章的目的而善意采取的任何行为或者程序中,不承担民事责任。

第 32-3903 条　委员会的权力和职责

A. 委员会应当:

1. 采用执行本章的必要规则。

2. 启动调查并采取纪律处分以执行本章。

3. 对申请人进行资格评估,符合条件的颁发执照。

4. 采取并使用印章认证委员会正式文件。

5. 根据第 32-3927 条确定费用。

6. 采用临床培训规则。

B. 委员会可以:

1. 根据《亚利桑那州议会法》注释版第 41 卷第 4 章第 4 节,雇用履行委员会职能所需的人员。

2. 为委员会的运作而购买、租赁、出租、出售或者以其他方式处置动产和不动产。

3. 批准执照考试。

第 32-3904 条　行政主管;人员;职责;报酬

A. 根据《亚利桑那州议会法》注释版第 41 卷第 4 章第 4 节,委员会可以任命一名行政主管,该行政主管响应委员会之意任职。行政主管不得为委员会成员。

B. 行政主管有资格在第 38-611 条所确定的范围内,获得委员会规定的报酬。

C. 行政主管应:

1. 履行委员会的行政职责。

2. 根据《亚利桑那州议会法》注释版第 41 卷第 4 章第 4 节,雇用履行委员会职能所需的人员。

3. 履行委员会指定的其他职责。

第 32-3905 条　针灸审查委员会基金

A. 针灸审查委员会基金按照第 32-3927 条的规定收取费用。基金由委员会管理。根据《亚利桑那州议会法》注释版第 35-146 条和第 35-147 条的规定,委员会应当将本章下收集的全部款项的百分之十存入本州的普通基金,其余百分之九十存入针灸审查委员会基金。

B. 按照《亚利桑那州议会法》注释版第 35-143.01 条的规定缴存针灸审查委员会基金内的税款。

第 32-3906 条　第三方补偿

本章不要求直接向依照本章获得执照的人提供第三方补偿。

第 2 节　执　　照

第 32-3921 条　执照;不受影响的行为和人员

A. 不具有依照本章颁发的执照的人员,不得从事针灸实践活动。

B. 本章不适用于:

1. 依照本章取得执照的卫生保健专业人员,在其执照范围内实践。

2. 在经委员会批准的针灸学校就读的学生,由根据本章颁发执照的针灸师直接监督指导,作为委员会批准的学习课程的一部分。

3. 经其他司法管辖区颁发执照或者认证从事针灸实践的人在本州的针灸实践,如果该人是在由委员会批准的针灸学校的正规教学过程中进行针灸实践,或者在由针灸专业组织批准的教育研讨会中进行针灸实践,此种情形下由根据本章获得执照的人员或者根据本卷执照的执业范围包括针灸的卫生专业人员直接监督针灸服务。

4. 居住在州外并被授权在该管辖区内从事针灸实践的针灸师,如果该人与在该州有执照的针灸师进行了一次或者不频繁的会诊,并且会诊涉及一个或者多个特定的患者。

5. 自行针灸的人员。

第32－3922条　针灸戒毒专家治疗化学药物依赖或者创伤;证书;要求;指纹;知情同意;定义

A. 委员会可以向以治疗酗酒、药物滥用、创伤或者化学药物依赖为目的的耳针治疗者颁发针灸戒毒专家证书,如果其具备以下所有条件:

1. 提供文件证明顺利完成了委员会批准的针灸治疗酗酒、药物滥用、创伤或者化学药物依赖的培训计划,且该课程达到或者超过了国家针灸戒毒协会或者委员会批准的团体制定的培训标准。

2. 提供委员会要求的文件,证明其顺利完成了委员会批准的洁针技术课程。

3. 提交委员会规定的申请和本章第32－3927条规定的费用。

4. 向委员会提交全套指纹,以便根据《亚利桑那州议会法》注释版第41－1750条和公法第92－544条获得州和联邦犯罪记录检查。公共安全部可以与联邦调查局交换这一指纹数据。

5. 在初次认证或者重新认证的申请中披露在本州或者美国其他州、地区或者准州颁发给申请人的所有其他有效和过去的专业卫生保健执照和证书。

B. 根据本节规定颁发的证书,允许证书持有者在根据本章规定获得执照的人的监督下从事耳针治疗。

C. 根据本条颁发的证书有效期为一年。如果证书持有人在证书到期前提交委员会规定的申请,并缴纳第32－3927条规定的费用,则证书可以由委员会续期。

D. 在对患者进行治疗之前,耳穴针灸师应当从患者那里获得一份经委员会批准的《知情同意书》。

E. 在本条中,"耳针疗法"系指在耳郭或者耳道上进行针灸,以治疗酗酒、药物滥用、创伤或者化学药物依赖性。

第32－3923条　持证人的称谓和缩写;禁止行为;张贴执照

A. 根据本章获得执照的人可以使用"执业针灸师"的称谓和缩写"L.Ac."。

B. 未按本章取得执照的人,不得使用任何称谓、缩写、文字、字母、符号或者数字来表明该人已按本章获得执照。

C. 根据本章持有执照本身并不赋予一个人使用"doctor"或者"physician"称谓的权利。

D. 依照本章规定取得执照的人员,应当将执照或者执照的正式副本张贴在办公设施接待区域的显著位置。

E. 根据本章获得执照的人不得向公众表示,根据该执照该人获准从事针灸以外其他形式的治疗。

第 32－3924 条　申请执照的资格

依照本章规定取得针灸执照的,应当按照委员会的规定提出申请。申请人应当在首次执照申请中披露其在本州或者美国其他州、地区或者领地获得的所有其他有效的和过去的专业卫生保健执照和证书。申请应当向委员会提交文件,证明申请人已经顺利完成委员会批准的洁针技术课程,并满足以下所有要求:

1. 符合任何一条:

（a）经 NCCAOM 或者其继受机构或者委员会批准的其他认证机构或者考试认证。

（b）通过了 NCCAOM 提供的穴位定位模块、东方医学模块基础、生物医学模块和针灸模块。

（c）获得另一州颁发的与本州标准相似的执照,且认证或者执照未被撤销。

2. 从委员会批准的针灸项目毕业或者完成培训,至少培训一千八百五十学时,其中包括至少八百学时的委员会批准的临床培训。

3. 自 2016 年 7 月 1 日起,为了根据《亚利桑那州议会法》注释版第 41－1750 条和公法第 92－544 条对州和联邦犯罪记录进行核查,向委员会提交了一套完整的指纹。公共安全部可以与联邦调查局交换这一指纹数据。

第 32－3925 条　执照续期;继续教育

A. 除了本法第 32－4301 条另有规定外,依据本章颁发的执照应当每年续期,否则有效期到期。

B. 行政主管应当至少在执照到期前六十日向每名持证人发送续期申请。

C. 持证人应当根据要求向委员会提交文件,证明持证人每年顺利完成了至少十五学时的委员会批准的继续教育。

D. 如果符合执照续期的规定,委员会可以恢复因未能续期而被取消的执照。

第 32－3926 条　客座教授证书

A. 对于在该州针灸学校任教的针灸师,如果其证明其具有至少五年的针灸实践经验并具有适当的技能和培训,委员会可以向其颁发客座教授证书。针灸师应当按委员会规定提交申请,并按照第 32－3927 条规定的收费标准提交申请。

B. 根据本条颁发的证书允许证书持有者只在与证书持有者的教师职位职责相关的范围内从事针灸实践。

C. 根据本条颁发的证书有效期为一年。如果证书持有人在证书有效期届满前至少三十日提出申请,委员会可以准予延期一年。委员会可以批准总共两次一年的延期。

第 32－3927 条　费用

A. 委员会应当在其年度会议上通过正式表决,确定不超过下列费用的不可退还费用:

1. 颁发初始执照,六百美元。

2. 申请执照或者证书,一百五十美元。

3. 执照续期,六百美元。

4. 执照逾期续期,额外支付一百美元。

5. 颁发执照或者证书副本,五十美元。

6. 颁发初始客座教授证书,六百美元。

7. 客座教授证书续期,六百美元。

8. 颁发初始耳穴针灸证书,二百五十美元。

9. 耳穴针灸证书续期,二百五十美元。

10. 复制记录、文件、信件、会议记录、申请和文件,每页二十五美分。

11. 本日历年度委员会会议的会议记录副本,每套会议记录二十五美元。

B. 委员会应当就本章未规定的,但委员会认为对执行本章是必要和适当的服务收取额外费用。费用不得超过提供这些服务的实际费用。

第 3 节 监   管

第 32 - 3951 条   拒绝授予、撤销或者吊销执照;听证;替代性制裁

A. 委员会可以采用下列任何理由拒绝授予、撤销或者吊销根据本章颁发的执照:

1. 涉及道德败坏的重罪或者轻罪的定罪。定罪记录或者由定罪发生地法院书记官或者由该法院法官发出的核证副本,足以作为定罪的证据。

2. 通过欺诈或者欺骗手段骗取本章规定的执照。

3. 持证人针灸实践中的违反职业道德的行为或者不称职行为。

4. 在持证人针灸实践中使用假名、化名的。

5. 违反本章或者委员会规则的。

B. 如果委员会根据听证会确定存在撤销或者吊销执照的理由,委员会可以永久或者在一定期限内实施该措施,并可以施加委员会规定的条件。委员会还可以对每项违反本章的行为处以不超过一万美元的民事处罚。委员会应当根据《亚利桑那州议会法》注释版第 35 - 146 条和第 35 - 147 条的规定,将根据本款收取的民事罚款存入该州的普通基金。

C. 委员会可以不举行听证会就拒绝颁发执照。申请人收到不予受理通知后,可以要求举行听证,对不予受理的申请进行复核。

D. 委员会应当根据《亚利桑那州议会法》注释版第 41 卷第 6 章第 10 节的规定举行撤销或者吊销执照的听证会,出席者均可以由律师代理。

E. 委员会可以提出关注函、发布谴责令、规定察看期或者限制或者约束持证人的执业,而不是拒绝授予、撤销或者吊销执照。委员会可以发布非纪律处分命令,要求持证人在委员会规定的一个或者多个区域完成规定学时的继续教育,以便向持证人提供对当前事态发展、技能、程序或者治疗的必要了解。

F. 如果行政主管对持证人实施纪律处分,委员会应当立即通知持证人的雇主。

G. 委员会可以指定一名调查员向委员会提供有关涉嫌违反本章规定的信息。

H. 委员会自行或者响应参与委员会调查或者诉讼的任何人的申请,可以发布传票,要

求证人出庭作证，或者要求出示与委员会调查或者诉讼有关的文件、报告、记录或者任何其他证据，以供检查或者复印。

第 32 - 3952 条　审查和复印证据的权利

关于根据本法第 32 - 3951 条进行的委员会调查，委员会有权在合理时间内审查和复印被调查人的任何文件、报告、记录或者其他物证，或者任何诊所、持证人办公室或者其他公共或者私人机构以及《亚利桑那州议会法》注释版第 36 - 401 条定义的卫生保健机构保存或者拥有的报告、记录和其他文件，如果委员会认为这些信息与持证人的违反职业道德的行为或者精神或者身体能力有关。

第 32 - 3953 条　禁令救济；保证金；送达

A. 除所有其他补救办法外，如果委员会有各种理由认为某人违反了本章或者委员会规则，委员会可以通过被指控发生违法行为的县的总检察长或者县律师，向该县的上级法院申请禁止该人从事违法行为的禁令。

B. 法院应当发布临时限制令、初步禁止令或者永久禁止令，而不要求委员会缴纳保证金。

C. 在发现被告的本州任何一个县，可以向被告送达诉讼文书。

第 32 - 3954 条　违规；分类

违反本章规定的，犯第 1 类轻罪。

第 32 - 3955 条　针灸助理；职责范围；注册要求；头衔的使用

A. 本章并不禁止针灸助理根据委员会通过的规则，在符合以下条件的情况下，协助执业针灸师：

1. 针灸助理可以：

（a）取出针灸针。

（b）监督针灸程序，如热敷或者艾灸。

（c）执行非关键性的职能，如收集患者的基本信息，测量血压和照顾患者治疗室。

2. 针灸助理不得插入针灸针或者评估、解释、设计或者修改既定的针灸护理治疗方案。

3. 针灸助理应当以委员会规定的表格向委员会申请注册。如果其违反本章有关针灸服务的任何规定，或者实施有损于公众健康或者安全的行为或者做法，委员会可以暂停或者撤销其注册。

B. 下列行为均属违法：

1. 从事针灸助理工作，除非该人是根据本章和委员会通过的规则，在执业针灸师的监督下工作。

2. 使用缩写"a.a."或者"针灸助理"的称谓，除非该人是根据本章和委员会通过的规则，在执业针灸师的监督下工作。

亚利桑那州针灸行政法[①]

第1节 一般规定

第 R4－8－101 条　定义

ARS 第 32－3901 条（即《亚利桑那州议会法》注释版第 32 卷第 39 章第 1 条，下同）中的定义适用于本章。

"ACAOM"系指针灸及东方医学教育审核委员会。

"针灸课程"系指经委员会批准的培训，旨在为学员参加 NCCAOM 考试和获得执照做准备。

"针灸学员"系指在针灸或者耳穴针灸培训计划中注册的个人。

"针灸师"系指经委员会颁发执照或者认证的在本州从事针灸实践的个人。

"行政完整性审查"系指委员会确定申请人是否提供了完整的申请资料的过程。

"申请人"系指向委员会申请初始或者续期执照或者证书的个人。

"申请资料包"系指委员会要求申请人或者代表申请人提交的费、表格、文件和附加信息。

"经批准的继续教育"系指委员会确定的符合第 R4－8－408 条标准的计划性教育履历。

"耳穴针灸"系指使用五针方案治疗酗酒、药物滥用或者化学药物依赖的一种疗法。

"洁针技术"系指为避免疾病和感染的传播，保护公众和患者，并符合州和联邦法律的针刺消毒和使用方式。

"临床时间"系指学员在根据本法第 R4－8－203 条或者第 R4－8－208 条获得执照的个人监督下提供患者护理的实际时间。

"课程"系指帮助学员获得与针灸实践相关的知识、技能和信息的系统学习经验。

"日"系指日历日。

"五针疗法"系指由国家针灸戒毒协会开发的用于治疗酗酒、药物滥用或者化学药物依赖的疗法，包括将五根针插入外耳的特定穴位。

"学时"系指至少五十分钟的课程参与。

"关注函"系指一种替代性制裁，通知持证人或者证书持有人，虽然证据不表明需要实施纪律处分，但委员会认为持证人或者证书持有人应当改变某些做法，否则，可能导致启动纪律处分。关注函是一份公开文件，可以在未来的纪律处分程序中使用。

"NADA"系指国家针灸戒毒协会。

"NCCAOM"系指国家针灸与东方医学认证委员会。

"答辩人"系指被指控违反《亚利桑那州议会法》注释版（ARS）第 32 卷第 39 章或者本章的个人。

[①]　根据《亚利桑那州行政法典》第 4 卷第 8 章"针灸审查委员会"译出。

"顺利完成洁针技术课程"系指课程参与者参加了该课程,以及在考试中获得合格分数,或者从课程提供者处获得其他证实,证明学员掌握了课程内容。

"督导"系指由委员会颁发执照的针灸师,负责监督和指导针灸学员或者证书持有人。

第 R4－8－102 条　文件的认证;翻译;核查

A. 申请人应当确保由其或者代表其提交给委员会的文件有官方或者政府的印章或者验证的书面证明。如果委员会确定申请人无法通过尽职调查获得印章或者证明,委员会应当免除这一要求。

B. 申请人应当确保文凭、成绩单、执照、证书、考试成绩或者其他申请所需文件的正式副本,能够由签发机构直接转交给委员会。

C. 申请人应当确保所提交的非英语文件附有英文原文翻译,该翻译由申请人以外的合格译员完成。申请人应当确保译文附有一份准确性宣誓书,在该宣誓书中,负责翻译或者核对译文的译员在宣誓后确认,整个文件已经翻译完毕,没有任何遗漏或者添加,而且译文是真实和正确的。只有当申请人提供了包括准确性声明在内的全部翻译件的复印件时,委员会才会将翻译件的原件退回给申请人。

D. 以下人员被认为是合格的翻译人员:

1. 官方翻译局或者政府机构的官员或者雇员。

2. 在美国经认证的学院或者大学中教授所翻译语言的教授或者讲师。该教授或者讲师应当确保准确性宣誓书包括所教课程的名称,使用学院或者大学的官方信笺,并经过公证。

3. 签发翻译文件的美国领事。如果是私人翻译,美国领事应当根据第(C)款的要求核实该译文以及翻译者的身份。

4. 派驻美国的总领事或者外交代表,或者外国政府机构的其他代表。如果是私人翻译,该代表应当根据第(C)款的要求核实译文和翻译者的身份。

第 R4－8－103 条　更改邮寄地址、电子邮件地址或者电话号码

委员会应当使用提供给委员会的联系信息与持证人、证书持有人或者获得委员会批准的人员进行沟通。为确保委员会的及时沟通,持证人、证书持有人或者获得委员会批准的人员应当在更改邮寄地址(包括新旧地址)、电子邮件地址或者住宅、商业或者移动电话号码的三十日内以书面形式通知委员会。

第 R4－8－104 条　到期

第 R4－8－105 条　执照、认证和获批的时间表

A. 为了 ARS 第 41－1073 条的目的,委员会制定了表 1 中所列的时间范围。申请人或者要求委员会批准的人和委员会负责人,可以书面同意延长实质性审查和整体时间范围安排,但不超过总体时间范围安排的百分之二十五。

B. 行政完整性审查时间范围,从委员会收到申请材料或者批准请求时开始。在行政完整性审查时间范围内,委员会应当通知申请人或者请求批准的人,申请材料或者批准请求是完整的还是不完整的。如果申请材料或者批准请求不完整,委员会应当在通知中说明缺少哪些信息。

C. 申请人或者请求批准的人,如果其申请材料或者批准请求不完整,应当在表 1 所列的完成时间内向委员会提交所缺信息。行政完整性审查和总体时间范围都从委员会根据(B)发出通知之日起暂停,直到委员会收到所有缺失的信息。

D. 在收到所有缺失的资料后,委员会应当通知申请人或者请求批准的人,申请资料或者批准请求已经完成。如果委员会在表1所列的行政完整性审查时间范围内授予或者拒绝颁发执照、证书或者批准,委员会不应当单独发送完整性通知。

E. 表1中所列的实质性审查时间范围从委员会发出行政完整性通知之日开始。

F. 如果委员会在实质性审查过程中确定需要补充资料,委员会应当向申请人或者要求批准的人发出一份全面的书面补充资料要求。

G. 收到第(F)款要求的申请人或者申请批准的人,应当在表1所列的答复时间内向委员会提交补充资料。实质性的审查和总体时间范围都从委员会的要求之日起暂停,直到委员会收到补充信息为止。

H. 申请人或者要求批准的人可以在时间到期前向委员会提供书面通知,将第(C)款或者第(G)款规定的时间延长三十日。如果请求批准的申请人或者个人未能在表1规定的时间内或者延长的时间内向委员会提交缺失的或者补充的信息,委员会应当关闭该申请人或者个人的档案。为获得进一步的审议,档案被关闭的申请人或者申请批准的人应当重新申请。

I. 在表1所列的总体时间范围内,委员会应当:

1. 如果委员会确定申请人或者要求批准的人符合《议会法》和本章规定的所有标准,则颁发执照、证书或者批准;或者

2. 如果委员会确定申请者或者要求批准的人不符合《议会法》和本章规定的所有标准,则拒绝颁发执照、证书或者批准。

J. 如果委员会拒绝颁发执照、证书或者批准,委员会应当向申请人或者请求批准的人发出书面通知,说明:

1. 拒绝的原因,并引用相关法律规定或者规则。

2. 申请人或者个人有权根据 ARS 第 41 卷第 6 章第 10 节对拒绝提出上诉。

3. 对拒绝提出上诉的时间。

4. 申请人或者个人要求召开非正式和解会议的权利。

K. 如果一个时间范围内的最后一日是星期六、星期日或者国家官方假日,那么下一个工作日就是该时间范围内的最后一日。

第 R4‑8‑105 条　表 1 时间范围(每日)

表1　时间范围(每日)

执照、证书或者批准的类型	授　　　权	行政完整性时间范围	完成时间	实质性审查时间范围	答复时间	总体时间范围
针灸执照	ARS 32‑3924;R4‑8‑203	20	30	40	30	60
客座教授证书	ARS 32‑3926;R4‑8‑208	20	30	40	30	60

执照、证书或者批准的类型	授　权	行政完整性时间范围	完成时间	实质性审查时间范围	答复时间	总体时间范围
耳穴针灸专业证书	ARS 32 - 3922;R4 - 8 - 301	20	30	40	30	60
耳穴针灸训练项目	ARS 32 - 3922;R4 - 8 - 401	20	30	40	30	60
针灸计划	ARS 32 - 3924(2);R4 - 8 - 403	20	30	40	30	60
临床培训计划	ARS 32 - 3924(2);R4 - 8 - 403	20	30	40	30	60
洁针技术课程	ARS 32 - 3924;R4 - 8 - 402	20	30	40	30	60
继续教育批准	ARS 32 - 3925;R4 - 8 - 409	20	30	40	30	60
续期执照或者证书	ARS 32 - 3925;R4 - 8 - 204 or R4 - 8 - 303	20	30	40	30	60
客座教授证书延期	ARS 32 - 3926(C);R4 - 8 - 208	20	30	40	30	60
执照恢复	ARS 32 - 3925(D);R4 - 8 - 205	20	30	40	30	60

第 R4 - 8 - 106 条　费用

A. 根据 ARS 第 32 - 3927 条的授权,委员会设立并收取以下费用:

1. 申请针灸执照:一百五十美元。

2. 首次颁发针灸执照:二百七十五美元。

3. 针灸执照续期:二百七十五美元。

4. 逾期续期针灸执照的额外费用:一百美元。

5. 申请耳穴针灸证书:七十五美元。

6. 首次颁发耳穴针灸证书:七十五美元。

7. 续期耳穴针灸证书:七十五美元。

8. 客座教授证书:六百美元。

9. 客座教授证书延期:六百美元。

10. 执照或者证书副本:五十美元。

B. 除第(B)款(1)项至第(B)款(3)项的规定或者 ARS 第 41 - 1077 条的要求外,所有费用均不退还。在以下情况下,委员会应当退还根据第(A)款(2)项或者第(A)款(6)项支付的费用:

1. 委员会拒绝向申请人颁发执照或者证书。

2. 委员会根据第 R4 - 8 - 105 条关闭了申请人的档案;或者

3. 申请人撤回申请。

第 R4－8－107 条　参考材料

A. 委员会将以下材料作为参考：

1.《NADA 注册培训师资源手册》,1999 年,由国家针灸戒毒协会出版,地址：华盛顿哥伦比亚特区西北区 N 街 3220 号 275 室,邮编 20007。

2.《针灸师洁针技术手册》,2004 年第 5 版,由全国针灸基金会出版,地址：康涅狄格州查普林镇,邮政信箱 137,邮编 06235。

3.《认证手册》,第一部,2005 年,由针灸和东方医学认证委员会出版,地址：马里兰州格林贝尔特市格林威中心大道 7501 号马里兰贸易中心 3 号楼 260 室,邮编 20770。

B. 根据第(A)款纳入的材料不包含后来的版本或者修正案,并在委员会存档。

第 2 节　针灸执照;客座教授证书

第 R4－8－201 条　已重新编号

第 R4－8－202 条　已重新编号

第 R4－8－203 条　针灸执照申请

A. 要获得针灸执照,申请人应当向委员会提交一份申请材料,其中包括：

1. 使用委员会提供的表格,提供关于申请人的下列信息：

a. 姓名。

b. 申请人的曾用名。

c. 出生日期。

d. 社会安全号码。

e. 家庭、营业和电子邮件地址。

f. 家庭、营业和移动电话号码。

g. 说明申请人是否曾依法在本州或者其他州、地区或者其他国家或者其部分地区从事卫生保健实践,如果是的话：

（i）申请人依法获得从事卫生保健实践的司法管辖区清单。

（ii）每张执照的编号。

（iii）每张执照的颁发日期。

（iv）每张执照到期或者逾期日期。

（v）每张执照的限制,如果有的话。

（vi）每张执照是否通过背书、审查或者其他方式授予。

h. 说明申请人是否获得 NCCAOM 的认证,如果已经获得,认证是否有效,以及颁发和到期的日期。

i. 如果没有获得 NCCAOM 的认证,说明申请人是否：

（i）已经通过 NCCAOM 的所有模块：穴位定位;东方医学基础;生物医学;和针灸;或者

（ii）已经通过加利福尼亚州的针灸执照考试。

j. 一份申请人是否完成了在美国或者其他国家或者其部分地区认证的针灸课程的声

明,如果是,则说明课程完成的日期。

k. 说明申请人是否曾被美国其他州、区或者准州,或者其他国家或者其他国家的分支部门的发证机构拒绝颁发针灸执照或者证书,如果是,请说明拒绝颁发执照或者证书的管辖区名称、拒绝日期,以及对情况的解释。

l. 声明申请人是否曾被美国其他州、地区或者准州,或者其他国家或者其部分地区发证机构撤销、吊销、限制,或者对申请人的针灸执照或者证书采取任何其他行动,如果是,则说明采取该行动的辖区名称、采取的行动、行动日期,以及对情况的解释。

m. 说明申请人是否曾被定罪,包括在药物或者酒精影响下驾驶,但不包括轻微的交通违法行为,如果是,请说明定罪的司法管辖区名称、犯罪性质、定罪日期以及目前的状况。

n. 说明申请人是否曾有不当行为的索赔或者对申请人提起诉讼,指控其在针灸服务中存在非专业行为或者过失,如果有,则说明索赔或者案件编号、索赔或者诉讼的日期、指控事项,以及该索赔或者诉讼是否仍在审理中或者以何种方式解决。

o. 说明申请人是否有可能影响其安全和熟练地从事针灸实践的状况,如果有,则说明该状况的性质和必要的适应措施。

p. 说明申请人是否曾在接受调查期间自愿或者非自愿地从医疗机构辞职,如果是,请说明医疗机构的名称、辞职日期以及对当时情况的解释。

q. 说明申请人是否曾被医疗机构终止、限制或者采取任何其他有关申请人就业、专业培训或者特权的行动,如果是,则说明医疗机构的名称、行动的日期以及对情况的解释。

2. 与申请人对(A)(1)(k)至(A)(1)(q)的解释有关的官方记录或者文件。

3. 下列情况之一的文件:

a. 来自 NCCAOM 或者其继受机构的认证。

b. 由委员会承认的其他认证机构的认证。

c. 通过针灸执照或者认证考试的认证;或者

d. 美国其他州、地区或者准州,或者其他国家或者其他国家的分支部门的法律授权,其执照标准与本章规定的标准基本相似,且未被撤销的针灸执照。

4. 顺利完成委员会批准的洁针技术课程的文件。要求显示课程名称以及完成课程的日期和地点的结业证书副本。

5. 过去一年内拍摄的 2 英寸×2 英寸照片,须显示申请人的正脸。

6. 填写完整的亚利桑那州公共福利的公民身份和外国人身份声明,该表格可以向委员会索取。

7. 一套符合联邦调查局标准的完整指纹,由执法机构或者其他合格单位采集。

8. 公共安全部为处理州和联邦犯罪记录检查的指纹而收取的费用。

9. 委员会根据第 R4 - 8 - 106 条(A)款(1)项和第 R4 - 8 - 106 条(A)款(2)项规定的申请费和初始执照费。

B. 除了第(A)款规定的材料外,申请人应当提供文件证明其完成了至少一千八百五十学时的针灸培训,包括至少八百学时的临床培训,直接向委员会提交申请人参加委员会批准的针灸课程的每所学校的正式成绩单,显示:

1. 学校的名称和地址。

2. 申请人在该校就读的日期。

3. 申请人完成的课程和临床培训。

4. 每个课程或者临床培训的学时数。

5. 申请人在每门课程或者临床培训中获得的成绩或者分数。

6. 申请人是否从该校获得了文凭或者学位。

C. 除了遵守第(A)和(B)款的规定外,申请人应当签署一份宣誓书,注明日期并进行公证,表明申请资料中提供的所有信息,包括由申请人或者其代表提交的任何附带文件,都是真实、完整和正确的。

第 R4－8－204 条 针灸执照续期

A. 针灸执照自颁发之日起满十二个月后失效。

B. 委员会应当在六十日内通知持证人需要续期。及时续期是持证人的责任。如果没有收到需要续期的通知,不能作为没有及时续期的理由。

C. 如果持证人未能在到期日或者之前提交第(D)款所述的续期申请资料,持证人应当停止针灸实践。

D. 为续期针灸执照,持证人应当向委员会提交:

1. 提供有关持证人的下列信息的续期申请:

a. 姓名。

b. 执照号码。

c. 企业名称。

d. 家庭、营业和电子邮件地址。

e. 家庭、营业和移动电话号码。

f. 说明在过去十二个月内,美国其他州、地区、准州或者其他国家及其执照授予机构是否拒绝向持证人颁发针灸执照或者证书,如果是,则说明拒绝颁发执照或者证书的管辖区名称、拒绝日期,以及对情况的解释。

g. 说明在过去十二个月中,美国其他州、地区或者准州或者其他国家或者其他国家部分地区的发证机构是否撤销、吊销、限制,或者对持证人的执照采取其他行动,如果是,则说明对执照采取行动的管辖区名称、采取的行动、行动的日期,以及对情况的解释。

h. 说明在过去十二个月中,持证人是否被定罪,包括在药物或者酒精影响下驾驶,但不包括轻微的交通违法行为,如果是,则说明定罪的司法管辖区名称,犯罪性质,定罪日期,以及目前的状况。

i. 说明在过去十二个月中,是否有针对持证人的不良行为索赔或者诉讼,指控其在针灸实践中存在渎职或者过失,如果是,则说明索赔或者案件编号、索赔或者诉讼日期、指控事项,以及该索赔或者诉讼是否仍在审理中或者以何种方式解决。

j. 说明在过去十二个月中,持证人是否有可能影响其安全和熟练地从事针灸实践的状况,如果是,则说明该状况的性质和必要的适应措施。

k. 说明在过去十二个月中,持证人是否在接受调查期间自愿或者非自愿地从一家医疗机构辞职,如果是,则说明该医疗机构的名称、辞职日期以及对情况的解释。

1. 说明在过去十二个月中,是否有医疗机构终止、限制或者采取任何其他有关执照人就业、专业培训或者特权的行动,如果有,则说明医疗机构的名称、行动的日期以及对情况的解释。

2. 申明持证人完成了第 R4－8－206 条规定的继续教育。

3. 申明持证人符合 ARS 第 32－3211 条的要求。

4. 填写完毕的《亚利桑那州公共福利公民身份和外国人身份声明》,该表格可以向委员会索取。

5. 第 R4－8－106 条第(A)(3)项规定的续期费。

6. 持证人的签名,确认所提供的信息是准确、真实和完整的。

第 R4－8－205 条　针灸执照恢复

A. 因未按照第 R4－8－204 条第(D)款规定及时续期而导致针灸执照到期的个人,可以在执照到期后六十日内向委员会申请恢复针灸执照:

1. 第 R4－8－204 条第(D)款所述的申请资料。

2. 一份宣誓书,证明该人在执照到期后没有从事过针灸实践。

3. 第 R4－8－106 条(A)款(4)项规定的针灸执照延期续期费用。

B. 如果针灸执照到期超过六十日,委员会不应当按照第(A)款的规定恢复原持证人的执照。如果针灸执照到期超过六十日,原持证人可按照第 R4－8－203 条的规定申请执照。

第 R4－8－206 条　继续教育要求

A. 持证人应当每年至少完成十五学时的经批准的继续教育。

B. 委员会应当按照以下方式授予经批准的继续教育学时:

1. 培训会或者研讨会:每面授一小时可以获得一学时的继续教育。

2. 经认证的教育机构的课程:每学期可以获得十五学时的继续教育。

3. 自学、在线或者函授课程:由课程提供者决定继续教育学时。

4. 教授经批准的继续教育课程:每教授一小时,可以获得一学时的继续教育。

5. 在同行评审的专业期刊或者教科书中发表过一篇关于针灸或者传统东亚医学的文章:可以获得十五学时的继续教育。

6. 参加委员会会议:在一年内参加一次会议,可以获得一学时的继续教育。

7. 出版一本与针灸或者传统东亚医学有关的教科书:可以获得十五学时的继续教育。

C. 委员会应当按照以下规定限制批准的继续教育学时:

1. 通过教授批准的继续教育获得的学时不得超过规定的百分之三十。每年只能通过教授某项经批准的继续教育获得一次学时。作为小组成员参加经批准的继续教育不得获得学时。

2. 超过一年中所要求的最高学时,不得转入下一年。

D. 持证人应当从参加的每项经批准的继续教育的提供者那里获得一份证书或者其他出席证明,其中包括以下内容:

1. 持证人的姓名。

2. 持证人的执照编号。

3. 经批准的继续教育的名称。

4. 继续教育提供者的名称。

5. 批准该继续教育的实体名称。

6. 批准的继续教育的日期、时间和地点。

7. 经批准的继续教育的学时数。

E. 持证人应当将第(D)款所述的出勤证明留存两年,并根据第 R4－8－207 条和本章其他要求向委员会提供这些证明文件。

第 R4－8－207 条　对不遵守继续教育要求的行为进行合规性审计和制裁

当提供需要续期执照的通知时,委员会也应当向随机抽选的持证人提供继续教育记录的审计通知。接受继续教育审计的持证人应当在提交第 R4－8－206 条第(D)款规定的文件的同时,提交第 R4－8－204 条第(D)款规定的续期申请材料。如果持证人未能在到期日之前随续期申请包提交所需的文件,则执照到期。

第 R4－8－208 条　申请客座教授证书;客座教授证书的延期

A. 为获得客座教授证书,申请人应当向委员会提交:

1. 第 R4－8－203 条第(A)款规定的申请表,以及一份签字,确认所提供的信息是准确、真实和完整的。

2. 第 R4－8－106 条第(A)款(8)项规定的费用。

3. 证明拥有至少五年从事针灸实践经验的文件。

4. 申请人在其将要教授的科目方面的技能和培训证明,包括以下内容之一:

a. 由学院或者大学出具的关于申请人将要教授的科目的经验、教育或者其他培训的文件。

b. 申请前两年内有教授相同或者类似科目内容的经验文件;或者

c. 申请前两年内有一年在申请人所任教的专业领域的经验的文件。

5. 一份客座教授职责的详细计划。

B. 客座教授证书的有效期为一年,自颁发之日起算。若要将客座教授证书再延长一年,证书持有人应当在证书到期前至少三十日向委员会提交延期申请。延期申请包括:

1. 第 R4－8－204 条(D)款(1)项中描述的延期申请表,包括一份签字,确认所提供的信息是准确、真实和完整的。

2. 由客座教授将要任教的针灸学院的官员出具的带有官方信笺抬头的信函,要求批准延期。

3. 第 R4－8－106 条(A)款(9)项条规定的费用。

C. 委员会不得为客座教授证书延期两次以上。

第 R4－8－209 条　废止

第 R4－8－210 条　废止

第 3 节　耳穴针灸认证

第 R4－8－301 条　耳穴针灸证书的申请

要获得耳穴针灸师证书,在委员会批准的酗酒、药物滥用或者化学药物依赖计划中提供

耳穴针灸实践,申请人应当向委员会提交申请材料,其中包括:

　　1. 使用委员会提供的表格,提供关于申请人的下列信息:

　　a. 姓名。

　　b. 申请人的其他名字。

　　c. 出生日期。

　　d. 社会安全号码。

　　e. 家庭、营业和电子邮件地址。

　　f. 家庭、营业和移动电话号码。

　　g. 说明申请人是否曾依法在美国其他州、准州、地区或者其他国家或者其部分地区从事耳穴针灸实践,如果是:

　　i. 列出申请人曾依法从事耳穴针灸实践的司法管辖区。

　　ii. 每张执照或者证书的编号。

　　iii. 每张执照或者证书的颁发日期。

　　iv. 每张执照或者证书到期或者逾期日期。

　　v. 每张执照或者证书的限制,如果有的话。

　　vi. 每张执照或者证书的现行状态。

　　vii. 每张执照或者证书是否通过背书、审查或者其他方式授予。

　　h. 一份声明,说明申请人是否曾被美国其他州、地区或者准州,或者其他国家或者其他国家的部分地区的发证机构拒绝颁发耳穴针灸执照或者证书,如果是,则说明拒绝颁发执照或者证书的管辖区名称,拒绝的日期,以及对情况的说明。

　　i. 一份声明,说明申请人是否曾被美国其他州、地区或者准州,或者其他国家或者其部分地区的发证机构撤销、吊销、限制、制约或者采取任何其他有关申请人的耳穴针灸执照或者证书的行动,如果是,则说明采取该行动的司法管辖区的名称,所采取的行动,行动的日期,以及对情况的说明。

　　j. 一份声明,说明申请人是否曾被定罪,包括在药物或者酒精影响下驾驶,但不包括轻微的交通违法行为,如果是,请说明定罪的司法管辖区名称、犯罪性质、定罪日期以及目前的状况。

　　k. 一份声明,说明申请人是否曾有渎职索赔或者对申请人提起诉讼,指控其在从事耳穴针灸实践中存在渎职或者过失,如果是,说明索赔或者案件编号、索赔或者诉讼的日期、指控的事项,以及该索赔或者诉讼是否仍在审理中或者以何种方式解决。

　　l. 一份声明,说明申请人是否有可能影响其安全和熟练地从事耳穴针灸实践的状况,如果是,则说明该状况的性质和必要的适应措施。

　　m. 一份声明,申请人是否曾在接受调查期间自愿或者非自愿地从医疗机构辞职,如果是,则说明该医疗机构的名称、辞职日期以及对当时情况的说明。

　　n. 一份声明,说明申请人是否曾被医疗机构终止、限制或者采取任何其他有关申请人就业、专业培训或者特权的行动,如果是,则说明医疗机构的名称、行动的日期以及对情况的说明。

2. 与申请人对第(1)(h)项至第(1)(n)项的解释有关的官方记录或者文件。

3. 委员会根据第 R4－8－106 条(A)款(5)项和第 R4－8－106 条(A)款(6)项规定的申请费和初始执照费。

4. 完成委员会批准的文件：

a. 耳穴针灸治疗酗酒、药物滥用或者化学药物依赖的培训计划。要求显示课程名称、日期和地点的结业证书副本。

b. 洁针技术课程。要求显示课程名称、日期和地点的结业证书副本。

5. 如果申请人获得认证，将对申请人进行监督的亚利桑那州执业针灸师的姓名、执照号码和电话号码。

6. 一张 2 英寸×2 英寸的照片，在过去一年内拍摄，显示申请人的正脸，申请人在照片背面或者周围的白框上签名。

7. 填写完整的《亚利桑那州公共福利公民身份和外国人身份声明》，该表格可以向委员会索取。

8. 申请人注明日期并经公证的签名，确认申请中提供的信息，包括由申请人或者代表申请人提交的任何附带文件，都是真实和完整的。

第 R4－8－302 条　耳穴针灸实践要求

A. 持有耳穴针灸证书的人只能在委员会、州政府或者联邦政府批准的防治酗酒、药物滥用或者化学药物依赖计划中提供耳穴针灸服务。

B. 耳穴针灸证书持有人只能在根据 A.R.S.(《亚利桑那州议会法》注释版，下同)第 32－3924 条和本法第 R4－8－203 条获得授权的个人的监督下提供耳穴针灸服务。

C. 委员会批准的防治酗酒、药物滥用或者化学药物依赖计划，并由亚利桑那州卫生服务部根据 A.R.S 第 36 卷第 4 章授权为行为保健机构。

第 R4－8－303 条　耳穴针灸证书的续期

A. 耳穴针灸证书自颁发之日起十二个月后失效。

B. 委员会应当提前六十日通知证书持有人是否需要续期。证书持有人有责任及时续期。如果没有收到需要续期的通知，不能作为没有及时续期的理由。

C. 如果证书持有人未能在到期日当天或者之前提交第(D)款所述的续期申请，则证书持有人应当停止耳穴针灸实践。

D. 为耳穴针灸证书续期，证书持有人应当向委员会提交：

1. 提供下列证书持有人信息的续期申请：

a. 姓名。

b. 证书编号。

c. 续期日期。

d. 证书持有人工作的酗酒、药物滥用或者化学药物依赖机构的名称、地址和电话号码。

e. 住宅和电子邮件地址。

f. 住宅和移动电话号码。

g. 一份声明，说明在过去十二个月内，在美国其他州、地区或者准州的分支机构是否拒绝向证书持有人颁发耳穴针灸执业执照或者证书,如果存在此种情形,拒绝颁发执照或者证书的管辖区名称、拒绝日期和情况说明。

h. 一份声明,说明在过去十二个月内,在美国其他州、地区或者领土的分支机构是否撤销、吊销、限制、制约或者采取了与证书持有人的执照或者证书有关的其他措施。如果存在此种情形,应当提供采取措施的管辖区名称、采取的措施、日期以及对情况的解释。

i. 一份声明,说明在过去十二个月中,证书持有人是否被判有罪,包括在药物或者酒精影响下驾驶,而非轻微的交通违法行为。如果存在此种情形,应当提供定罪的司法辖区名称、犯罪性质、定罪日期和当前状态等信息。

j. 一份声明,说明在过去十二个月内是否有针对证书持有人的渎职索赔或者诉讼,指控其在耳穴针灸实践中的渎职或者过失。如果存在此种情形,应当提供案件编号、索赔或者诉讼的日期、指控的事项,以及索赔或者诉讼是否仍未解决或者其解决方式。

k. 一份声明,说明证书持有人在过去十二个月内是否存在可能损害证书持有人安全和熟练地练习耳穴针灸的能力的情况。如果存在,应当说明情况的性质和必要的适应措施。

l. 一份声明,说明在过去十二个月中,证书持有人是否在接受调查期间自愿或者非自愿地从保健机构辞职,如果是,应当提供保健机构的名称、辞职日期以及对情况的解释。

m. 一份声明,说明在过去十二个月内,证书持有人是否有医疗机构终止、限制证书持有人的就业、专业培训等权利,或者对持证人采取任何其他措施。如果存在,应当提供医疗机构的名称、行动日期,以及对情况的解释。

n. 监督证书持有人的执业针灸师的姓名、执照号码和电话号码。

2. 根据针灸审查委员会提供的表格,完整填写的亚利桑那州公民身份和外国人身份的声明。

3. 第 R4－8－106 条第(A)款(7)项规定的续期费。

4. 证书持有人的日期签名,确认所提供的信息准确、真实和完整。

E. 委员会无权恢复到期的耳穴针灸证书。因未能根据本条(D)款及时续期而导致耳穴针灸认证到期的个人,可通过遵守第 R4－8－301 条申请认证。

第 R4－8－304 条　督导变更通知

A. 证书持有人应当在下列情况发生后十日内向委员会提供书面通知:

1. 证书持有人从一个批准的防治酗酒、药物滥用和化学药物依赖计划转换到另一个项目。

2. 证书持有人不再作为耳穴针灸医师执业。

3. 监督证书持证人的执业针灸师更换。

B. 根据第(A)款的规定提供通知的证书持有人,应当在通知中包括以下信息:

1. 证书持有人的姓名和证书号码。

2. 证书持有人受雇的经批准的防治酗酒、药物滥用和化学药物依赖计划的名称和地址。

3. 监督证书持证人的执业针灸师的姓名、执照号码和电话号码。

4. 证书持有人不作为耳穴针灸医师执业的声明。

第 R4－8－305 条　重新编纂

第 R4－8－306 条　重新编纂

第 R4‑8‑307 条　重新编纂

第 R4‑8‑308 条　重新编纂

第 R4‑8‑309 条　重新编纂

第 R4‑8‑310 条　重新编纂

第 R4‑8‑311 条　重新编纂

第 R4‑8‑312 条　重新编纂

第 4 节　培训计划和继续教育

第 R4‑8‑401 条　耳穴针灸培训计划审批

A. 委员会批准了一个被 NADA 认可的耳穴针灸培训计划。

B. 要获得委员会对未根据第(A)款获得批准的耳穴针灸培训计划的批准,培训计划的提供者应当向委员会提交证据,证明该计划符合以下条件:

1. 根据参照第 R4‑8‑107 条编制的《NADA 注册培训师资源手册》进行。

2. 由另一个委员会批准的针灸认证机构批准。

第 R4‑8‑402 条　洁针技术课程认证

为了获得委员会的批准,建议进行洁针技术课程的人员应当向委员会提交证明,证明该课程是根据参考第 R4‑8‑107 条规定编写的《针灸师洁针手册》进行的。

第 R4‑8‑403 条　针灸或者临床培训计划的批准

A. 为了获得委员会的批准,针灸专业的提供者应当向委员会提交:

1. 针灸专业是认证的候选项目或者已通过 ACAOM 认证,并提供至少一千八百五十学时的培训,包括至少八百学时的临床培训的文件;

2. 证明针灸专业符合第 R4‑8‑404 条第(A)款规定的标准的文件。

B. 为了获得委员会的批准,针灸临床培训计划的提供者应当向委员会提交:

1. 证明临床培训计划是针灸专业的一部分的文件,该针灸专业是认证的候选人或者通过 ACAOM 获得认证,或者本身是认证的候选人或者通过 ACAOM 获得认证;或者

2. 证明该临床计划符合第 R4‑8‑404 条第(B)款规定的标准的文件。

第 R4‑8‑404 条　针灸或者临床培训计划的标准

A. 委员会应当批准不符合第 R4‑8‑403 条第(A)款(1)项标准的针灸专业,前提是该专业:

1. 至少持续三年。

2. 符合参考第 R4‑8‑107 条编制的"认证手册"第一部分的基本要求和附带标准。

3. 提供以下课程内容和最少学时:

a. 传统的东亚医学理论、诊断、针灸治疗技术及相关研究:六百九十学时。

b. 临床培训:八百学时。

c. 生物医学临床科学:三百六十学时。

B. 委员会应批准不符合第 R4‑8‑403 条第(B)款(1)项规定的标准的针灸临床培训计划,前提是该临床培训计划:

131

1. 由一名拥有并经营针灸诊所的个人经营的。

2. 在针灸诊所提供至少百分之七十五的临床指导。

3. 在以下方面与患者直接接触:

a. 针灸临床的监督观察,包括病例介绍和讨论。

b. 东西方诊断程序在评估患者中的应用。

c. 用针灸技术对患者进行临床治疗。

第 R4 - 8 - 405 条　批准所需的文件

为了获得委员会对第 R4 - 8 - 404 条下针灸或者临床培训计划的批准,该计划的提供者应当向委员会提交或者让计划记录的保管人提交证明该计划符合第 R4 - 8 - 404 条标准的文件和其他证明。这些文件和其他证据可能包括目录、课程描述、课程计划和研究报告。

第 R4 - 8 - 406 条　废止

第 R4 - 8 - 407 条　计划的监控;记录;报告

A. 经批准的针灸或者临床培训计划的提供者,应当在计划财政年度结束后的六十日内向委员会提交一封信函,证明针灸或者临床培训计划继续符合第 R4 - 8 - 403 条或者第 R4 - 8 - 404 条的标准,并提交一份课程目录,包括:

1. 下一年拟议课程中的课程说明。

2. 学院计划、行政部门和管理机构的成员名单。

3. 对计划设施的描述。

B. 委员会代表可以对批准的针灸或者临床培训计划进行现场访问,以审查和评估计划的状态。经批准的计划的提供者应当补偿委员会进行审查和评估所产生的直接费用。

C. 经批准的针灸或者临床培训计划的提供者,应当确保所有的学生记录都用英文保存。

D. 经批准的针灸或者临床培训计划的提供者,应当在三十日内向委员会报告任何不符合第 R4 - 8 - 403 条或者第 R4 - 8 - 404 条标准的情况。

第 R4 - 8 - 408 条　批准继续教育

A. 只有当继续教育满足以下条件时,委员会才应当批准继续教育:

1. 与用于安全和胜任地运用针灸的知识或者技术技能相关。

2. 与直接或者间接针灸患者护理有关,包括执业管理、医学伦理或者汉语。

3. 包括继续教育参与者评估的方法:

a. 继续教育达到其既定目标的程度。

b. 教师对所教科目知识的充分性。

c. 使用适当的教学方法。

d. 所提供信息的适用性或者有用性。

4. 向继续教育参与者提供符合第 R4 - 8 - 206 条第(D)款要求的出勤证明。

B. 如果继续教育符合以下条件,委员会应当批准继续教育,无须根据第 R4 - 8 - 409 条申请:

1. 由另一个州的针灸执照委员会批准。

2. 由全国继续教育委员会提供;或者

3. 由委员会批准的针灸或者临床培训计划提供。

第 R4－8－409 条　继续教育批准申请

A. 为取得委员会对继续教育的批准,继续教育的提供者应当在教授继续教育前至少四十五日向委员会提交:

1. 可从委员会获得的表格,包含以下信息:

a. 继续教育的名称。

b. 继续教育提供者的名称和地址。

c. 继续教育提供者联系人的姓名、电话和传真号码。

d. 继续教育的日期、时间和地点。

e. 继续教育的主题。

f. 教学方法。

g. 要求的继续教育学时数。

2. 下列文件:

a. 继续教育教师的简历。

b. 继续教育的目标。

c. 继续教育的详细大纲。

d. 继续教育日程,显示教学时间和每个学时的主题。

e. 参与者评估继续教育的方法。

f. 符合第 R4－8－206 条第(D)款要求的出席证明。

B. 未经第 R4－8－408 条第(B)款批准的继续教育的提供者,不得宣传该继续教育已被委员会批准,直到委员会对根据第(A)款提交的申请做出决定。

C. 委员会对继续教育的批准在一年内有效,除非科目、教师或者教学时间有变化。在一年结束时或者当科目、教师或者教学时间有变化时,继续教育提供者应当再次申请批准。

第 R4－8－410 条　废止

第 R4－8－411 条　师承制培训标准——到期

第 R4－8－412 条　师承制培训计划督导的批准——到期

第 5 节　监督;记录保存

第 R4－8－501 条　针灸学生对患者治疗;监督

A. 在针灸导师允许针灸学生治疗患者之前,针灸导师应当:

1. 向针灸学生咨询要提供的治疗。

2. 确保针灸学生具备提供安全有效治疗所需的培训水平。

3. 确保从患者处获得《知情同意》的书面证据,表明患者知道学生将对其进行治疗。

4. 确保在针灸学生对患者进行治疗的过程中,督导人员亲自出现在诊所。

B. 如果一名针灸学生治疗一名患者,针灸导师应当确保记录保存:

1. 按照第 R4－8－502 条的要求进行维护。

2. 包括第（A）款（3）项要求的书面知情同意证明。

3. 指出针灸导师和针灸学生的姓名。

第 R4-8-502 条　保留记录

A. 针灸师应当：

1. 完整、清晰、准确地记录每位接受针灸治疗的患者。针灸师应当确保病历为英文，包括：

a. 患者姓名。

b. 病史。

c. 治疗日期。

d. 给予的治疗。

e. 针灸治疗的进展。

2. 在患者最后一次治疗后或者按照 ARS 第 12-2297 条的规定，将病历保存六年，以较晚的日期为准。

B. 针灸、耳穴针灸或者临床培训计划的提供者应当：

1. 准确完整地记录以下内容：

a. 符合第 4 条中的计划标准。

b. 参加这个计划的学生。提供者应确保学生记录表明：

i. 学生姓名。

ii. 登记日期。

iii. 选修的课程。

iv. 每门课程的成绩。

v. 计划完成或者学生停止参与的日期。

vi. 学生是否被授予文凭、学位或者结业证书。

2. 保存本条（B）款（1）（a）项要求的记录六年。

3. 将本条（B）款（1）（b）项要求的记录保留二十五年，直至学生完成或者最后一次参加该计划，或者根据 ARS 第 32-3001 条及以下要求。和私立中学后教育委员会的规则，以时间较长者为准。

C. 经批准的继续教育的提供者应当：

1. 准确完整地记录以下内容：

a. 委员会对继续教育的批准。

b. 继续教育的日期、时间和地点。

c. 每次继续教育讲座的参加者。

2. 保存第（C）款（1）项要求的记录两年。

第 R4-8-503 条　耳穴针灸医师的监督

监督耳穴针灸证书持有人的获得执照针灸师应当：

1. 在正常工作时间内，及时通过电话或者电子方式向耳穴针灸持证人咨询。

2. 确保耳穴针灸证书持有人安全有效地进行耳穴针灸治疗，并遵守耳穴针灸相关法律。

第 R4 – 8 – 504 条　重新编纂

第 R4 – 8 – 505 条　重新编纂

第 R4 – 8 – 506 条　重新编纂

第 6 节　投诉;听证程序;惩戒

第 R4 – 8 – 601 条　提出控诉

A. 包括委员会在内的所有人都可以提出控诉,声称违反了 ARS 第 32 卷第 39 章或者本章。

B. 控诉针对以下情况提出:

1. 根据 ARS 第 32 – 3921 条和本法第 R4 – 8 – 203 条获得执照的个人。

2. 根据 ARS 第 32 – 3922 条和第 R4 – 8 – 301 条认证的个人。

3. 根据 ARS 第 32 – 3926 条和第 R4 – 8 – 208 条认证的个人;或者

4. 根据 ARS 第 32 – 3921(B)条未获得豁免,且被认为在没有根据 ARS 第 32 卷第 39 章和本章颁发的执照或者证书的情况下从事针灸实践的个人。

C. 为提出控诉,个人应当以口头或者书面形式向委员会提供以下信息:

1. 日期。

2. 被申诉人的姓名、地址和电话号码。

3. 申诉人的姓名、地址和电话号码。

4. 如果申诉书是代表第三方提交的,第三方的名称和地址。

5. 与被控诉的个人或者相关企业的代表最后一次讨论控诉的日期:

a. 一份关于最后一次控诉讨论是通过电话还是当面进行的声明。

b. 最后一次讨论控诉的个人姓名。

6. 包括日期在内的事件的详细描述,这些事件被指控为违反了 ARS 第 32 卷第 39 章或者本章。

D. 申诉人应在声称构成违 ARS 第 32 卷第 39 章或者本章的事件发生后九十日内提出投诉。

E. 申诉人可随时向委员会发出通知,撤回控诉。

第 R4 – 8 – 602 条　控诉程序

A. 委员会应当审查控诉,以确定其是否符合第 R4 – 8 – 601 条的要求。如果控诉不符合第 R4 – 8 – 601 条的要求,委员会应当向控诉人提供书面通知,告知控诉被驳回,无须采取进一步行动。

B. 如果委员会确定控诉符合第 R4 – 8 – 601 条的要求,委员会应当评估控诉是否声称违反了 ARS 第 32 卷第 39 章或者本章的规定,并且:

1. 如果委员会确定指控属实,不构成违反 ARS 第 32 卷第 39 章或者本章,则驳回控诉,并向申诉人提供驳回的书面通知。

2. 如果委员会确定指控属实,则向被申诉人送达一份申诉书副本,该申诉书副本构成对 ARS 第 32 卷第 39 章或者本章的违反,并给被申诉人二十日时间提交:

a. 个人承认、否认或者进一步解释控诉中的每项指控的回应。

b. 与控诉相关的记录。

C. 如果被申诉人对申诉做出答复，委员会应当向申诉人发送一份答复副本，并给申诉人五日时间提交反驳意见。

D. 当本条第（B）款（2）项和第（C）款规定的时间到期时，委员会应当进行调查，并准备一份报告，概述控诉和调查结果。委员会应当：

1. 向申诉人和被申诉人提供调查报告的副本。

2. 向申诉人和被申诉人提供书面通知，告知将考虑控诉的委员会会议的日期、时间和地点。

E. 申诉人和被申诉人都可以由律师代表出席审议控诉的委员会会议。

F. 在考虑控诉的委员会会议上，委员会应当：

1. 向申诉人和被申诉人提供向委员会陈述、出示证据和问询证人的机会。

2. 通过公平谈判、公正地解决控诉中提出的问题。

3. 将控诉提交正式听证会。

第 R4－8－603 条　听证程序

委员会应根据 ARS 第 41 卷第 6 章第 10 节规定的程序举行法律要求的听证会。

第 R4－8－604 条　重新听证或者审查决定

A. 委员会应当根据 ARS 第 41 卷第 6 章第 10 节的规定，对其决定进行重新听证和审查。

B. 除本条第（I）款另有规定的情况外，一方当事人必须提出动议，要求重新听证或者审查委员会的决定，以用尽该方当事人的行政救济。

C. 在仲裁委员会对动议做出裁决之前，任何一方均可随时修改动议，要求重新听证或者审核。

D. 委员会可以因以下任何一种对一方权利有重大影响的原因而批准重新听证或者审查：

1. 委员会的程序不规范或任何命令或滥用酌处权剥夺了提出动议的当事方获得公平听证的机会。

2. 委员会、其工作人员或者行政法法官的不端行为。

3. 事故或者意外是普通谨慎无法避免的。

4. 新发现的重要证据，即使尽了合理的努力也无法在听证会上发现和出示。

5. 处罚过重或者不足。

6. 在审理过程中或者诉讼过程中出现的证据采信或者拒绝采信错误或者其他法律错误。

7. 事实的裁决或者决定没有证据证明是正当的，或者违反法律。

E. 委员会可以出于本条第（D）款所列的理由，确认或者修改一项决定，准许所有或者部分当事方就全部或者部分问题进行重审或者复审。修改决定或者准予重新听证或者审查的命令应具体说明命令的理由。如果批准重新听证或者审查，则重新听证或者审查应仅涵盖命令中规定的事项。

F. 在作出决定之日起三十日内,在通知当事各方并有机会陈述意见之后,委员会可以主动下令重新听证或者审查其决定,理由是它可能已准许对一方当事人的动议进行重新听证或者审查。委员会可以及时批准重新听证或者审查动议,理由无须在动议中说明。准予重新听证或者审查的命令应具体说明理由。

G. 当要求重新听证的动议是基于书面陈述时,书面陈述应与动议一起送达。对方当事人可在送达后十五日内送达反对宣誓书。根据第(H)款所述的正当理由或者双方的书面规定,委员会可将该期限最多延长二十日。答辩宣誓书可能是允许的。

H. 在有正当理由的情况下,委员会可以延长本节中列出的所有时限。一方有正当理由证明,该方的动议或者其他行动的依据无法通过适当勤勉及时获知,并且对该动议的裁决将做如下处理:

1. 进一步提供行政便利、快捷或者经济性。

2. 避免对任何一方造成不当损害。

I. 如果在特定决定中,委员会作出具体裁定,认为该决定的立即生效对于维护公众健康、安全或者福利是必要的,并且对该决定的重新听证或者审查是不切实际的、不必要的或者违背公共利益的,则该决定可以作为最终决定发布,而没有机会进行重新听证或者审查。如果对决定提出司法审查申请,则应当根据 ARS 第 12‑901 条及其后各项规定提出。

第 R4‑8‑605 条　纪律处分

在审议控诉的委员会会议或者听证会确定被许可人或者证书持有人违反了 ARS 第 39 卷第 32 章或者本章之后,委员会应当考虑以下因素,以确定根据 ARS 第 32‑3951 条施加的纪律处分程度:

1. 导致纪律处分的先前行为。

2. 不诚实或者自私的动机。

3. 作为经验丰富的针灸师。

4. 故意不遵守委员会的规则或者命令,恶意阻挠纪律处分程序。

5. 在调查或者纪律处分过程中提交虚假证据、虚假陈述或者其他欺骗行为。

6. 拒绝承认行为的错误性质。

7. 行为造成的损害程度。

8. 行为造成的损害是否得到了补救。

第7节　公众参与程序

第 R4‑8‑701 条　到期

第 R4‑8‑702 条　规则制定呈请书;审查机构惯例或者实质性政策声明;对基于经济、小型企业或者消费者影响的规则的异议

A. 个人可以根据 ARS 第 41‑1033 条向委员会申请:

1. 与委员会规则相关的规则制定行动,包括制定新规则或者修订或者废除现有规则;或者

2. 对声称构成规则的现有委员会惯例或者实质性政策声明的审查。

B. 个人可以根据 ARS 第 41‑1056.01 条向委员会申请,反对全部或者部分委员会规则,因为该规则的实际经济、小企业或者消费者影响:

1. 超出该规则对经济、小型企业或者消费者的预期影响;或者

2. 未作预估,给受该规则约束的人带来沉重负担。

C. 根据 ARS 第 41‑1033 条或者第 41‑1056.01 条和本条的规定,个人应当向委员会提交一份书面申请,包括以下信息:

1. 呈请人的姓名、住所或者营业地址、电子邮件地址、电话和传真号码。

2. 呈请人所代表的姓名。

3. 如果请求规则制定行动:

a. 所寻求的规则制定行动的声明,包括《亚利桑那州行政法典》(A.A.C.)对所有现有规则的引用,以及新规则或者规则修正案的具体语言。

b. 规则制定行动的原因,包括解释为什么现有规则不充分、不合理、过于繁琐或者不合法。

4. 如果请求审查现有的委员会惯例或者实质性政策声明:

a. 现有惯例或者实质性政策声明的主题。

b. 现有惯例或者实质性政策声明构成规则的原因。

5. 如果反对该规则是因为其对经济、小型企业和消费者影响声明:

a. 被提出异议的规则的 A.A.C.。

b. 描述该规则对经济、小型企业或者消费者的实际影响如何不同于估计的影响;或者

c. 说明该规则对经济、小企业或者消费者的实际影响,并评估受该规则约束的人所承受的负担。

6. 呈请人签名日期。

D. 个人可以在呈请书中提交支持信息。

第 R4‑8‑703 条　到期

第 R4‑8‑704 条　口头程序

A. 如 ARS 第 41‑1023 条第(C)款所述,请求口头诉讼的人应当:

1. 向委员会提出申请。

2. 包括提出请求者的姓名和当前地址。

3. 请参阅拟议规则,并包括(如果已知)发布拟议规则通知的亚利桑那州行政登记簿的日期和问题。

B. 委员会应当记录口头程序。委员会应当将口头诉讼期间提交的任何材料作为正式规则制定记录的一部分。

C. 审裁官应当遵循下列准则进行口头程序:

1. 与会者登记。与会者的登记是自愿的。

2. 有意发言人士的登记。希望发言的人应当在委员会提供的表格上提供以下信息:

a. 姓名。

b. 代表身份(如果适用)。

c. 该人是支持还是反对拟议规则。

d. 此人希望发言的大致时间。

3. 记录开始。审裁官应当在会议开始时确定所要审议的规则以及会议的地点、日期、时间和目的,并提出议程。

4. 一份委员会代表的声明。委员会代表应当解释拟议规则的背景和一般内容。

5. 公众口头意见征询期。任何人均可以在口头诉讼中发言。发言人应当就拟议规则发言。发言人可以就拟议规则提出问题,并就拟议规则提出口头论点、数据和观点。审裁官可限制分配给每个发言人的时间,避免不必要的重复。

6. 结束语。审裁官应当宣布就拟议规则提交书面意见的地点和截止日期。

第 R4-8-705 条　到期

第 R4-8-706 条　对规则的书面批评

A. 个人可以向委员会提交对现有规则的书面批评。

B. 对规章提出书面批评的人应当根据行政法规的引用来确定该规章,并说明为什么该规章是不充分的、不适当的、不合理的。

C. 委员会应当在十五日内确认收到批评意见,并将批评意见记录在正式记录中,以供委员会根据 ARS 第 41-1056 条进行审查。

WEST'S ALASKA

WEST'S ALASKA STATUTES ANNOTATED

§ 08.06.010. Practice of acupuncture without license prohibited

A person may not practice acupuncture without a license.

§ 08.06.020. Application for license

A person desiring to practice acupuncture shall apply in writing to the department.

§ 08.06.030. License to practice acupuncture

(a) A person is qualified to receive a license to practice acupuncture if the person

(1) is of good moral character;

(2) is at least 21 years of age;

(3) either

(A) has completed a course of study consistent with the core curriculum and guidelines of the Accreditation Commission for Acupuncture and Oriental Medicine at a school of acupuncture approved by the department; or

(B) is licensed to practice acupuncture in another jurisdiction that has acupuncture licensing requirements equivalent to those of this state;

(4) is qualified for certification by the National Certification Commission for Acupuncture and Oriental Medicine as a diplomate in acupuncture;

(5) does not have a disciplinary proceeding or unresolved complaint pending at the time of application; and

(6) has not had a license to practice acupuncture suspended or revoked in this state or in another jurisdiction.

(b) The department shall issue a license to practice acupuncture to each person who is qualified and who pays the appropriate fee.

(c) Each person licensed to practice acupuncture under this chapter shall display the license in a conspicuous place where the licensee practices.

§ 08.06.040. Renewal of license

The department may not renew a license under this chapter unless the applicant demonstrates continued competence as an acupuncturist in a manner established by the department in regulations.

§ 08.06.050. Disclosure

(a) A person who practices acupuncture shall disclose that the person's training and practice are in acupuncture

(1) to each patient; and

(2) on all material used in the practice of acupuncture and made available to patients or to the public.

(b) A person who practices acupuncture without being covered by malpractice insurance shall disclose to each patient that the person does not have the insurance.

§ 08.06.060. Restrictions on practice of acupuncture

A person who practices acupuncture may not

(1) give, prescribe, or recommend in the practice a

(A) prescription drug;

(B) controlled substance;

(C) poison;

(2) engage in surgery; or

(3) use the word "physician" in the person's title unless the person is also licensed as a physician.

§ 08.06.070. Grounds for imposition of disciplinary sanctions

After a hearing, the department may impose a disciplinary sanction on a person licensed under this chapter when the department finds that the licensee

(1) secured a license through deceit, fraud, or intentional misrepresentation;

(2) engaged in deceit, fraud, or intentional misrepresentation in the course of providing professional services or engaging in professional activities;

(3) advertised professional services in a false or misleading manner;

(4) has been convicted of a felony or other crime that affects the licensee's ability to continue to practice competently and safely;

(5) intentionally or negligently engaged in patient care, or permitted the performance of patient care by persons under the licensee's supervision, that does not conform to minimum professional standards regardless of whether actual injury to the patient occurred;

(6) failed to comply with this chapter, with a regulation adopted under this chapter, or with an order of the department;

(7) continued to practice after becoming unfit due to

(A) professional incompetence;

(B) failure to keep informed of current professional practices;

(C) addiction to or severe dependency on alcohol or other drugs that impairs the ability to practice safely;

(D) physical or mental disability; or

(8) engaged in lewd or immoral conduct in connection with the delivery of professional service to patients.

§ 08.06.080. Exemption

This chapter does not apply to a person who practices acupuncture under AS 08.36 or AS 08.64.

§ 08.06.090. Penalty

A person who violates this chapter or a regulation adopted under this chapter is guilty of a class B misdemeanor.

§ 08.06.100. Regulations

The department may adopt regulations to implement this chapter, including regulations establishing

(1) standards for the practice of acupuncture;

(2) standards for continuing education and training;

(3) a code of ethics for the practice of acupuncture.

§ 08.06.190. Definitions

In this chapter,

(1) "acupuncture" means a form of healing developed from traditional Chinese medical concepts that uses the stimulation of certain points on or near the surface of the body by the insertion of needles to prevent or modify the perception of pain or to normalize physiological functions;

(2) "department" means the Department of Commerce, Community, and Economic Development;

(3) "practice of acupuncture" means the insertion of sterile acupuncture needles and the application of moxibustion to specific areas of the human body based upon acupuncture diagnosis; the practice of acupuncture includes adjunctive therapies involving mechanical, thermal, electrical, and electromagnetic treatment and the recommendation of dietary guidelines and therapeutic exercise.

ALASKA ADMINISTRATIVE CODE

Article 1. Licensing

12 AAC 05.100. Application requirements.

(a) An applicant for a license to practice acupuncture shall apply on a form provided by the department and pay the applicable fees in 12 AAC 02.108.

(b) An applicant for a license to practice acupuncture shall document compliance with the requirements in AS 08.06.030(a) by submitting.

(1) two letters of reference attesting to the applicant's good moral character;

(2) if applicable, a certified copy of a transcript from an approved school of acupuncture verifying the applicant's course of study;

(3) official verification of a license sent directly to the department from each jurisdiction where the applicant holds or has ever held a license to practice acupuncture; the verification must include information on any disciplinary proceedings or unresolved complaints against the applicant;

(4) a certified copy of the applicant's diplomate of acupuncture certificate issued by the National Certification Commission for Acupuncture and Oriental Medicine (NCCAOM) or a letter from the NCCAOM verifying that the applicant is qualified for a diplomate of acupuncture certificate.

12 AAC 05.110. Approved school of acupuncture.

To be approved by the department, a school of acupuncture must be recognized by the Council of Colleges of Acupuncture and Oriental Medicine (CCAOM) or the Accreditation Commission for Acupuncture and Oriental Medicine (ACAOM).

Article 2. License Renewal and Continuing Competency

12 AAC 05.200. License renewal.

(a) A license to practice acupuncture expires on September 30 of even-numbered years.

(b) A licensee applying for license renewal shall

(1) complete a renewal application on a form provided by the department;

(2) pay the license renewal fee established in 12 AAC 02.108;

(3) repealed 12/25/2019;

(4) submit a sworn statement of contact hours of continuing competency activities completed during the concluding licensing period, if required by 12 AAC 05.210.

12 AAC 05.210. Continuing competency requirements.

(a) An applicant for renewal of a license to practice acupuncture shall document completion of one of the following:

(1) certification as a diplomate in acupuncture by the NCCAOM during the entire concluding licensing period; or

(2) 15 Professional Development Activity points earned solely in core competency activities in acupuncture as defined by the NCCAOM during the concluding licensing period.

(b) An applicant for renewal of a license to practice acupuncture who has been licensed less than 12 months is exempt from the requirements of this section.

（c）Repealed 12/25/2019.

12 AAC 05.220. Approved continuing competency activities.

To be accepted by the department, continuing competency activities under 12 AAC 05.210 (a)(2) must be designated a Core Competency Professional Development Activity in acupuncture by the National Certification Commission for Acupuncture and Oriental Medicine (NCCAOM).

12 AAC 05.230. Audit of continuing competency requirements.

（a）The department will audit renewal applications in accordance with 12 AAC 02.960, to monitor compliance with the continuing competency requirements of 12 AAC 05.210 and 12 AAC 05.220.

Article 3. Practice Standards

12 AAC 05.300. Disclosure.

（a）A licensee shall disclose to each patient that the licensee's training and practice is in acupuncture by posting a conspicuous notice in the patient waiting room and including the disclosure on all written material made available to patients or the public.

（b）A licensee who is not covered by malpractice insurance shall

（1）post a conspicuous notice in the patient waiting room that states the licensee does not have malpractice insurance; or

（2）require each patient or the patient's legal guardian to sign a statement acknowledging that the patient or the patient's guardian has been informed that the licensee is not covered by malpractice insurance.

（c）If the licensee has a patient who is blind or otherwise not able to read the written disclosure required by this section, the licensee shall

（1）verbally disclose to the patient or the patient's legal guardian at the initial visit that the licensee's training and practice is in acupuncture; and

（2）if the licensee is not covered by malpractice insurance, verbally disclose that fact to the patient or the patient's legal guardian at the initial visit and at least once each year that the patient receives care from the licensee.

Article 4. General Provisions

12 AAC 05.990. Definitions.

In this chapter and in AS 08.06, unless the context otherwise requires,

（1）"department" means the Department of Commerce, Community, and Economic Development;

（2）"NCCAOM" means the National Certification Commission For Acupuncture and Oriental Medicine.

（3）repealed 12/25/2019.

OKLAHOMA

OKLAHOMA ADMINISTRATIVE CODE

140: 15 - 10 - 1.　Registration from the Board

No chiropractic physician shall represent to the public that he/she is a specialist in the practice of Acupuncture and/or Meridian Therapy unless said chiropractic physician holds a registration issued by the Board stating that the chiropractic physician is proficient in Acupuncture and/or Meridian Therapy. The Board shall maintain a registry listing all chiropractic physicians who are authorized by the Board. This rule does not apply to chiropractic physicians licensed to practice chiropractic in Oklahoma who graduated from a chiropractic institution on or before January 1, 2000.

140: 15 - 10 - 2.　Application for registration; educational requirements

(a) Any chiropractic physician who desires to represent to the public he/she is a specialist in Acupuncture and/or Meridian Therapy shall make application, on a form prescribed by the Board, for registration for such purpose. Each such chiropractic physician shall submit to the Board documentary evidence of satisfactory completion of at least one hundred (100) hours of education in Acupuncture and/or Meridian Therapy. Such education shall be obtained through an educational program which is subject to or has been approved by the Board and meets the following criteria:

(1) Is conducted under the auspices of and taught by the postgraduate faculty of a fully accredited chiropractic college or institution, by a school of acupuncture recognized by the National Council of Acupuncture Schools and Colleges or by a school of acupuncture recognized by the Accreditation Commission for Acupuncture and Oriental Medicine.

(2) Requires completion of a certification examination approved by the Board; and

(3) Meets other such criteria as the Board deems appropriate.

(b) Upon successful demonstration of these requirements, the Board shall list the chiropractic physician's name on the registry.

VERNON'S TEXAS

VERNON'S TEXAS STATUTES AND CODES ANNOTATED

Subchapter A.   General Provisions

§ 205.001.   Definitions

In this chapter:

(1) "Acudetox specialist" means a person certified under Section 205.303.

(2) "Acupuncture" means:

(A) the nonsurgical, nonincisive insertion of an acupuncture needle and the application of moxibustion to specific areas of the human body as a primary mode of therapy to treat and mitigate a human condition, including evaluation and assessment of the condition; and

(B) the administration of thermal or electrical treatments or the recommendation of dietary guidelines, energy flow exercise, or dietary or herbal supplements in conjunction with the treatment described by Paragraph (A).

(3) "Acupuncture board" means the Texas State Board of Acupuncture Examiners.

(4) "Acupuncturist" means a person who:

(A) practices acupuncture; and

(B) directly or indirectly charges a fee for the performance of acupuncture services.

(5) "Chiropractor" means a person licensed to practice chiropractic by the Texas Board of Chiropractic Examiners.

(6) "Executive director" means the executive director of the Texas Medical Board.

(7) "Medical board" means the Texas Medical Board.

(8) "Physician" means a person licensed to practice medicine by the Texas Medical Board.

§ 205.002.   Repealed by Acts 2005, 79th Leg., ch. 269, § 3.35, eff. Sept. 1, 2005

§ 205.003.   Exemption; Limitation

(a) This chapter does not apply to a health care professional licensed under another statute of this state and acting within the scope of the license.

(b) This chapter does not:

(1) limit the practice of medicine by a physician;

(2) permit the unauthorized practice of medicine; or

(3) permit a person to dispense, administer, or supply a controlled substance, narcotic, or dangerous drug unless the person is authorized by other law to do so.

Subchapter B.   Texas State Board of Acupuncture Examiners

§ 205.051.   Board; Membership

(a) The Texas State Board of Acupuncture Examiners consists of nine members appointed by the governor with the advice and consent of the senate as follows:

(1) four acupuncturist members who have at least five years of experience in the practice of acupuncture in this state and who are not physicians;

(2) two physician members experienced in the practice of acupuncture; and

(3) three members of the general public who are not licensed or trained in a health care profession.

(b) Appointments to the acupuncture board shall be made without regard to the race, color, disability, sex, religion, age, or national origin of the appointee.

§ 205.052.   Public Member Eligibility

A person is not eligible for appointment as a public member of the acupuncture board if the person or the person's spouse:

(1) is registered, certified, or licensed by an occupational regulatory agency in the field of health care;

(2) is employed by or participates in the management of a business entity or other organization regulated by the medical board or receiving funds from the medical board or acupuncture board;

(3) owns or controls, directly or indirectly, more than a 10 percent interest in a business entity or other organization regulated by the medical board or acupuncture board or receiving funds from the medical board;

(4) uses or receives a substantial amount of tangible goods, services, or funds from the medical board or acupuncture board, other than compensation or reimbursement authorized by law for acupuncture board membership, attendance, or expenses; or

(5) owns, operates, or has a financial interest in a school of acupuncture.

§ 205.053. Membership and Employee Restrictions

(a) In this section, "Texas trade association" means a cooperative and voluntarily joined statewide association of business or professional competitors in this state designed to assist its members and its industry or profession in dealing with mutual business or professional problems and in promoting their common interest.

(b) An officer, board member, employee, or paid consultant of a Texas trade association in the field of health care may not be a member of the acupuncture board or an employee of the medical board who is exempt from the state's position classification plan or is compensated at or above the amount prescribed by the General Appropriations Act for step 1, salary group A17, of the position classification salary schedule.

(c) A person may not be a member of the acupuncture board and may not be a medical board employee in a "bona fide executive, administrative, or professional capacity," as that phrase is used for purposes of establishing an exemption to the overtime provisions of the federal Fair Labor Standards Act of 1938 (29 U.S.C. Section 201 et seq.), if:

(1) the person is an officer, employee, or paid consultant of a Texas trade association in the field of health care; or

(2) the person's spouse is an officer, manager, or paid consultant of a Texas trade association in the field of health care.

(d) A person may not be a member of the acupuncture board or act as general counsel to the acupuncture board or the medical board if the person is required to register as a lobbyist under Chapter 305, Government Code, because of the person's activities for compensation on behalf of a profession related to the operation of the medical board or acupuncture board.

(e) A person may not serve on the acupuncture board if the person owns, operates, or has a financial interest in a school of acupuncture

§ 205.054. Terms; Vacancies

(a) Members of the acupuncture board serve staggered six-year terms. The terms of three members expire on January 31 of each odd-numbered year.

(b) A vacancy on the acupuncture board shall be filled by appointment of the governor.

§ 205.055. Presiding Officer

The governor shall designate an acupuncturist member of the acupuncture board as presiding officer. The presiding officer serves in that capacity at the will of the governor.

§ 205.056. Grounds for Removal

(a) It is a ground for removal from the acupuncture board that a member:

(1) does not have at the time of appointment the qualifications required by Sections 205.051 and 205.052;

(2) does not maintain during service on the acupuncture board the qualifications required by Sections 205.051 and 205.052;

(3) violates a prohibition established by Section 205.053;

(4) cannot, because of illness or disability, discharge the member's duties for a substantial part of the member's term; or

(5) is absent from more than half of the regularly scheduled acupuncture board meetings that the member is eligible to attend during a calendar year.

(b) The validity of an action of the acupuncture board is not affected by the fact that it is taken when a ground for removal of an acupuncture board member exists.

(c) If the executive director has knowledge that a potential ground for removal of an acupuncture board member exists, the executive director shall notify the presiding officer of the acupuncture board of the potential ground. The presiding officer shall then notify the governor and the attorney general that a potential ground for removal exists. If the potential ground for removal involves the presiding officer, the executive director shall notify the next highest officer of the acupuncture board, who shall notify the governor and the attorney general that a potential ground for removal exists.

§ 205.057.   Training

(a) A person who is appointed to and qualifies for office as a member of the acupuncture board may not vote, deliberate, or be counted as a member in attendance at a meeting of the acupuncture board until the person completes a training program that complies with this section.

(b) The training program must provide the person with information regarding:

(1) the law governing acupuncture board operations;

(2) the programs, functions, rules, and budget of the acupuncture board;

(3) the scope of and limitations on the rulemaking authority of the acupuncture board;

(4) the types of acupuncture board rules, interpretations, and enforcement actions that may implicate federal antitrust law by limiting competition or impacting prices charged by persons engaged in a profession or business the acupuncture board regulates, including any rule, interpretation, or enforcement action that:

(A) regulates the scope of practice of persons in a profession or business the acupuncture board regulates;

(B) restricts advertising by persons in a profession or business the acupuncture board regulates;

(C) affects the price of goods or services provided by persons in a profession or business the acupuncture board regulates; or

(D) restricts participation in a profession or business the acupuncture board regulates;

(5) the results of the most recent formal audit of the acupuncture board;

(6) the requirements of:

(A) laws relating to open meetings, public information, administrative procedure, and disclosure of conflicts of interest; and

(B) other laws applicable to members of the acupuncture board in performing their duties; and

(7) any applicable ethics policies adopted by the acupuncture board or the Texas Ethics Commission.

(c) A person appointed to the acupuncture board is entitled to reimbursement, as provided by the General Appropriations Act, for the travel expenses incurred in attending the training program regardless of whether the attendance at the program occurs before or after the person qualifies for office.

(d) The executive director shall create a training manual that includes the information required by Subsection (b). The executive director shall distribute a copy of the training manual annually to each acupuncture board member. Each board member shall sign and submit to the executive director a statement acknowledging that the member received and has reviewed the training manual.

§ 205.058. Qualifications and Standards of Conduct Information

The executive director or the executive director's designee shall provide, as often as necessary, to members of the acupuncture board information regarding their:

(1) qualifications for office under this chapter; and

(2) responsibilities under applicable laws relating to standards of conduct for state officers.

§ 205.059. Compensation; Per Diem

An acupuncture board member may not receive compensation for service on the acupuncture board but is entitled to receive a per diem as set by legislative appropriation for transportation and related expenses incurred for each day that the member engages in the acupuncture board's business.

§ 205.060. Application of Open Meetings, Open Records, and Administrative Procedure Laws

Except as provided by this chapter, the acupuncture board is subject to Chapters 551, 552, and 2001, Government Code.

Subchapter C. Powers and Duties of Acupuncture Board and Medical Board

§ 205.101. General Powers and Duties of Acupuncture Board

(a) Subject to the advice and approval of the medical board, the acupuncture board shall:

(1) establish qualifications for an acupuncturist to practice in this state;

(2) establish minimum education and training requirements necessary for the acupuncture board to recommend that the medical board issue a license to practice acupuncture;

(3) administer an examination that is validated by independent testing professionals for a license to practice acupuncture;

(4) develop requirements for licensure by endorsement of other states;

(5) prescribe the application form for a license to practice acupuncture;

(6) recommend rules to establish licensing and other fees;

(7) establish the requirements for a tutorial program for acupuncture students who have completed at least 48 semester hours of college; and

(8) recommend additional rules as are necessary to administer and enforce this chapter.

(b) The acupuncture board does not have independent rulemaking authority. A rule adopted by the acupuncture board is subject to medical board approval.

(c) The acupuncture board shall:

(1) review and approve or reject each application for the issuance or renewal of a license;

(2) issue each license; and

(3) deny, suspend, or revoke a license or otherwise discipline a license holder.

§ 205.102. Assistance by Medical Board

(a) The medical board shall provide administrative and clerical employees as necessary to enable the acupuncture board to administer this chapter.

(b) Subject to the advice and approval of the medical board, the acupuncture board shall develop and implement policies that clearly separate the policy-making responsibilities of the acupuncture board and the management responsibilities of the executive director and the staff of the medical board.

§ 205.103. Fees

The medical board shall set and collect fees in amounts that are reasonable and necessary to cover the costs of administering and enforcing this chapter without the use of any other funds generated by the medical board.

§ 205.104. Rules Restricting Advertising or Competitive Bidding

(a) The medical board may not adopt rules under this chapter restricting advertising or competitive bidding by a license holder except to prohibit false, misleading, or deceptive practices.

(b) In its rules to prohibit false, misleading, or deceptive practices, the medical board may not include a rule that:

(1) restricts the use of any medium for advertising;

(2) restricts the use of a license holder's personal appearance or voice in an advertisement;

(3) relates to the size or duration of an advertisement by the license holder; or

(4) restricts the license holder's advertisement under a trade name.

§ 205.1041. Guidelines for Early Involvement in Rulemaking Process

(a) The acupuncture board shall develop guidelines to establish procedures for receiving input during the rulemaking process from individuals and groups that have an interest in matters under the acupuncture board's jurisdiction. The guidelines must provide an opportunity for those individuals and groups to provide input before the acupuncture board submits the rule to the medical board for approval.

(b) A rule adopted by the acupuncture board may not be challenged on the grounds that the board did not comply with this section. If the acupuncture board was unable to solicit a significant amount of input from the public or affected persons early in the rulemaking process, the board shall state in writing the reasons why the board was unable to do so.

§ 205.1045. Rules on Consequences of Criminal Conviction

The acupuncture board shall adopt rules and guidelines as necessary to comply with Chapter 53, except to the extent the requirements of this chapter are stricter than the requirements of Chapter 53.

§ 205.105. Repealed by Acts 2011, 82nd Leg., ch. 1083 (S.B. 1179), § 25(139), eff. June 17, 2011

§ 205.106. Use of Technology

Subject to the advice and approval of the medical board, the acupuncture board shall implement a policy requiring the acupuncture board to use appropriate technological solutions to improve the acupuncture board's ability to perform its functions. The policy must ensure that the public is able to interact with the acupuncture board on the Internet.

§ 205.107. Negotiated Rulemaking and Alternative Dispute Resolution Policy

(a) Subject to the advice and approval of the medical board, the acupuncture board shall develop and implement a policy to encourage the use of:

(1) negotiated rulemaking procedures under Chapter 2008, Government Code, for the adoption of acupuncture board rules; and

(2) appropriate alternative dispute resolution procedures under Chapter 2009, Government Code, to assist in the resolution of internal and external disputes under the acupuncture board's jurisdiction.

(b) The acupuncture board procedures relating to alternative dispute resolution must conform, to the extent possible, to any model guidelines issued by the State Office of Administrative Hearings for the use of alternative dispute resolution by state agencies.

(c) The acupuncture board shall designate a trained person to:

(1) coordinate the implementation of the policy adopted under Subsection (a);

(2) serve as a resource for any training needed to implement the procedures for negotiated rulemaking or alternative dispute resolution; and

(3) collect data concerning the effectiveness of those procedures, as implemented by the acupuncture board.

Subchapter D. Public Access and Information and Complaint Procedures

§ 205.151. Public Interest Information

(a) The acupuncture board shall prepare information of public interest describing the functions of the acupuncture board and the procedures by which complaints are filed with and resolved by the acupuncture board.

(b) The acupuncture board shall make the information available to the public and appropriate state agencies.

§ 205.152. Complaints

(a) The acupuncture board by rule shall establish methods by which consumers and service recipients are notified of the name, mailing address, and telephone number of the acupuncture board for the purpose of directing a complaint to the acupuncture board. The acupuncture board may provide for that notification:

(1) on each registration form, application, or written contract for services of a person regulated under this chapter;

(2) on a sign prominently displayed in the place of business of each person regulated under this chapter; or

(3) in a bill for service provided by a person regulated under this chapter.

(b) The acupuncture board shall keep information about each complaint filed with the acupuncture board. The information shall include:

(1) the date the complaint is received;

(2) the name of the complainant;

(3) the subject matter of the complaint;

(4) a record of all persons contacted in relation to the complaint;

(5) a summary of the results of the review or investigation of the complaint; and

(6) for a complaint for which the acupuncture board took no action, an explanation of the reason the complaint was closed without action.

(c) The acupuncture board shall keep a file about each written complaint filed with the acupuncture board that the acupuncture board has authority to resolve. The acupuncture board shall provide to the person filing the complaint and each person who is the subject of the complaint the acupuncture board's policies and procedures pertaining to complaint investigation and resolution.

(d) The acupuncture board, at least quarterly and until final disposition of the complaint, shall notify the person filing the complaint and each person who is the subject of the complaint of the status of the complaint unless the notice would jeopardize an investigation.

§ 205.1521. Conduct of Investigation

The acupuncture board shall complete a preliminary investigation of a complaint received by the acupuncture board not later than the 30th day after the date of receiving the complaint. The acupuncture board shall first determine whether the acupuncturist constitutes a continuing threat to the public welfare. On completion of the preliminary investigation, the acupuncture board shall determine whether to officially proceed on the complaint. If the acupuncture board fails to complete the preliminary investigation in the time required by this section, the acupuncture board's official investigation of the complaint is considered to commence on that date.

§ 205.153.   Public Participation

(a) Subject to the advice and approval of the medical board, the acupuncture board shall develop and implement policies that provide the public with a reasonable opportunity to appear before the acupuncture board and to speak on any issue under the acupuncture board's jurisdiction.

(b) The executive director shall prepare and maintain a written plan that describes how a person who does not speak English may be provided reasonable access to the acupuncture board's programs and services.

Subchapter E.   License Requirements

§ 205.201.   License Required

Except as provided by Section 205.303, a person may not practice acupuncture in this state unless the person holds a license to practice acupuncture issued by the acupuncture board under this chapter.

§ 205.202.   Issuance of License

(a) The acupuncture board shall issue a license to practice acupuncture in this state to a person who meets the requirements of this chapter and the rules adopted under this chapter.

(b) The acupuncture board may delegate authority to medical board employees to issue licenses under this chapter to applicants who clearly meet all licensing requirements. If the medical board employees determine that the applicant does not clearly meet all licensing requirements, the application shall be returned to the acupuncture board. A license issued under this subsection does not require formal acupuncture board approval.

§ 205.2025.   Criminal History Record Information Requirement for License Issuance

(a) The acupuncture board shall require that an applicant for a license submit a complete and legible set of fingerprints, on a form prescribed by the board, to the board or to the Department of Public Safety for the purpose of obtaining criminal history record information from the Department of Public Safety and the Federal Bureau of Investigation.

(b) The acupuncture board may not issue a license to a person who does not comply with the requirement of Subsection (a).

(c) The acupuncture board shall conduct a criminal history record information check of each applicant for a license using information:

(1) provided by the individual under this section; and

(2) made available to the board by the Department of Public Safety, the Federal Bureau of Investigation, and any other criminal justice agency under Chapter 411, Government Code.

(d) The acupuncture board may:

(1) enter into an agreement with the Department of Public Safety to administer a criminal

history record information check required under this section; and

(2) authorize the Department of Public Safety to collect from each applicant the costs incurred by the Department of Public Safety in conducting the criminal history record information check.

§ 205.203.   License Examination

(a) An applicant for a license to practice acupuncture must pass an acupuncture examination and a jurisprudence examination approved by the acupuncture board as provided by this section.

(b) To be eligible for the examination, an applicant must:

(1) be at least 21 years of age;

(2) have completed at least 60 semester hours of college courses, including basic science courses as determined by the acupuncture board; and

(3) be a graduate of an acupuncture school with entrance requirements and a course of instruction that meet standards set under Section 205.206.

(c) The acupuncture examination shall be conducted on practical and theoretical acupuncture and other subjects required by the acupuncture board.

(c - 1) The jurisprudence examination shall be conducted on the licensing requirements and other laws, rules, or regulations applicable to the professional practice of acupuncture in this state.

(d) The examination may be in writing, by a practical demonstration of the applicant's skill, or both, as required by the acupuncture board.

(e) The medical board shall notify each applicant of the time and place of the examination.

(f) The acupuncture board shall adopt rules for the jurisprudence examination under Subsection (c - 1) regarding:

(1) the development of the examination;

(2) applicable fees;

(3) administration of the examination;

(4) reexamination procedures;

(5) grading procedures; and

(6) notice of results.

§ 205.204.   Application for Examination

An application for examination must be:

(1) in writing on a form prescribed by the acupuncture board;

(2) verified by affidavit;

(3) filed with the executive director; and

(4) accompanied by a fee in an amount set by the medical board.

§ 205.2045.   Appearance of Applicant Before Acupuncture Board

An applicant for a license to practice acupuncture may not be required to appear before the acupuncture board or a committee of the acupuncture board unless the application raises questions concerning:

（1）a physical or mental impairment of the applicant;

（2）a criminal conviction of the applicant; or

（3）revocation of a professional license held by the applicant.

§ 205.205.　Examination Results

（a）Not later than the 30th day after the date a licensing examination is administered under this chapter, the acupuncture board shall notify each examinee of the results of the examination. If an examination is graded or reviewed by a national testing service, the acupuncture board shall notify examinees of the results of the examination not later than the 14th day after the date the acupuncture board receives the results from the testing service.

（b）If the notice of examination results graded or reviewed by a national testing service will be delayed for longer than 90 days after the examination date, the acupuncture board shall notify the examinee of the reason for the delay before the 90th day. The acupuncture board may require a testing service to notify examinees of the results of an examination.

（c）If requested in writing by a person who fails a licensing examination administered under this chapter, the acupuncture board shall furnish the person with an analysis of the person's performance on the examination if an analysis is available from the national testing service.

§ 205.206.　Acupuncture Schools

（a）A reputable acupuncture school, in addition to meeting standards set by the acupuncture board, must:

（1）maintain a resident course of instruction equivalent to not less than six terms of four months each for a total of not less than 1,800 instructional hours;

（2）provide supervised patient treatment for at least two terms of the resident course of instruction;

（3）maintain a course of instruction in anatomy-histology, bacteriology, physiology, symptomatology, pathology, meridian and point locations, hygiene, and public health; and

（4）have the necessary teaching force and facilities for proper instruction in required subjects.

（b）In establishing standards for the entrance requirements and course of instruction of an acupuncture school, the acupuncture board may consider the standards set by the National Accreditation Commission for Schools and Colleges of Acupuncture and Oriental Medicine.

（c）In addition to the other requirements of this section, an acupuncture school or degree program is subject to approval by the Texas Higher Education Coordinating Board unless the school or program qualifies for an exemption under Section 61.303, Education Code.

（d）In reviewing an acupuncture school or degree program as required by Subsection（c）， the Texas Higher Education Coordinating Board shall seek input from the acupuncture board regarding the standards to be used for assessing whether a school or degree program adequately prepares an individual for the practice of acupuncture.

§ 205.207. Reciprocal License

The medical board may waive any license requirement for an applicant after reviewing the applicant's credentials and determining that the applicant holds a license from another state that has license requirements substantially equivalent to those of this state.

§ 205.208. Temporary License

(a) The acupuncture board may, through the executive director, issue a temporary license to practice acupuncture to an applicant who:

(1) submits an application on a form prescribed by the acupuncture board;

(2) has passed a national or other examination recognized by the acupuncture board relating to the practice of acupuncture;

(3) pays the appropriate fee;

(4) if licensed in another state, is in good standing as an acupuncturist; and

(5) meets all the qualifications for a license under this chapter but is waiting for the next scheduled meeting of the medical board for the license to be issued.

(b) A temporary license is valid for 100 days after the date issued and may be extended only for another 30 days after the date the initial temporary license expires.

Subchapter F.   License Renewal

§ 205.251. Renewal Required

(a) The medical board by rule shall provide for the annual or biennial renewal of a license to practice acupuncture.

(b) The medical board by rule may adopt a system under which licenses expire on various dates during the year. For the year in which the license expiration date is changed, license fees shall be prorated on a monthly basis so that each license holder pays only that portion of the license fee that is allocable to the number of months during which the license is valid. On renewal of the license on the new expiration date, the total license renewal fee is payable.

§ 205.2515. Criminal History Record Information Requirement for Renewal

(a) An applicant for renewal of a license issued under this chapter shall submit a complete and legible set of fingerprints for purposes of performing a criminal history record information check of the applicant as provided by Section 205.2025.

(b) The acupuncture board may administratively suspend or refuse to renew the license of a person who does not comply with the requirement of Subsection (a).

(c) A license holder is not required to submit fingerprints under this section for the renewal of the license if the holder has previously submitted fingerprints under:

（1）Section 205.2025 for the initial issuance of the license; or

（2）this section as part of a prior renewal of a license.

§ 205.252. Notice of License Expiration

Not later than the 30th day before the expiration date of a person's license, the medical board shall send written notice of the impending license expiration to the person at the person's last known address according to the records of the medical board.

§ 205.253. Procedure for Renewal

（a）A person who is otherwise eligible to renew a license may renew an unexpired license by paying the required renewal fee to the medical board before the expiration date of the license. A person whose license has expired may not engage in activities that require a license until the license has been renewed under this section or Section 205.254.

（b）If the person's license has been expired for 90 days or less, the person may renew the license by paying to the medical board a fee in an amount equal to one and one-half times the required renewal fee.

（c）If the person's license has been expired for longer than 90 days but less than one year, the person may renew the license by paying to the medical board a fee in an amount equal to two times the required renewal fee.

（d）If the person's license has been expired for one year or longer, the person may not renew the license. The person may obtain a new license by submitting to reexamination and complying with the requirements and procedures for obtaining an original license.

§ 205.254. Renewal of Expired License by Out-of-State Practitioner

（a）The medical board may renew without reexamination the license of a person who was licensed to practice acupuncture in this state, moved to another state, and is currently licensed and has been in practice in the other state for the two years preceding application.

（b）The person must pay to the medical board a fee in an amount equal to two times the required renewal fee for the license.

§ 205.255. Continuing Education

（a）The acupuncture board by rule may require a license holder to complete a certain number of hours of continuing education courses approved by the acupuncture board to renew a license.

（a-1）The acupuncture board shall establish written guidelines for granting continuing education credit that specify:

（1）procedural requirements;

（2）the qualifications needed to be considered a preferred provider of continuing education; and

（3）course content requirements.

（b）The acupuncture board shall consider the approval of a course conducted by:

(1) a knowledgeable health care provider; or

(2) a reputable school, state, or professional organization.

(c) After guidelines are established under Subsection (a-1), the acupuncture board shall delegate to medical board employees the authority to approve course applications for courses that clearly meet the guidelines. Medical board employees shall refer any courses that are not clearly within the guidelines to the acupuncture board for review and approval.

§ 205.256. Refusal for Violation of Board Order

The acupuncture board may refuse to renew a license issued under this chapter if the license holder is in violation of an acupuncture board order.

Subchapter G.   Practice by License Holder

§ 205.301. Referral by Other Health Care Practitioner Required

(a) A license holder may perform acupuncture on a person only if the person was:

(1) evaluated by a physician or dentist, as appropriate, for the condition being treated within six months before the date acupuncture is performed; or

(2) referred by a chiropractor within 30 days before the date acupuncture is performed.

(b) A license holder acting under Subsection (a)(1) must obtain reasonable documentation that the required evaluation has taken place. If the license holder is unable to determine that an evaluation has taken place, the license holder must obtain a written statement signed by the person on a form prescribed by the acupuncture board that states the person has been evaluated by a physician or dentist within the prescribed time. The form must contain a clear statement that the person should be evaluated by a physician or dentist for the condition being treated by the license holder.

(c) A license holder acting under Subsection (a)(2) shall refer the person to a physician after performing acupuncture 20 times or for 30 days, whichever occurs first, if substantial improvement does not occur in the person's condition for which the referral was made.

(d) The medical board, with advice from the acupuncture board, by rule may modify:

(1) the scope of the evaluation under Subsection (a)(1);

(2) the period during which treatment must begin under Subsection (a)(1) or (2); or

(3) the number of treatments or days before referral to a physician is required under Subsection (c).

§ 205.302. Authorized Practice Without Referral

(a) After notice and public hearing, the medical board shall determine by rule whether an acupuncturist may treat a patient for alcoholism or chronic pain without a referral from a physician, dentist, or chiropractor. The medical board shall make the determination based on clinical evidence and what the medical board determines to be in the best interest of affected patients.

(b) Notwithstanding Section 205.301, a license holder may, without a referral from a physician, dentist, or chiropractor, perform acupuncture on a person for:

(1) smoking addiction;

(2) weight loss; or

(3) substance abuse, to the extent permitted by medical board rule adopted with advice from the acupuncture board.

§ 205.303. Acudetox Specialist

(a) The medical board may certify a person as an acudetox specialist under this section if the person:

(1) provides to the medical board documentation that the person:

(A) is a licensed social worker, licensed professional counselor, licensed psychologist, licensed chemical dependency counselor, licensed vocational nurse, or licensed registered nurse; and

(B) has successfully completed a training program in acupuncture detoxification that meets guidelines approved by the medical board; and

(2) pays a certification fee in an amount set by the medical board.

(b) An acudetox specialist may practice acupuncture only:

(1) to the extent allowed by rules adopted by the medical board for the treatment of alcoholism, substance abuse, or chemical dependency; and

(2) under the supervision of a licensed acupuncturist or physician.

(c) A program that includes the services of an acudetox specialist shall:

(1) notify each participant in the program of the qualifications of the acudetox specialist and of the procedure for registering a complaint regarding the acudetox specialist with the medical board; and

(2) keep a record of each client's name, the date the client received the acudetox specialist's services, and the name, signature, and certification number of the acudetox specialist.

(d) The medical board may annually renew the certification of an acudetox specialist under this section if the person:

(1) provides to the medical board documentation that:

(A) the certification or license required under Subsection (a)(1)(A) is in effect; and

(B) the person has successfully met continuing education requirements established by the medical board under Subsection (e); and

(2) pays a certification renewal fee in an amount set by the medical board.

(e) The medical board shall establish continuing education requirements for an acudetox specialist that, at a minimum, include six hours of education in the practice of acupuncture and a course in either clean needle technique or universal infection control precaution procedures.

§ 205.304. Professional Review Action

Sections 160.002, 160.003, 160.006, 160.007(d), 160.013, 160.014, and 160.015 apply to professional review actions relating to the practice of acupuncture by an acupuncturist or acupuncturist student.

§ 205.305. License Holder Information

(a) Each license holder shall file with the acupuncture board:

(1) the license holder's mailing address;

(2) the address of the license holder's residence;

(3) the mailing address of each office of the license holder; and

(4) the address for the location of each office of the license holder that has an address different from the office's mailing address.

(b) A license holder shall:

(1) notify the acupuncture board of a change of the license holder's residence or business address; and

(2) provide the acupuncture board with the license holder's new address not later than the 30th day after the date the address change occurs.

Subchapter H. Disciplinary Procedures

§ 205.351. Grounds for License Denial or Disciplinary Action

(a) A license to practice acupuncture may be denied or, after notice and hearing, a license holder may be subject to disciplinary action under Section 205.352 if the license applicant or license holder:

(1) intemperately uses drugs or intoxicating liquors to an extent that, in the opinion of the board, could endanger the lives of patients;

(2) obtains or attempts to obtain a license by fraud or deception;

(3) has been adjudged mentally incompetent by a court;

(4) has a mental or physical condition that renders the person unable to perform safely as an acupuncturist;

(5) fails to practice acupuncture in an acceptable manner consistent with public health and welfare;

(6) violates this chapter or a rule adopted under this chapter;

(7) has been convicted of a crime involving moral turpitude or a felony or is the subject of deferred adjudication or pretrial diversion for such an offense;

(8) holds the person out as a physician or surgeon or any combination or derivative of those terms unless the person is also licensed by the medical board as a physician or surgeon;

(9) fraudulently or deceptively uses a license;

(10) engages in unprofessional or dishonorable conduct that is likely to deceive, defraud,

or injure a member of the public;

(11) commits an act in violation of state law if the act is connected with the person's practice as an acupuncturist;

(12) fails to adequately supervise the activities of a person acting under the supervision of the license holder;

(13) directly or indirectly aids or abets the practice of acupuncture by any person not licensed to practice acupuncture by the acupuncture board;

(14) is unable to practice acupuncture with reasonable skill and with safety to patients because of illness, drunkenness, or excessive use of drugs, narcotics, chemicals, or any other type of material or because of any mental or physical condition;

(15) is the subject of repeated or recurring meritorious health-care liability claims that in the opinion of the acupuncture board evidence professional incompetence likely to injure the public;

(16) has had a license to practice acupuncture suspended, revoked, or restricted by another state or has been subject to other disciplinary action by another state or by the uniformed services of the United States regarding practice as an acupuncturist; or

(17) sexually abuses or exploits another person through the license holder's practice as an acupuncturist.

(b) If the acupuncture board proposes to suspend, revoke, or refuse to renew a person's license, the person is entitled to a hearing conducted by the State Office of Administrative Hearings.

(c) A complaint, indictment, or conviction of a violation of law is not necessary for an action under Subsection (a)(11). Proof of the commission of the act while in the practice of acupuncture or under the guise of the practice of acupuncture is sufficient for action by the acupuncture board.

(d) A certified copy of the record of the state or uniformed services of the United States taking an action is conclusive evidence of the action for purposes of Subsection (a)(16).

§ 205.352. Disciplinary Powers of Acupuncture Board

(a) On finding that grounds exist to deny a license or take disciplinary action against a license holder, the acupuncture board by order may:

(1) deny the person's application for a license, license renewal, or certificate to practice acupuncture or revoke the person's license or certificate to practice acupuncture;

(2) require the person to submit to the care, counseling, or treatment of a health care practitioner designated by the acupuncture board as a condition for the issuance, continuance, or renewal of a license or certificate to practice acupuncture;

(3) require the person to participate in a program of education or counseling prescribed by the acupuncture board;

(4) suspend, limit, or restrict the person's license or certificate to practice acupuncture, including limiting the practice of the person to, or excluding from the practice, one or more specified activities of acupuncture or stipulating periodic review by the acupuncture board;

(5) require the person to practice under the direction of an acupuncturist designated by the acupuncture board for a specified period of time;

(6) assess an administrative penalty against the person as provided by Subchapter J

(7) require the person to perform public service considered appropriate by the acupuncture board;

(8) stay enforcement of an order and place the person on probation with the acupuncture board retaining the right to vacate the probationary stay and enforce the original order for noncompliance with the terms of probation or impose any other remedial measure or sanction authorized by this section;

(9) require the person to continue or review professional education until the person attains a degree of skill satisfactory to the acupuncture board in those areas that are the basis of the probation under Subdivision (8);

(10) require the person to report regularly to the acupuncture board on matters that are the basis of the probation under Subdivision (8); or

(11) administer a public reprimand.

(b) The acupuncture board may reinstate or reissue a license or remove any disciplinary or corrective measure that the acupuncture board has imposed under this section.

§ 205.3522. Surrender of License

(a) The acupuncture board may accept the voluntary surrender of a license.

(b) A surrendered license may not be returned to the license holder unless the acupuncture board determines, under acupuncture board rules, that the former holder of the license is competent to resume practice.

(c) The acupuncture board shall recommend rules to the medical board for determining the competency of a former license holder to return to practice.

§ 205.3523. Physical or Mental Examination

(a) The acupuncture board shall adopt guidelines, in conjunction with persons interested in or affected by this section, to enable the board to evaluate circumstances in which an acupuncturist or applicant may be required to submit to an examination for mental or physical health conditions, alcohol and substance abuse, or professional behavior problems.

(b) The acupuncture board shall refer an acupuncturist or applicant with a physical or mental health condition to the most appropriate medical specialist. The acupuncture board may not require an acupuncturist or applicant to submit to an examination by a physician having a specialty specified by the board unless medically indicated. The acupuncture board may not require an acupuncturist or applicant to submit to an examination to be conducted an unreasonable distance from the person's home or place of business unless the acupuncturist or applicant resides and works in an area in which there are a limited number of physicians able to perform an appropriate examination.

(c) The guidelines adopted under this section do not impair or remove the acupuncture board's power to make an independent licensing decision.

§ 205.353. Repealed by Acts 2005, 79th Leg., ch. 269, § 3.35, eff. Sept. 1, 2005

§ 205.354. Rules for Disciplinary Proceedings

Rules of practice adopted by the medical board under Section 2001.004, Government Code, applicable to the proceedings for a disciplinary action may not conflict with rules adopted by the State Office of Administrative Hearings.

§ 205.3541. Informal Proceedings

(a) The acupuncture board by rule shall adopt procedures governing:

(1) informal disposition of a contested case under Section 2001.056, Government Code; and

(2) informal proceedings held in compliance with Section 2001.054, Government Code.

(b) Rules adopted under this section must require that:

(1) an informal meeting in compliance with Section 2001.054, Government Code, be scheduled not later than the 180th day after the date the complaint is filed with the acupuncture board, unless good cause is shown by the acupuncture board for scheduling the informal meeting after that date;

(2) the acupuncture board give notice to the license holder of the time and place of the meeting not later than the 30th day before the date the meeting is held;

(3) the complainant and the license holder be provided an opportunity to be heard;

(4) at least one of the acupuncture board members participating in the informal meeting as a panelist be a member who represents the public;

(5) the acupuncture board's legal counsel or a representative of the attorney general be present to advise the acupuncture board or the medical board's staff; and

(6) an employee of the medical board be at the meeting to present to the acupuncture board's representative the facts the medical board staff reasonably believes it could prove by competent evidence or qualified witnesses at a hearing.

(c) An affected acupuncturist is entitled, orally or in writing, to:

(1) reply to the staff's presentation; and

(2) present the facts the acupuncturist reasonably believes the acupuncturist could prove by competent evidence or qualified witnesses at a hearing.

(d) After ample time is given for the presentations, the acupuncture board panel shall recommend that the investigation be closed or shall attempt to mediate the disputed matters and make a recommendation regarding the disposition of the case in the absence of a hearing under applicable law concerning contested cases.

(e) If the license holder has previously been the subject of disciplinary action by the acupuncture board, the acupuncture board shall schedule the informal meeting as soon as practicable but not later than the deadline prescribed by Subsection (b)(1).

§ 205.3542. Acupuncture Board Representation in Informal Proceedings

(a) In an informal proceeding under Section 205.3541, at least two panelists shall be appointed to determine whether an informal disposition is appropriate.

(b) Notwithstanding Subsection (a) and Section 205.3541(b)(4), an informal proceeding may be conducted by one panelist if the affected acupuncturist waives the requirement that at least two panelists conduct the informal proceeding. If the acupuncturist waives that requirement, the panelist may be any member of the acupuncture board.

(c) The panel requirements described by Subsection (a) apply to an informal proceeding conducted by the acupuncture board under Section 205.3541, including a proceeding to:

(1) consider a disciplinary case to determine if a violation has occurred; or

(2) request modification or termination of an order.

(d) The panel requirements described by Subsection (a) do not apply to an informal proceeding conducted by the acupuncture board under Section 205.3541 to show compliance with an order of the acupuncture board.

§ 205.3543. Roles and Responsibilities of Participants in Informal Proceedings

(a) An acupuncture board member that serves as a panelist at an informal meeting under Section 205.3541 shall make recommendations for the disposition of a complaint or allegation. The member may request the assistance of a medical board employee at any time.

(b) Medical board employees shall present a summary of the allegations against the affected acupuncturist and of the facts pertaining to the allegation that the employees reasonably believe may be proven by competent evidence at a formal hearing.

(c) An acupuncture board or medical board attorney shall act as counsel to the panel and, notwithstanding Subsection (e), shall be present during the informal meeting and the panel's deliberations to advise the panel on legal issues that arise during the proceeding. The attorney may ask questions of participants in the informal meeting to clarify any statement made by the participant. The attorney shall provide to the panel a historical perspective on comparable cases that have appeared before the acupuncture board or medical board, keep the proceedings focused on the case being discussed, and ensure that the medical board's employees and the affected acupuncturist have an opportunity to present information related to the case. During the panel's deliberation, the attorney may be present only to advise the panel on legal issues and to provide information on comparable cases that have appeared before the acupuncture board or medical board.

(d) The panel and medical board employees shall provide an opportunity for the affected acupuncturist and the acupuncturist's authorized representative to reply to the board employees' presentation and to present oral and written statements and facts that the acupuncturist and representative reasonably believe could be proven by competent evidence at a formal hearing.

(e) An employee of the medical board who participated in the presentation of the allegation or information gathered in the investigation of the complaint, the affected acupuncturist, the acupuncturist's authorized representative, the complainant, the witnesses, and members of the public may not be present during the deliberations of the panel. Only the members of the panel and the attorney serving as counsel to the panel may be present during the deliberations.

(f) The panel shall recommend the dismissal of the complaint or allegations or, if the panel determines that the affected acupuncturist has violated a statute or acupuncture board rule, the panel may recommend board action and terms for an informal settlement of the case.

(g) The panel's recommendations under Subsection (f) must be made in a written order and presented to the affected acupuncturist and the acupuncturist's authorized representative. The acupuncturist may accept the proposed settlement within the time established by the panel at the informal meeting. If the acupuncturist rejects the proposed settlement or does not act within the required time, the acupuncture board may proceed with the filing of a formal complaint with the State Office of Administrative Hearings.

§ 205.3544.　Limit on Access to Investigation Files

The acupuncture board shall prohibit or limit access to an investigation file relating to a license holder in an informal proceeding in the manner provided by Section 164.007(c).

§ 205.355.　Required Disciplinary Action for Failure to Obtain Referral

Except as provided by Section 205.301(a)(2), a license to practice acupuncture shall be denied or, after notice and hearing, revoked if the applicant or license holder violates Section 205.301(a)(1).

§ 205.356.　Rehabilitation Order

(a) The acupuncture board, through an agreed order or after a contested proceeding, may impose a nondisciplinary rehabilitation order on an applicant, as a prerequisite for issuing a license, or on a license holder based on:

(1) the person's intemperate use of drugs or alcohol directly resulting from habituation or addiction caused by medical care or treatment provided by a physician;

(2) the person's intemperate use of drugs or alcohol during the five years preceding the date of the report that could adversely affect the person's ability to safely practice as an acupuncturist, if the person:

(A) reported the use;

(B) has not previously been the subject of a substance abuse related order of the acupuncture board; and

(C) did not violate the standard of care as a result of the impairment;

(3) a judgment by a court that the person is of unsound mind; or

(4) the results of a mental or physical examination, or an admission by the person, indicating that the person suffers from a potentially dangerous limitation or an inability to practice as an acupuncturist with reasonable skill and safety by reason of illness or as a result of any physical or mental condition.

(b) The acupuncture board may not issue an order under this section if, before the individual signs the proposed order, the board receives a valid complaint with regard to the individual based on the individual's intemperate use of drugs or alcohol in a manner affecting the standard of care.

(c) The acupuncture board must determine whether an individual has committed a standard of care violation described by Subsection (a)(2) before imposing an order under this section.

(d) The acupuncture board may disclose a rehabilitation order to a local or statewide private acupuncture association only as provided by Section 205.3562.

§ 205.3561. Expert Immunity

An expert who assists the acupuncture board is immune from suit and judgment and may not be subjected to a suit for damages for any investigation, report, recommendation, statement, evaluation, finding, or other action taken without fraud or malice in the course of assisting the board in a disciplinary proceeding. The attorney general shall represent the expert in any suit resulting from a service provided by the expert in good faith to the acupuncture board.

§ 205.3562. Responsibilities of Private Associations

(a) If a rehabilitation order imposed under Section 205.356 requires a license holder to participate in activities or programs provided by a local or statewide private acupuncture association, the acupuncture board shall inform the association of the license holder's duties under the order. The information provided under this section must include specific guidance to enable the association to comply with any requirements necessary to assist in the acupuncturist's rehabilitation.

(b) The acupuncture board may provide to the association any information that the board determines to be necessary, including a copy of the rehabilitation order. Any information received by the association remains confidential, is not subject to discovery, subpoena, or other means of legal compulsion, and may be disclosed only to the acupuncture board.

§ 205.357. Effect of Rehabilitation Order

(a) A rehabilitation order imposed under Section 205.356 is a nondisciplinary private order. If entered by agreement, the order is an agreed disposition or settlement agreement for purposes of civil litigation and is exempt from the open records law.

(b) A rehabilitation order imposed under Section 205.356 must contain findings of fact and conclusions of law. The order may impose a revocation, cancellation, suspension, period of probation or restriction, or any other term authorized by this chapter or agreed to by the acupuncture board and the person subject to the order.

(c) A violation of a rehabilitation order may result in disciplinary action under the provisions of this chapter for contested matters or the terms of the agreed order.

(d) A violation of a rehabilitation order is grounds for disciplinary action based on:

(1) unprofessional or dishonorable conduct; or

(2) any provision of this chapter that applies to the conduct resulting in the violation.

§ 205.358.　Audit of Rehabilitation Order

(a) The acupuncture board shall keep rehabilitation orders imposed under Section 205.356 in a confidential file. The file is subject to an independent audit to ensure that only qualified license holders are subject to rehabilitation orders. The audit shall be conducted by a state auditor or private auditor with whom the acupuncture board contracts to perform the audit.

(b) An audit may be performed at any time at the direction of the acupuncture board. The acupuncture board shall ensure that an audit is performed at least once in each three-year period.

(c) The audit results are a matter of public record and shall be reported in a manner that maintains the confidentiality of each license holder who is subject to a rehabilitation order.

§ 205.359.　Subpoena

(a) On behalf of the acupuncture board, the executive director of the medical board or the presiding officer of the acupuncture board may issue a subpoena or subpoena duces tecum:

(1) for purposes of an investigation or contested proceeding related to:

(A) alleged misconduct by an acupuncturist; or

(B) an alleged violation of this chapter or other law related to practice as an acupuncturist or to the provision of health care under the authority of this chapter; and

(2) to determine whether to:

(A) issue, suspend, restrict, revoke, or cancel a license authorized by this chapter; or

(B) deny or grant an application for a license under this chapter.

(b) Failure to timely comply with a subpoena issued under this section is a ground for:

(1) disciplinary action by the acupuncture board or any other licensing or regulatory agency with jurisdiction over the individual or entity subject to the subpoena; and

(2) denial of a license application.

§ 205.360.　Delegation of Certain Complaint Dispositions

(a) The acupuncture board may delegate to a committee of medical board employees the authority to dismiss or enter into an agreed settlement of a complaint that does not relate directly to patient care or that involves only administrative violations. The disposition determined by the committee must be approved by the acupuncture board at a public meeting.

(b) A complaint delegated under this section shall be referred for informal proceedings under Section 205.3541 if:

(1) the committee of employees determines that the complaint should not be dismissed or

settled;

(2) the committee is unable to reach an agreed settlement; or

(3) the affected acupuncturist requests that the complaint be referred for informal proceedings.

§ 205.361. Temporary Suspension

(a) The presiding officer of the acupuncture board, with that board's approval, shall appoint a three-member disciplinary panel consisting of acupuncture board members to determine whether a person's license to practice as an acupuncturist should be temporarily suspended.

(b) If the disciplinary panel determines from the information presented to the panel that a person licensed to practice as an acupuncturist would, by the person's continuation in practice, constitute a continuing threat to the public welfare, the disciplinary panel shall temporarily suspend the license of that person.

(c) A license may be suspended under this section without notice or hearing on the complaint if:

(1) institution of proceedings for a hearing before the acupuncture board is initiated simultaneously with the temporary suspension; and

(2) a hearing is held under Chapter 2001, Government Code, and this chapter as soon as possible.

(d) Notwithstanding Chapter 551, Government Code, the disciplinary panel may hold a meeting by telephone conference call if immediate action is required and convening of the panel at one location is inconvenient for any member of the disciplinary panel.

§ 205.362. Cease and Desist Order

(a) If it appears to the acupuncture board that a person who is not licensed under this chapter is violating this chapter, a rule adopted under this chapter, or another state statute or rule relating to the practice of acupuncture, the board, after notice and opportunity for a hearing, may issue a cease and desist order prohibiting the person from engaging in the activity.

(b) A violation of an order under this section constitutes grounds for imposing an administrative penalty under Section 205.352.

§ 205.363. Refund

(a) Subject to Subsection (b), the acupuncture board may order a license holder to pay a refund to a consumer as provided in an agreement resulting from an informal settlement conference instead of or in addition to imposing an administrative penalty under this subchapter.

(b) The amount of a refund ordered under Subsection (a) may not exceed the amount the consumer paid to the license holder for a service regulated by this chapter. The acupuncture board may not require payment of other damages or estimate harm in a refund order.

§ 205.364. Modification of Findings or Rulings by Administrative Law Judge

The acupuncture board may change a finding of fact or conclusion of law or vacate or modify an order of an administrative law judge only if the acupuncture board makes a determination required by Section 2001.058(e), Government Code.

Subchapter I. Criminal Penalties and Other Enforcement Provisions

§ 205.401. Criminal Penalty

(a) Except as provided by Section 205.303, a person commits an offense if the person practices acupuncture in this state without a license issued under this chapter.

(b) Each day a person practices acupuncture in violation of Subsection (a) constitutes a separate offense.

(c) An offense under Subsection (a) is a felony of the third degree.

§ 205.402. Injunctive Relief; Civil Penalty

(a) The acupuncture board, the attorney general, or a district or county attorney may bring a civil action to compel compliance with this chapter or to enforce a rule adopted under this chapter.

(b) In addition to injunctive relief or any other remedy provided by law, a person who violates this chapter or a rule adopted under this chapter is liable to the state for a civil penalty in an amount not to exceed $2,000 for each violation.

(c) Each day a violation continues or occurs is a separate violation for purposes of imposing a civil penalty.

(d) The attorney general, at the request of the acupuncture board or on the attorney general's own initiative, may bring a civil action to collect a civil penalty.

Subchapter J. Administrative Penalties

§ 205.451. Imposition of Administrative Penalty

The acupuncture board by order may impose an administrative penalty against a person licensed or regulated under this chapter who violates this chapter or a rule or order adopted under this chapter.

§ 205.452. Procedure

(a) The acupuncture board by rule shall prescribe the procedure by which it may impose an administrative penalty.

(b) A proceeding under this subchapter is subject to Chapter 2001, Government Code.

§ 205.453. Amount of Penalty

(a) The amount of an administrative penalty may not exceed $5,000 for each violation. Each day a violation continues or occurs is a separate violation for purposes of imposing a penalty.

(b) The amount of the penalty shall be based on:

(1) the seriousness of the violation, including:

(A) the nature, circumstances, extent, and gravity of any prohibited act; and

(B) the hazard or potential hazard created to the health, safety, or economic welfare of the public;

(2) the economic harm to property or the environment caused by the violation;

(3) the history of previous violations;

(4) the amount necessary to deter a future violation;

(5) efforts to correct the violation; and

(6) any other matter that justice may require.

§ 205.454. Notice of Violation and Penalty

(a) If the acupuncture board by order determines that a violation has occurred and imposes an administrative penalty, the acupuncture board shall notify the affected person of the board's order.

(b) The notice must include a statement of the right of the person to judicial review of the order.

§ 205.455. Options Following Decision: Pay or Appeal

(a) Not later than the 30th day after the date the acupuncture board's order imposing the administrative penalty is final, the person shall:

(1) pay the penalty;

(2) pay the penalty and file a petition for judicial review contesting the occurrence of the violation, the amount of the penalty, or both; or

(3) without paying the penalty, file a petition for judicial review contesting the occurrence of the violation, the amount of the penalty, or both.

(b) Within the 30-day period, a person who acts under Subsection (a)(3) may:

(1) stay enforcement of the penalty by:

(A) paying the penalty to the court for placement in an escrow account; or

(B) giving to the court a supersedeas bond approved by the court for the amount of the penalty and that is effective until all judicial review of the acupuncture board's order is final; or

(2) request the court to stay enforcement of the penalty by:

(A) filing with the court an affidavit of the person stating that the person is financially unable to pay the penalty and is financially unable to give the supersedeas bond; and

(B) giving a copy of the affidavit to the presiding officer of the acupuncture board by certified mail.

(c) If the presiding officer of the acupuncture board receives a copy of an affidavit under Subsection (b)(2), the presiding officer may file with the court a contest to the affidavit not later than the fifth day after the date the copy is received.

(d) The court shall hold a hearing on the facts alleged in the affidavit as soon as practicable and shall stay the enforcement of the penalty on finding that the alleged facts are true. The person who files an affidavit has the burden of proving that the person is financially unable to pay the penalty and to give a supersedeas bond.

§ 205.456. Collection of Penalty

If the person does not pay the administrative penalty and the enforcement of the penalty is not stayed, the presiding officer of the acupuncture board may refer the matter to the attorney general for collection of the penalty.

§ 205.457. Determination by Court

(a) If on appeal the court sustains the determination that a violation occurred, the court may uphold or reduce the amount of the administrative penalty and order the person to pay the full or reduced penalty.

(b) If the court does not sustain the determination that a violation occurred, the court shall order that a penalty is not owed.

§ 205.458. Remittance of Penalty and Interest

(a) If after judicial review the administrative penalty is reduced or not imposed by the court, the court shall, after the judgment becomes final:

(1) order that the appropriate amount, plus accrued interest, be remitted to the person if the person paid the penalty; or

(2) order the release of the bond in full if the penalty is not imposed or order the release of the bond after the person pays the penalty imposed if the person posted a supersedeas bond.

(b) The interest paid under Subsection (a)(1) is the rate charged on loans to depository institutions by the New York Federal Reserve Bank. The interest is paid for the period beginning on the date the penalty is paid and ending on the date the penalty is remitted.

TEXAS ADMINISTRATIVE CODE

§ 183.1. Purpose

(a) These rules are promulgated under the authority of the Medical Practice Act, Title 3 Subtitle B Tex. Occ. Code and the Acupuncture Act, Chapter 205 Tex. Occ. Code, to establish procedures and standards for the training, education, licensing, and discipline of persons performing acupuncture in this State so as to establish an orderly system of regulating the practice of acupuncture in a manner which protects the health, safety, and welfare of the public.

(b) The Acupuncture board's functions include but are not limited to the following:

(1) Establish standards for the practice of acupuncture.

(2) Regulate the practice of acupuncture through the licensure and discipline of acupuncturists.

(3) Interpret the Acupuncture Act and the Acupuncture board Rules acupuncturists and the

public to ensure informed professionals, allied health professionals, and consumers.

(4) Receive complaints and investigate possible violations of the Acupuncture Act and the Acupuncture board Rules.

(5) Discipline violators through appropriate legal action to enforce the Acupuncture Act and the Acupuncture board Rules.

(6) Provide a mechanism for public comment with regard to the Acupuncture Act and the Acupuncture board Rules.

(7) Review and modify the Acupuncture board rules when necessary and appropriate, subject to approval of the Medical Board.

(8) Examine and license qualified applicants to practice acupuncture in Texas in a manner that ensures that applicable standards are maintained.

(9) Provide recommendations to the legislature concerning appropriate changes to the Acupuncture Act to ensure that the acts are current and applicable to changing needs and practices.

(10) Provide informal public information on licensees.

(11) Maintain data concerning the practice of acupuncture.

§ 183.2. Definitions

The following words and terms, when used in this chapter, shall have the following meanings, unless the content clearly indicates otherwise.

(1) Ability to communicate in the English language — An applicant who has met the requirements set out in § 183.4(a)(8) of this title (relating to Licensure).

(2) Acceptable approved acupuncture school — Effective January 1, 1996, and in addition to and consistent with the requirements of § 205.206 of the Tex. Occ. Code:

(A) a school of acupuncture located in the United States or Canada which, at the time of the applicant's graduation, was a candidate for accreditation by the Accreditation Commission for Acupuncture and Oriental Medicine (ACAOM) or another accrediting body recognized by the Texas Higher Education Coordinating Board, provides certification that the curriculum at the time of the applicant's graduation was equivalent to the curriculum upon which accreditation granted, offered a masters degree or a professional certificate or diploma upon graduation, and had a curriculum of 1,800 hours with at least 450 hours of herbal studies which at a minimum included the following:

(i) basic herbology including recognition, nomenclature, functions, temperature, taste, contraindications, and therapeutic combinations of herbs;

(ii) herbal formulas including traditional herbal formulas and their modifications or variations based on traditional methods of herbal therapy;

(iii) patent herbs including the names of the more common patent herbal medications and their uses; and

(ⅳ) clinical training emphasizing herbal uses; or

(B) a school of acupuncture located in the United States or Canada which, at the time of the applicant's graduation, was accredited by ACAOM or another accrediting body recognized by the Texas Higher Education Coordinating Board, offered a masters degree or a professional certificate or diploma upon graduation, and had a curriculum of 1,800 hours with at least 450 hours of herbal studies which at a minimum included the following:

(ⅰ) basic herbology including recognition, nomenclature, functions, temperature, taste, contraindications, and therapeutic combinations of herbs;

(ⅱ) herbal formulas including traditional herbal formulas and their modifications or variations based on traditional methods of herbal therapy;

(ⅲ) patent herbs including the names of the more common patent herbal medications and their uses; and

(ⅳ) clinical training emphasizing herbal uses; or

(C) a school of acupuncture located outside the United States or Canada that is determined by the board to be substantially equivalent to a Texas acupuncture school or a school defined in subparagraph (B) of this paragraph. An evaluation by the American Association of Collegiate Registrars and Admissions Officers (AACRAO) or an evaluation requested by the board may be utilized when making a determination of substantial equivalence.

(3) Acupuncture Act or "the Act" — Chapter 205 of the Texas Occupations Code.

(4) Acupuncture —

(A) The insertion of an acupuncture needle and the application of moxibustion to specific areas of the human body as a primary mode of therapy to treat and mitigate a human condition, including the evaluation and assessment of the condition; and

(B) the administration of thermal or electrical treatments or the recommendation of dietary guidelines, energy flow exercise, or dietary or herbal supplements in conjunction with the treatment described by subparagraph (A) of this paragraph.

(5) Acupuncture board or "board" — The Texas State Board of Acupuncture Examiners.

(6) Acupuncturist — A licensee of the acupuncture board who directly or indirectly charges a fee for the performance of acupuncture services.

(7) Agency — The divisions, departments, and employees of the Texas Medical Board, the Texas Physician Assistant Board, and the Texas State Board of Acupuncture Examiners.

(8) APA — The Administrative Procedure Act, Government Code, § 2001.001 et seq.

(9) Applicant — A party seeking a license from the board.

(10) Application — An application is all documents and information necessary to complete an applicant's request for licensure including the following:

(A) forms furnished by the board, completed by the applicant:

(ⅰ) all forms and addenda requiring a written response must be printed in ink or typed;

(ii) photographs must meet United States Government passport standards;

(B) a fingerprint card, furnished by the acupuncture board, completed by the applicant, that must be readable by the Texas Department of Public Safety;

(C) all documents required under § 183. 4 (c) of this title (relating to Licensure Documentation); and

(D) the required fee, payable by check through a United States bank.

(11) Assistant Presiding Officer — A member of the acupuncture board elected by the acupuncture board to fulfill the duties of the presiding officer in the event the presiding officer is incapacitated or absent, or the presiding officer's duly qualified successor under Robert's Rules of Order Newly Revised or board rules.

(12) Board member — One of the members of the acupuncture board, appointed and qualified pursuant to §§ 205.051 – 205.053 of the Act.

(13) Chiropractor — A licensee of the Texas State Board of Chiropractic Examiners.

(14) Contested case — A proceeding, including but not restricted to, licensing, in which the legal rights, duties, or privileges of a party are to be determined by the board after an opportunity for adjudicative hearing.

(15) Documents — Applications, petitions, complaints, motions, protests, replies, exceptions, answers, notices, or other written instruments filed with the medical board or acupuncture board in a licensure proceeding or by a party in a contested case.

(16) Eligible for legal practice and/or licensure in country of graduation — An applicant who has completed all requirements for legal practice of acupuncture and/or licensure in the country in which the school is located except for any citizenship requirements.

(17) Executive Director — The executive director of the agency or the authorized designee of the executive director.

(18) Full force — Applicants for licensure who possess a license in another jurisdiction must have it in full force and not restricted, canceled, suspended or revoked. An acupuncturist with a license in full force may include an acupuncturist who does not have a current, active, valid annual permit in another jurisdiction because that jurisdiction requires the acupuncturist to practice in the jurisdiction before the annual permit is current.

(19) Full NCCAOM examination — The National Certification Commission for Acupuncture and Oriental Medicine examination, consisting of the following:

(A) if taken before June 1, 2004: the Comprehensive Written Exam (CWE), the Clean Needle Technique Portion (CNTP), the Practical Examination of Point Location Skills (PEPLS), and the Chinese Herbology Exam; or

(B) if taken on or after June 1, 2004: the NCCAOM Foundation of Oriental Medicine Module, Acupuncture Module, Point Location Module, the Chinese Herbology Module, and the Biomedicine Module.

(20) Good professional character — An applicant for licensure must not be in violation of or have committed any act described in the Act, § 205.351.

(21) Administrative Law Judge (ALJ) — An individual appointed to preside over administrative hearings pursuant to the APA.

(22) License — Includes the whole or part of any board permit, certificate, approval, registration, or similar form of permission required by law; specifically, a license and a registration.

(23) Licensing — Includes the medical board's and acupuncture board's process respecting the granting, denial, renewal, revocation, suspension, annulment, withdrawal, or amendment of a license.

(24) Medical board — The Texas Medical Board.

(25) Misdemeanors involving moral turpitude — Any misdemeanor of which fraud, dishonesty, or deceit is an essential element; burglary; robbery; sexual offense; theft; child molesting; substance diversion or substance abuse; an offense involving baseness, vileness, or depravity in the private social duties one owes to others or to society in general; or an offense committed with knowing disregard for justice or honesty.

(26) Party — The acupuncture board and each person named or admitted as a party in a SOAH hearing or contested case before the acupuncture board.

(27) Person — Any individual, partnership, corporation, association, governmental subdivision, or public or private organization of any character.

(28) Physician — A licensee of the medical board.

(29) Pleading — Written documents filed by parties concerning their respective claims.

(30) Presiding officer — The member of the acupuncture board appointed by the governor to preside over acupuncture board proceedings or the presiding officer's duly qualified successor in accordance with Robert's Rules of Order Newly Revised or board rules.

(31) Register — The Texas Register.

(32) Rule — Any agency statement of general applicability that implements, interprets, or prescribes law or policy, or describes the procedures or practice requirements of this board. The term includes the amendment or repeal of a prior section but does not include statements concerning only the internal management or organization of any agency and not affecting private rights or procedures. This definition includes substantive regulations.

(33) Secretary — The secretary-treasurer of the acupuncture board.

(34) Substantially equivalent to a Texas acupuncture school — A school or college of acupuncture that is an institution of higher learning designed to select and educate acupuncture students; provide students with the opportunity to acquire a sound basic acupuncture education through training; to develop programs of acupuncture education to produce practitioners, teachers, and researchers; and to afford opportunity for postgraduate and continuing medical education. The school must provide resources, including faculty and facilities, sufficient to

support a curriculum offered in an intellectual and practical environment that enables the program to meet these standards. The faculty of the school shall actively contribute to the development and transmission of new knowledge. The school of acupuncture shall contribute to the advancement of knowledge and to the intellectual growth of its students and faculty through scholarly activity, including research. The school of acupuncture shall include, but not be limited to, the following characteristics:

(A) the facilities for didactic and clinical training (i.e., laboratories, hospitals, library, etc.) shall be adequate to ensure opportunity for proper education.

(B) the admissions standards shall be substantially equivalent to a Texas school of acupuncture.

(C) the basic curriculum shall include courses substantially equivalent to those delineated in the Accreditation Commission for Acupuncture and Oriental Medicine (ACAOM) core curriculum at the time of applicant's graduation.

(D) the curriculum shall be of at least 1800 hours in duration.

(35) Military service member — A person who is on active duty.

(36) Military spouse — A person who is married to a military service member.

(37) Military veteran — A person who served on active duty and who was discharged or released from active duty.

(38) Active duty — A person who is currently serving as full-time military service member in the armed forces of the United States or active duty military service as a member of the Texas military forces, as defined by § 437.001, Government Code, or similar military service of another state.

(39) Armed forces of the United States — Army, Navy, Air Force, Coast Guard, or Marine Corps of the United States or a reserve unit of one of those branches of the armed forces.

§ 183.3. Meetings

(a) The acupuncture board may meet up to four times a year to carry out the mandates of the Act.

(b) Special meetings may be called by the presiding officer of the acupuncture board, by resolution of the acupuncture board, or upon written request to the presiding officer of the acupuncture board signed by at least three members of the board.

(c) Acupuncture board and committee meetings shall, to the extent possible, be conducted pursuant to the provisions of Robert's Rules of Order Newly Revised unless, by rule, the acupuncture board adopts a different procedure.

(d) All elections and any other issues requiring a vote of the acupuncture board shall be decided by a simple majority of the members present. A quorum for transaction of any business by the acupuncture board shall be one more than half the acupuncture board's membership at the time of the meeting. If more than two candidates contest an election or if no candidate receives a majority of the votes cast on the first ballot, a second ballot shall be conducted between the two candidates receiving the highest number of votes.

(e) The acupuncture board, at a regular meeting or special meeting, may elect from its membership an assistant presiding officer and a secretary-treasurer to serve a term of one year or for a term of a set duration established by majority vote of the acupuncture board.

(f) The acupuncture board, at a regular meeting or special meeting, upon majority vote of the members present may remove the assistant presiding officer or secretary-treasurer from office.

(g) The following are standing and permanent committees of the acupuncture board. Each committee, with the exception of the Executive Committee, shall consist of at least one board member who is a licensed physician, one board member who is a licensed acupuncturist, and one public board member. In the event that a committee does not have a representative of one or more of these groups, the presiding officer shall appoint additional members as necessary to maintain this composition. The Executive Committee shall include the presiding officer, the assistant presiding officer, and the secretary-treasurer, plus additional members so that the committee consists of a minimum of two board members who are licensed acupuncturists, one board member who is a licensed physician, and one public board member. The responsibilities and authority of these committees shall include those duties and powers as set forth below and such other responsibilities and authority which the acupuncture board may from time to time delegate to these committees.

(1) Licensure Committee:

(A) draft and review proposed rules regarding licensure, and make recommendations to the acupuncture board regarding changes or implementation of such rules;

(B) draft and review proposed application forms for licensure, and make recommendations to the acupuncture board regarding changes or implementation of such rules;

(C) oversee the application process for licensure;

(D) receive and review applications for licensure;

(E) make determinations of eligibility, present the results of reviews of applications for licensure and make recommendations to the acupuncture board regarding licensure of applicants;

(F) oversee and make recommendations to the acupuncture board regarding any aspect of the examination process including the approval of an appropriate licensure examination and the administration of such an examination and documentation and verification of records from all applicants for licensure;

(G) draft and review proposed rules regarding any aspect of the examination;

(H) maintain communication with Texas acupuncture schools;

(I) make recommendations to the acupuncture board regarding matters brought to the attention of the Licensure Committee.

(2) Discipline and Ethics Committee:

(A) draft and review proposed rules regarding the discipline of acupuncturists and enforcement of Subchapter H of the Act;

(B) oversee the disciplinary process and give guidance to the acupuncture board and staff regarding methods to improve the disciplinary process and more effectively enforce Subchapter H of the Act;

(C) monitor the effectiveness, appropriateness, and timeliness of the disciplinary process;

(D) make recommendations regarding resolution and disposition of specific cases and approve, adopt, modify, or reject recommendations from staff or representatives of the acupuncture board regarding actions to be taken on pending cases. Approve dismissals of complaints and closure of investigations;

(E) draft and review proposed ethics guidelines and rules for the practice of acupuncture, and make recommendations to the acupuncture board regarding the adoption of such ethics guidelines and rules;

(F) make recommendations to the acupuncture board and staff regarding policies, priorities, budget, and any other matters related to the disciplinary process and enforcement of Subchapter H of the Act; and

(G) make recommendations to the acupuncture board regarding matters brought to the attention of the Discipline and Ethics Committee.

(3) Education Committee:

(A) draft and propose rules regarding educational requirements for licensure in Texas and make recommendations to the acupuncture board regarding changes or implementation of such rules;

(B) draft and propose rules regarding training required for licensure in Texas and make recommendations to the acupuncture board regarding changes or implementation of such rules;

(C) draft and propose rules regarding continuing education requirements for renewal of a Texas license and make recommendations to the acupuncture board regarding changes or implementation of such rules;

(D) consult with the Texas Higher Education Coordinating Board regarding educational requirements for schools of acupuncture, oversight responsibilities of each entity, degrees which may be offered by schools of acupuncture;

(E) maintain communication with acupuncture schools;

(F) plan and make visits to acupuncture schools at specified intervals, with the goal of promoting opportunities to meet with the students so they may become aware of the board and its functions;

(G) develop information regarding foreign acupuncture schools in the areas of curriculum, faculty, facilities, academic resources, and performance of graduates;

(H) draft and propose rules which would set the requirements for degree programs in acupuncture;

(I) be available for assistance with problems relating to acupuncture school issues which may arise within the purview of the board;

(J) offer assistance to the Licensure Committee in determining eligibility of graduates of foreign acupuncture schools for licensure;

(K) study and make recommendations regarding documentation and verification of records from foreign acupuncture schools;

(L) make recommendations to the acupuncture board regarding matters brought to the attention of the Education Committee.

(4) Executive Committee:

(A) review agenda for board meetings;

(B) ensure records are maintained of all committee actions;

(C) review requests from the public to appear before the board and to speak regarding issues relating to acupuncture;

(D) review inquiries regarding policy or administrative procedures;

(E) delegate tasks to other committees;

(F) take action on matters of urgency that may arise between board meetings;

(G) assist the medical board in the organization, preparation, and delivery of information and testimony to the Legislature and committees of the Legislature;

(H) formulate and make recommendations to the board concerning future board goals and objectives and the establishment of priorities and methods for their accomplishment;

(I) study and make recommendations to the board regarding the role and responsibility of the board offices and committees;

(J) study and make recommendations to the board regarding ways to improve the efficiency and effectiveness of the administration of the board pursuant to the Occupations Code, § 205.102(b);

(K) make recommendations to the board regarding matters brought to the attention of the executive committee.

(h) Meetings of the acupuncture board and of its committees are open to the public unless such meetings are conducted in executive session pursuant to the Open Meetings Act and the Act. In order that board meetings may be conducted safely, efficiently, and with decorum, members of the public shall refrain at all times from smoking or using tobacco products, eating, or reading newspapers and magazines. Members of the public may not engage in disruptive activity that interferes with board proceedings, including, but not limited to, excessive movement within the meeting room, noise or loud talking, and resting of feet on tables and chairs. The public shall remain within those areas of the board's offices designated as open to the public. Members of the public shall not address or question board members during meetings unless recognized by the board's presiding officer pursuant to a published agenda item.

(i) Journalists have the same right of access as other members of the public to acupuncture board meetings conducted in open session, and are also subject to the rules of conduct described in subsection (h) of this section. Observers of any board meeting may make audio or visual recordings of such proceedings conducted in open session subject to the following limitations: the acupuncture board's presiding officer may request periodically that camera operators extinguish their artificial lights to allow excessive heat to dissipate; camera operators may not assemble or disassemble their equipment while the board is in session and conducting business; persons seeking to position microphones for recording board proceedings may not disrupt the meeting or disturb participants; journalists may conduct interviews in the reception area of the board's offices or, at the discretion of the acupuncture board's presiding officer, in the meeting room after recess or adjournment; no interview may be conducted in the hallways of the board's offices; and the acupuncture board's presiding officer may exclude from a meeting any person who, after being duly warned, persists in conduct described in this subsection and subsection (h) of this section.

(j) The assistant presiding officer of the acupuncture board shall assume the duties of the presiding officer in the event of the presiding officer's absence or incapacity.

(k) In the absence or incapacity of both the presiding officer and the assistant presiding officer, the secretary-treasurer shall assume the duties of the presiding officer.

(1) In the event of the absence or incapacity of the presiding officer, the assistant presiding officer, and secretary-treasurer, the members of the acupuncture board may elect another member to act as the presiding officer of a board meeting or may elect an interim acting presiding officer for the duration of the absences or incapacity or until another presiding officer is appointed by the governor.

(m) Upon the death, resignation, or permanent incapacity of the assistant presiding officer or the secretary-treasurer, the acupuncture board shall elect from its membership an officer to fill the vacant position. Such an election shall be conducted as soon as practicable at a regular or special meeting of the acupuncture board.

(n) Committee minutes shall be approved by the full board with a quorum of the committee members present to vote on approval of the minutes.

§ 183.4.   Licensure

(a) Qualifications. An applicant must present satisfactory proof to the acupuncture board that the applicant meets the following requirements:

(1) is at least 21 years of age;

(2) is of good professional character as defined in § 183.2 of this chapter (relating to Definitions);

(3) has successfully completed 60 semester hours of general academic college level courses,

other than in acupuncture school, that are not remedial and would be acceptable at the time they were completed for credit on an academic degree at a two or four year institution of higher education within the United States accredited by an agency recognized by the Higher Education Coordinating Board or its equivalent in other states as a regional accrediting body. Coursework completed as a part of a degree program in acupuncture or Oriental medicine may be accepted by the acupuncture board if, in the opinion of the acupuncture board, such coursework is substantially equivalent to the required hours of general academic college level coursework;

(4) is a graduate of an acceptable approved acupuncture school;

(5) has taken and passed, within five attempts, each component of the full National Certification Commission for Acupuncture and Oriental Medicine (NCCAOM) examination:

(A) If an applicant submits to multiple attempts on a component before and on or after June 1, 2004, the number of attempts shall be combined based on the subject matter tested;

(B) An applicant who is unable to pass each component of the NCCAOM examination, within five attempts, may be allowed to appear before the Licensure Committee of the board to reconsider applicant's ineligibility if the applicant:

(i) is allowed a 6th attempt by NCCAOM;

(ii) passes on the 6th attempt; and

(iii) presents satisfactory evidence to the board as to why the applicant required an additional examination attempt and demonstrates good cause as to why applicant's determination of ineligibility should be reconsidered.

(C) A decision to reconsider an applicant's ineligibility based on subparagraph (B) of this paragraph shall be a discretionary decision of the board;

(6) has taken and passed the CCAOM (Council of Colleges of Acupuncture and Oriental Medicine) Clean Needle Technique (CNT) course and practical examination;

(7) has taken and passed a jurisprudence examination ("JP exam"), which shall be conducted on the licensing requirements and other laws, rules, or regulations applicable to the acupuncture profession in this state. The jurisprudence examination shall be developed and administered as follows:

(A) Questions for the JP Exam shall be prepared by agency staff with input from the Acupuncture board and the agency staff shall make arrangements for a facility by which applicants can take the examination.

(B) Applicants must pass the JP exam with a score of 75 or better.

(C) An examinee shall not be permitted to bring medical books, compends, notes, medical journals, calculators or other help into the examination room, nor be allowed to communicate by word or sign with another examinee while the examination is in progress without permission of the presiding examiner, nor be allowed to leave the examination room except when so permitted by the presiding examiner.

(D) Irregularities during an examination such as giving or obtaining unauthorized information or aid as evidenced by observation or subsequent statistical analysis of answer sheets shall be sufficient cause to terminate an applicant's participation in an examination, invalidate the applicant's examination results, or take other appropriate action.

(E) A person who has passed the JP Exam shall not be required to retake the Exam for another or similar license, except as a specific requirement of the board;

(8) is able to communicate in English as demonstrated by one of the following:

(A) passage of the NCCAOM examination taken in English;

(B) passage of the TOEFL (Test of English as a Foreign Language) with a score of at least "intermediate" on the Reading and Listening sections and a score of at least "fair" on the Speaking and Writing sections of the Internet Based Test (iBT®), or a score of 550 or higher on the paper based test (PBT);

(C) passage of the TSE (Test of Spoken English) with a score of 45 or higher;

(D) passage of the TOEIC (Test of English for International Communication) with a score of 500 or higher;

(E) graduation from an acceptable approved school of acupuncture located in the United States or Canada; or

(F) at the discretion of the acupuncture board, passage of any other similar, validated exam testing English competency given by a testing service with results reported directly to the acupuncture board or with results otherwise subject to verification by direct contact between the testing service and the acupuncture board; and

(9) can demonstrate current competence through the active practice of acupuncture as follows:

(A) All applicants for licensure shall provide sufficient documentation to the board that the applicant has, on a full-time basis, actively treated persons, been a student at an acceptable approved acupuncture school, or been on the active teaching faculty of an acceptable approved acupuncture school, within either of the last two years preceding receipt of an application for licensure.

(B) The term "full-time basis," for purposes of this section, shall mean at least 20 hours per week for 40 weeks duration during a given year.

(C) Applicants who do not meet the requirements of subparagraphs (A) and (B) of this paragraph may, in the discretion of the executive director or board, be eligible for an unrestricted license or a restricted license subject to one or more of the following conditions or restrictions:

(i) limitation of the practice of the applicant to specified components of the practice of acupuncture and/or exclusion of specified components of the practice of acupuncture; or

(ii) remedial education including, but not limited to, enrollment, as a student, and successful completion of 240 hours of clinical practice at an acceptable approved acupuncture school or other structured program approved by the board.

(10) Alternative License Procedure for Military Service Members, Military Veterans and Military Spouses.

(A) An applicant who is a military service member, military veteran or military spouse may be eligible for alternative demonstrations of competency for certain licensure requirements. Unless specifically allowed in this subsection, an applicant must meet the requirements for licensure as specified in this chapter.

(B) To be eligible, an applicant must be a military service member, military veteran or military spouse and meet one of the following requirements:

(i) holds an active unrestricted acupuncture license issued by another state that has licensing requirements that are substantially equivalent to the requirements for a Texas acupuncture license; or

(ii) within the five years preceding the application date held an acupuncture license in this state.

(C) The executive director may waive any prerequisite to obtaining a license for an applicant described by this subsection after reviewing the applicant's credentials.

(D) Applications for licensure from applicants qualifying under this subsection shall be expedited by the board's licensure division.

(E) Alternative Demonstrations of Competency Allowed. Applicants qualifying under this subsection:

(i) are not required to comply with subsection (c)(1) of this section; and

(ii) notwithstanding the one year expiration in subsection (b)(1)(B) of this section, are allowed an additional 6 months to complete the application prior to it becoming inactive; and

(iii) notwithstanding the 60 day deadline in subsection (b)(1)(G) of this section, may be considered for permanent licensure up to 5 days prior to the board meeting.

(F) Applicants with Military Experience.

(i) For applications filed on or after March 1, 2014, the board shall, with respect to an applicant who is a military service member or military veteran as defined in §183.2 of this chapter, credit verified military service, training, or education toward the licensing requirements, other than an examination requirement, for a license issued by the board.

(ii) This section does not apply to an applicant who:

(I) has had an acupuncture license suspended or revoked by another state or a Canadian province;

(II) holds an acupuncture license issued by another state or a Canadian province that is subject to a restriction, disciplinary order, or probationary order; or

(III) has an unacceptable criminal history.

(b) Procedural rules for licensure applicants. The following provisions shall apply to all licensure applicants.

(1) Applicants for licensure:

(A) whose documentation indicates any name other than the name under which the applicant has applied must furnish proof of the name change;

(B) whose applications have been filed with the board in excess of one year will be considered expired. Any fee previously submitted with that application shall be forfeited unless otherwise provided by § 175.5 of this title (relating to Payment of Fees or Penalties). Any further request for licensure will require submission of a new application and inclusion of the current licensure fee. An extension to an application may be granted under certain circumstances, including:

(i) Delay by board staff in processing an application;

(ii) Application requires Licensure Committee review after completion of all other processing and will expire prior to the next scheduled meeting;

(iii) Licensure Committee requires an applicant to meet specific additional requirements for licensure and the application will expire prior to deadline established by the Committee;

(iv) Applicant requires a reasonable, limited additional period of time to obtain documentation after completing all other requirements and demonstrating diligence in attempting to provide the required documentation;

(v) Applicant is delayed due to unanticipated military assignments, medical reasons, or catastrophic events;

(C) who in any way falsify the application may be required to appear before the acupuncture board. It will be at the discretion of the acupuncture board whether or not the applicant will be issued a Texas acupuncture license;

(D) on whom adverse information is received by the acupuncture board may be required to appear before the acupuncture board. It will be at the discretion of the acupuncture board whether or not the applicant will be issued a Texas license;

(E) shall be required to comply with the acupuncture board's rules and regulations which are in effect at the time the completed application form and fee are filed with the board;

(F) may be required to sit for additional oral, written, or practical examinations or demonstrations that, in the opinion of the acupuncture board, are necessary to determine competency of the applicant;

(G) must have the application for licensure completed and legible in every detail 60 days prior to the acupuncture board meeting in which they are to be considered for licensure unless otherwise determined by the acupuncture board based on good cause.

(2) Applicants for licensure who wish to request reasonable accommodation due to a disability must submit the request at the time of filing the application.

（3）Applicants who have been licensed in any other state, province, or country shall complete a notarized oath or other verified sworn statement in regard to the following:

（A）whether the license, certificate, or authority has been the subject of proceedings against the applicant for the restriction for cause, cancellation for cause, suspension for cause, or revocation of the license, certificate, or authority to practice in the state, province, or country, and if so, the status of such proceedings and any resulting action; and

（B）whether an investigation in regard to the applicant is pending in any jurisdiction or a prosecution is pending against the applicant in any state, federal, national, local, or provincial court for any offense that under the laws of the state of Texas is a felony, and if so, the status of such prosecution or investigation.

（4）An applicant for a license to practice acupuncture may not be required to appear before the acupuncture board or any of its committees unless the application raises questions about the applicant's:

（A）physical or mental impairment;

（B）criminal conviction; or

（C）revocation of a professional license.

（c）Licensure documentation.

（1）Original documents/interview. Upon request, any applicant must appear for a personal interview at the board offices and present original documents to a representative of the board for inspection. Original documents may include, but are not limited to, those listed in paragraph （2）of this subsection.

（2）Required documentation. Documentation required of all applicants for licensure shall include the following:

（A）Birth certificate/proof of age. Each applicant for licensure must provide a copy of a birth certificate, and translation if necessary, to prove that the applicant is at least 21 years of age. In instances where a birth certificate is not available, the applicant must provide copies of a passport or other suitable alternate documentation.

（B）Name change. Any applicant who submits documentation showing a name other than the name under which the applicant has applied must present copies of marriage licenses, divorce decrees, or court orders stating the name change. In cases where the applicant's name has been changed by naturalization the applicant must submit the original naturalization certificate by hand delivery or by certified mail to the board office for inspection.

（C）Examination scores. Each applicant for licensure must have a certified transcript of grades submitted directly from the appropriate testing service to the acupuncture board for all examinations used in Texas for purposes of licensure in Texas.

（D）Dean's certification. Each applicant for licensure must have a certificate of graduation submitted directly from the school of acupuncture on a form provided by the acupuncture board.

The applicant shall attach to the form a recent photograph, meeting United States Government passport standards, before submitting it to the school of acupuncture. The school shall have the Dean or the designated appointee sign the form attesting to the information on the form and placing the school seal over the photograph.

(E) Diploma or certificate. All applicants for licensure must submit a copy of their diploma or certificate of graduation.

(F) Evaluations. All applicants must provide, on a form furnished by the acupuncture board, evaluations of their professional affiliations for the past ten years or since graduation from acupuncture school, whichever is the shorter period.

(G) Preacupuncture school transcript. Each applicant must have the appropriate school or schools submit a copy of the record of their undergraduate education directly to the acupuncture board. Transcripts must show courses taken and grades obtained. If determined that the documentation submitted by the applicant is not sufficient to show proof of the completion of 60 semester hours of college courses other than in acupuncture school, the applicant must obtain coursework verification by submitting documentation to the acupuncture board for a determination as to the adequacy of such education or to a two or four year institution of higher education within the United States. The institution must be preapproved by the board's executive director and accredited by an agency recognized as a regional accrediting body by the Texas Higher Education Coordinating Board or its equivalent in another state.

(H) School of acupuncture transcript. Each applicant must have his or her acupuncture school submit a transcript of courses taken and grades obtained directly to the acupuncture board. Transcripts must clearly demonstrate completion of 1,800 instructional hours, with at least 450 hours of herbal studies.

(I) Fingerprint card. Each applicant must submit his or her fingerprints according to the procedure prescribed by the board.

(J) Other verification. For good cause shown, with the approval of the acupuncture board, verification of any information required by this subsection may be made by a means not otherwise provided for in this subsection.

(3) Additional documentation. Applicants may be required to submit other documentation, including but not limited to the following:

(A) Translations. An accurate certified translation of any document that is in a language other than the English language must be submitted along with the original document or a certified copy of the original document which has been translated.

(B) Arrest Records. If an applicant has ever been arrested, a copy of the arrest and arrest disposition from the arresting authority and must be submitted by that authority directly to the acupuncture board.

(C) Malpractice. If an applicant has ever been named in a malpractice claim filed with any liability carrier or if an applicant has ever been named in a malpractice suit, the applicant shall submit the following:

(ⅰ) a completed liability carrier form furnished by the acupuncture board regarding each claim filed against the applicant's insurance;

(ⅱ) for each claim that becomes a malpractice suit, a letter from the attorney representing the applicant directly to this board explaining the allegation, dates of the allegation, and current status of the suit. If the suit has been closed, the attorney must state the disposition of the suit, and if any money was paid, the amount of the settlement, unless release of such information is prohibited by law or an order of a court with competent jurisdiction. If such letter is not available, the applicant will be required to furnish a notarized affidavit explaining why this letter cannot be provided; and

(ⅲ) a statement, composed by the applicant, explaining the circumstances pertaining to patient care in defense of the allegations.

(D) Inpatient treatment for alcohol/substance abuse or mental illness. Each applicant that has been admitted to an inpatient facility within the last five years for the treatment of alcohol/substance abuse or mental illness must submit the following:

(ⅰ) an applicant's statement explaining the circumstances of the hospitalization;

(ⅱ) an admitting summary and discharge summary, submitted directly from the inpatient facility;

(ⅲ) a statement from the applicant's treating physician/psychotherapist as to diagnosis, prognosis, medications prescribed, and follow-up treatment recommended; and

(ⅳ) a copy of any contracts or agreements signed with any licensing authority.

(E) Outpatient treatment for alcohol/substance abuse or mental illness. Each applicant that has been treated on an outpatient basis within the last five years for alcohol/substance abuse or mental illness must submit the following:

(ⅰ) an applicant's statement explaining the circumstances of the outpatient treatment;

(ⅱ) a statement from the applicant's treating physician/psychotherapist as to diagnosis, prognosis, medications prescribed, and follow-up treatment recommended; and

(ⅲ) a copy of any contracts or agreements signed with any licensing authority.

(F) Additional documentation. Additional documentation as is deemed necessary to facilitate the investigation of any application for licensure.

(G) DD214. A copy of the DD214 indicating separation from any branch of the United States military must be submitted.

(H) Other verification. For good cause shown, with the approval of the acupuncture board, verification of any information required by this subsection may be made by a means not otherwise provided for in this subsection.

(I) False documentation. Falsification of any affidavit or submission of false information to obtain a license may subject an acupuncturist to denial of a license or to discipline pursuant to the Act, § 205.351.

(4) Substitute documents/proof. The acupuncture board may, at its discretion, allow substitute documents where proof of exhaustive efforts on the applicant's part to secure the required documents is presented. These exceptions are reviewed by the acupuncture board, a board committee, or the board's executive director on an individual case-by-case basis.

(d) Temporary license.

(1) Issuance. The acupuncture board may, through the executive director of the agency, issue a temporary license to a licensure applicant who:

(A) appears to meet all the qualifications for an acupuncture license under the Act, but is waiting for the next scheduled meeting of the acupuncture board for review and for the license to be issued; or

(B) has not, on a full-time basis, actively practiced as an acupuncturist as defined under subsection (a)(9) of this section but meets all other requirements for licensure.

(2) Duration/renewal. A temporary license shall be valid for 100 days from the date issued and may be extended only for another 30 days after the date the initial temporary license expires. Issuance of a temporary license may be subject to restrictions at the discretion of the executive director and shall not be deemed dispositive in regard to the decision by the acupuncture board to grant or deny an application for a permanent license.

(e) Distinguished professor temporary license.

(1) Issuance. The acupuncture board may issue a distinguished professor temporary license to an acupuncturist who:

(A) holds a substantially equivalent license, certificate, or authority to practice acupuncture in another state, province, or country;

(B) agrees to and limits any acupuncture practice in this state to acupuncture practice for demonstration or teaching purposes for acupuncture students and/or instructors, and in direct affiliation with an acupuncture school that is a candidate for accreditation or has accreditation through the Accreditation Commission for Acupuncture and Oriental Medicine (ACAOM) at which the students are trained and/or the instructors teach;

(C) agrees to and limits practice to demonstrations or instruction under the direct supervision of a licensed Texas acupuncturist who holds an unrestricted license to practice acupuncture in this state;

(D) pays any required fees for issuance of the distinguished professor temporary license; and

(E) passes the JP Exam, as provided in subsection (a)(7) of this section.

(2) Duration. The distinguished professor temporary license shall be valid for a continuous one-year period; however, the permit is revocable at any time the board deems necessary. The

distinguished professor temporary license shall automatically expire one year after the date of issuance. The distinguished professor temporary license may not be renewed or reissued.

(3) Disciplinary action. A distinguished professor temporary license may be denied, terminated, canceled, suspended, or revoked for any violation of acupuncture board rules or the Act, Subchapter H.

(f) Relicensure. If an acupuncturist's license has been expired for one year, it is considered to have been canceled, and the acupuncturist may not renew the license. The acupuncturist may submit an application for relicensure and must comply with the requirements and procedures for obtaining an original license.

§ 183.5.　Biennial Renewal of License

(a) Acupuncturists licensed under the Act shall register biennially and pay a fee. An acupuncturist may renew an unexpired license by submitting the required form and by paying the required renewal fee to the acupuncture board on or before the expiration date. The fee shall accompany a written application which legibly sets forth the licensee's name, mailing address, the place or places where the licensee is engaged in the practice of acupuncture, and other necessary information prescribed by the acupuncture board.

(b) Falsification of an affidavit or submission of false information to obtain renewal of a license shall subject an acupuncturist to denial of a license renewal or to discipline pursuant to § 205.351 of the Act.

(c) If the renewal fee and completed application form are not received on or before the expiration date, penalty fees will be imposed as outlined in § 175.3(3) of this title (relating to Penalties).

(d) If an acupuncturist's permit has been expired for 90 days or less, the acupuncturist may obtain a new permit by submitting to the board a completed permit application, the registration fee, as defined in § 175.2(3) of this title (relating to Registration and Renewal Fees) and the penalty fee, as defined in § 175.3(3)(A) of this title.

(e) If an acupuncturist's permit has been expired for more than 90 days, but less than one year, the acupuncturist may obtain a new permit by submitting to the board a completed permit application, the registration fee, as defined in § 175.2(3) of this title and the penalty fee, as defined in § 175.3(3)(B) of this title.

(f) If an acupuncturist's registration permit has been expired for one year or longer, the acupuncturist's license is automatically canceled, unless an investigation is pending, and the acupuncturist may not register for a new permit.

(g) Practicing acupuncture after an acupuncturist's permit has expired under subsection (c) of this section, without obtaining a new registration permit for the current registration period, has the same effect as, and is subject to all penalties of, practicing acupuncture without a license.

(h) A military service member who holds an acupuncture license in Texas is entitled to two years of additional time to complete any other requirement related to the renewal of the military service member's license.

§ 183.6. Denial of License; Discipline of Licensee

(a) An applicant for a license under the Act shall be subject to denial of the application pursuant to the provisions of § 205.351 of the Act.

(b) An acupuncturist who holds a license issued under authority of the Act shall be subject to discipline, including revocation of license, pursuant to § 205.351 of the Act.

(c) The denial of licensure or the imposition of disciplinary action by the acupuncture board pursuant to § 205.351 of the Act shall be in accordance with the Act, the procedures set forth in Chapters 187 and 190 of this title (relating to Procedural Rules and Disciplinary Guidelines), the Administrative Procedure Act, and the rules of the State Office of Administrative Hearings. Chapters 187 and 190 of this title (relating to Procedural Rules and Disciplinary Guidelines) shall be applied to acupuncturists to the extent applicable. If the provisions of Chapter 187 or Chapter 190 conflict with the Act or rules under this chapter, the Act and provisions of this chapter shall control.

(d) Disciplinary guidelines.

(1) Chapter 190 of this title (relating to Disciplinary Guidelines) shall apply to acupuncturists regulated under this chapter and be used as guidelines for the following areas as they relate to the denial of licensure or disciplinary action of a licensee:

(A) practice inconsistent with public health and welfare;

(B) unprofessional or dishonorable conduct;

(C) disciplinary actions by state boards and peer groups;

(D) repeated and recurring meritorious health care liability claims;

(E) aggravating and mitigating factors; and

(F) criminal convictions.

(2) If the provisions of Chapter 190 conflict with the Act or rules under this chapter, the Act and provisions of this chapter shall control.

(e) Pursuant to § 205.352 of the Act, § 187.9 of this title (relating to Board Actions), and § 187.13 of this title (relating to Informal Board Proceedings Relating to Licensure Eligibility) the Board may impose a nondisciplinary remedial plan to resolve an investigation of a complaint or as a condition for licensure.

§ 183.7. Scope of Practice

(a) An acupuncturist may perform acupuncture on a person who has been evaluated by a physician or dentist, as appropriate, for the condition being treated within twelve months before the date acupuncture was performed.

(b) The holder of a license may perform acupuncture on a person who was referred by a doctor licensed to practice chiropractic by the Texas Board of Chiropractic Examiners if the licensee commences the treatment within 30 days of the date of the referral. The licensee shall refer the person to a physician after performing acupuncture 20 times or for two months, whichever occurs first, if no substantial improvement occurs in the person's condition for which the referral was made.

(c) Notwithstanding subsections (a) and (b) of this section, an acupuncturist holding a current and valid license may without an evaluation or a referral from a physician, dentist, or chiropractor perform acupuncture on a person for smoking addiction, weight loss, alcoholism, chronic pain, or substance abuse.

(d) A licensed acupuncturist must recommend an evaluation by a licensed Texas physician or dentist, if after performing acupuncture 20 times or for two months, whichever occurs first, there is no substantial improvement of the patient's chronic pain.

(e) A licensed acupuncturist shall recommend an evaluation by a licensed Texas physician or dentist, as appropriate, if after performing acupuncture 20 times or for two months, whichever occurs first, there is no substantial improvement of the patient's alcoholism or substance abuse.

§ 183.8. Investigations

(a) Confidentiality. All complaints, adverse reports, investigation files, other investigation reports, and other investigative information in the possession of, received, or gathered by the board shall be confidential and no employee, agent, or member of the board may disclose information contained in such files except in the following circumstances:

(1) to the appropriate licensing authorities in other states, the District of Columbia, or a territory or country in which the acupuncturist is licensed;

(2) to appropriate law enforcement agencies if the investigative information indicates a crime may have been committed;

(3) to a health care entity upon receipt of written request. Disclosures by the board to a health care entity shall include only information about a complaint filed against an acupuncturist that was resolved after investigation by a disciplinary order of the board or by an agreed settlement, and the basis of and current status of any complaint under active investigation; and

(4) to other persons if required during the conduct of the investigation.

(b) Request for Information and Records.

(1) Patient records. Upon the request of the board or board representatives, a licensee shall furnish to the board legible copies of patient records in English or the original records within 14 days of the date of the request.

(2) Renewal of licenses. A licensee shall furnish a written explanation of his or her answer to any question asked on the application for license renewal, if requested by the medical board or acupuncture board. This explanation shall include all details as the medical board or acupuncture board may request and shall be furnished within 14 days of the date of the medical

or acupuncture board's request.

(c) Professional Liability Suits and Claims. Following receipt of a notice of claim letter or a complaint filed in court against a licensee that is reported to the acupuncture board, the licensee shall furnish to the medical or acupuncture board the following information within 14 days of the date of receipt of the medical or acupuncture board's request for said information:

(1) a completed questionnaire to provide summary information concerning the suit or claim;

(2) a completed questionnaire to provide information deemed necessary in assessing the licensee's competency;

(3) true, legible, and complete copies of the licensee's office patient records and hospital records, if applicable, concerning the patient on whose behalf damages are sought; and

(4) current information on the status of any suit or claim previously reported to either board.

(d) Investigation of Professional Review Actions. A written report of a professional review action taken by a peer review committee or a health care entity provided to the acupuncture board must contain the results and circumstances of the professional review action. Such results and circumstances shall include:

(1) the specific basis for the professional review action, whether or not such action was directly related to care of individual patients; and

(2) the specific limitations imposed upon the acupuncturist's clinical privileges, upon membership in the professional society or association, and the duration of such limitations.

(e) Other Reports.

(1) Relevant information shall be reported to the acupuncture board indicating that an acupuncturist's practice poses a continuing threat to the public welfare shall include a narrative statement describing the time, date, and place of the acts or omissions on which the report is based.

(2) A report that an acupuncturist's practice constitutes a continuing threat to the public welfare shall be made to the acupuncture board as soon as possible after the peer review committee, licensed acupuncturist or acupuncture student involved reaches that conclusion and is able to assemble the relevant information.

(f) Reporting Professional Liability Claims.

(1) Reporting responsibilities. The reporting form must be completed and forwarded to the acupuncture board for each defendant acupuncturist against whom a professional liability claim or complaint has been filed. The information is to be reported by insurers or other entities providing professional liability insurance for an acupuncturist. If a nonadmitted insurance carrier does not report or if the acupuncturist has no insurance carrier, reporting shall be the responsibility of the acupuncturist.

（2）Separate reports required and identifying information. One separate report shall be filed for each defendant acupuncturist insured. When Part II is filed, it shall be accompanied by the completed Part I or other identifying information as described in paragraph （4）（A） of this subsection.

（3）Timeframes and attachments. The information in Part I of the form must be provided within 30 days of receipt of the claim or suit. A copy of the claim letter or petition must be attached. The information in Part II must be reported within 105 days after disposition of the claim. Disposed claims shall be defined as those claims where a court order has been entered, a settlement agreement has been reached, or the complaint has been dropped or dismissed.

（4）Alternate reporting formats. The information may be reported either on the form provided or in any other legible format which contains at least the requested data.

（A）If the reporter elects to use a reporting format other than the acupuncture board's form for data required in Part II, there must be enough identification data available to board staff to match the closure report to the original file. The data required to accomplish this include:

（i）name and license number of defendant acupuncturist（s）; and

（ii）name of plaintiff.

（B）A court order or settlement agreement is an acceptable alternative submission for Part II. An order or settlement agreement should contain the necessary information to match the closure information to the original file. If the order or agreement is lacking some of the required data, the additional information may be legibly written on the order or agreement.

（5）Penalty. Failure by a licensed insurer to report under this section shall be referred to the State Board of Insurance. Sanctions under the Insurance Code, Article 1.10, section 7, may be imposed for failure to report.

（6）Definition. For the purposes of this subsection a professional liability claim or complaint shall be defined as a cause of action against an acupuncturist for treatment, lack of treatment, or other claimed departure from accepted standards of health care or safety which proximately results in injury to or death of the patient, whether the patient's claim or cause of action sounds in tort or contract.

（7）Claims not required to be reported. Examples of claims that are not required to be reported under this chapter but which may be reported include, but are not limited to, the following:

（A）product liability claims （i. e. where an acupuncturist invented a device which may have injured a patient but the acupuncturist has had no personal acupuncturist-patient relationship with the specific patient claiming injury by the device）;

（B）antitrust allegations;

（C）allegations involving improper peer review activities;

（D）civil rights violations; or

(E) allegations of liability for injuries occurring on an acupuncturist's property, but not involving a breach of duty to the patient (i.e. slip and fall accidents).

(8) Claims that are not required to be reported under this chapter may, however, be voluntarily reported.

(9) The reporting form shall be as follows:

Tabular or graphic material set at this point is not displayable.

PART II. COMPLETE AFTER DISPOSITION OF THE CLAIM AS DEFINED IN 22 TAC § 183.8 (f), INCLUDING DISMISSALS OR SETTLEMENTS. FILE WITH T. S. B. A. E. WITHIN 105 DAYS AFTER DISPOSITION OF THE CLAIM. A COPY OF COURT ORDER OR SETTLEMENT AGREEMENT MAY BE USED AS PROVIDED IN TAC § 183.8(f).

8. Date of disposition:

9. Type of Disposition:

_____(1) Settlement

_____(2) Judgement after trial

_____(3) Other (please specify)

_____

10. Amount of indemnity agreed upon or ordered on behalf of this defendant:

$_____. Note: If percentage of fault was not determined by the court or insurer in the case of multiple defendants, the insurer may report the total amount paid for the claim followed by a slash and the number of insured defendants. (Example: $100,000/3)

11. Appeal, if known: _____ Yes _____ No. If yes, which party:

_____

_____

Person completing this report _____ Phone number _____

§ 183.9. Impaired Acupuncturists

(a) Mental or physical examination requirement.

(1) The board may require a licensee or applicant to submit to a mental and/or physical examination by a physician or physicians designated by the board if the board has probable cause to believe that the licensee or applicant is impaired. Impairment is present if one appears to be unable to practice with reasonable skill and safety to patients by reason of age, illness, drunkenness, excessive use of drugs, narcotics, chemicals, or any other type of material; or as a result of any mental or physical condition.

(2) Probable cause may include, but is not limited to, any one of the following:

(A) sworn statements from two people, willing to testify before the acupuncture board, or the State Office of Administrative Hearings that a certain licensee or applicant is impaired;

(B) a sworn statement from an official representative of the Texas Association of Acupuncturists or the Texas Association of Acupuncture and Oriental Medicine stating that the representative is willing to testify before the board that a certain licensee or applicant is impaired;

(C) evidence that a licensee or applicant left a treatment program for alcohol or chemical dependency before completion of that program;

(D) evidence that a licensee or applicant is guilty of intemperate use of drugs or alcohol;

(E) evidence of repeated arrests of a licensee or applicant for intoxication;

(F) evidence of recurring temporary commitments of a licensee or applicant to a mental institution; or

(G) medical records indicating that a licensee or applicant has an illness or condition which results in the inability to function properly in his or her practice.

(H) actions or statements by a licensee or applicant at a hearing conducted by the Board that gives the Board reason to believe that the licensee or applicant has an impairment.

(3) Upon presentation to the Executive Director of probable cause, the Board authorizes the Executive Director to write the licensee/applicant requesting that the licensee/applicant submit to a physical or mental examination within 30 days of the receipt of the letter from the Executive Director. The letter shall state the reasons for the request for the mental or physical examination, the medical specialists the Executive Director has approved to conduct such examinations, and the date by which the examination and the results are to be received by the Board.

(4) If the licensee/applicant to whom a letter requiring a mental or physical examination is sent refuses to submit to the examination, the Board, through its Executive Director, shall issue an order requiring the licensee/applicant to show cause why the licensee/applicant should not be required to submit to the examination and shall schedule a hearing on the order not later than the 30 days after the date on which the notice of the hearing is provided to the licensee. The licensee/applicant shall be notified by either personal service or certified mail with return receipt requested.

(5) At the show cause hearing provided in for in paragraph (4) of this subsection, a panel of the Board's representatives shall determine whether the licensee/applicant shall submit to an evaluation or that the matter shall be closed with no examination required.

(A) At the hearing, the licensee/applicant and the licensee/applicant's attorney, if any, are entitled to present testimony and other evidence showing that the licensee/applicant should not be required to submit to the examination.

(B) If, after consideration of the evidence presented at the show cause hearing, the panel determines that the licensee/applicant shall submit to an examination, the Board's representatives shall, through its Executive Director, issue an order requiring the examination within 60 days after the date of the entry of the order requiring examination. A licensee is entitled to cross-examine an expert who offers testimony at hearing before the Board.

(C) If the panel determines that no such examination is necessary, the panel will withdraw the request for examination.

(D) The results of any Board-ordered mental or physical examination are confidential shall be presented to the Board under seal for it to take whatever action is deemed necessary and appropriate based on the results of the mental or physical examination. A licensee shall be provided the results of an examination and given the opportunity to provide a response at least 30 days before the Board takes action.

(6) In fulfilling its obligations under Section 205.3523 of the Act, the Board shall refer the licensee/applicant to the most appropriate medical specialist for evaluation. The Board may not require a licensee/applicant to submit to an examination by a physician having a specialty specified by the Board unless medically indicated. The Board may not require a licensee/applicant to submit to an examination to be conducted an unreasonable distance from the person's home or place of business unless the licensee/applicant resides and works in an area in which there are a limited number of physicians able to perform an appropriate examination.

(7) The guidelines adopted under this subsection do not impair or remove the Board's power to make an independent licensing or disciplinary decision unless a temporary suspension is convened.

(b) Chapter 180 of this title (relating to Texas Physician Health Program and Rehabilitation Orders) shall be applied to acupuncturists who are believed to be impaired and eligible for the Texas Physician Health Program. Rehabilitation orders entered into on or before January 1, 2010 shall be governed by law as it existed immediately before that date.

§ 183.10. Patient Records

(a) Acupuncturists licensed under the Act shall keep and maintain adequate records of all patient visits or consultations which shall, at a minimum, be written in English and include:

(1) the patient's name and address;

(2) vital signs to include body temperature, pulse or heart rate, respiratory rate, and blood pressure upon initial presentation of the patient, and those vital signs as deemed appropriate by the practitioner for follow-up treatment;

(3) the chief complaint of the patient;

(4) a patient history;

(5) a treatment plan for each patient visit or consultation;

(6) a notation of any herbal medications, including amounts and forms, and other modalities used in the course of treatment with corresponding dates for such treatment;

(7) a system of billing records which accurately reflect patient names, services rendered, the date of the services rendered, and the amount charged or billed for each service rendered;

(8) a written record regarding whether or not a patient was evaluated by a physician or dentist, as appropriate, for the condition being treated within 12 months before the date

acupuncture was performed as required by §183.7(a) of this title (relating to Scope of Practice);

(9) a written record regarding whether or not a patient was referred to a physician after the acupuncturist performed acupuncture 20 times or for two months whichever occurs first, as required by §183.7(b) of this title (relating to Scope of Practice) in regard to treatment of patients upon referral by a doctor licensed to practice chiropractic by the Texas Board of Chiropractic Examiners;

(10) in the case of referrals to the acupuncturist of a patient by a doctor licensed to practice chiropractic by the Texas Board of Chiropractic Examiners, the acupuncturist shall record the date of the referral and the most recent date of chiropractic treatment prior to acupuncture treatment; and,

(11) reasonable documentation that the evaluation required by §183.7 of this title (relating to Scope of Practice) was performed or, in the event that the licensee is unable to determine that the evaluation took place, a written statement signed by the patient stating that the patient has been evaluated by a physician within the required time frame on a copy of the following form:

(b) Pursuant to §205.302 of the Act, an acupuncturist shall not be required to keep and maintain the documentation set forth in subsection (a)(11) of this section when performing acupuncture on a patient only for smoking addiction, substance abuse, alcoholism, chronic pain, or weight loss.

(c) Maintenance of Medical and Billing Records.

(1) A licensed acupuncturist shall maintain adequate medical and billing records of a patient for a minimum of five years from the anniversary date of the date of last treatment by the acupuncturist.

(2) If a patient was younger than 18 years of age when last treated by the acupuncturist, the medical and billing records of the patient shall be maintained by the acupuncturist until the patient reaches age 21 or for five years from the date of last treatment, whichever is longer.

(3) Acupuncturists shall retain medical and billing records for such longer length of time than that imposed herein when mandated by other federal or state statute or regulation.

(4) An acupuncturist may destroy medical and billing records that relate to any civil, criminal or administrative proceeding only if the physician knows the proceeding has been finally resolved and the records have been maintained at least as long as required by paragraphs (1)–(3) of this subsection.

(d) Consent for the release of confidential information must be in writing and signed by the patient, or a parent or legal guardian if the patient is a minor, or a legal guardian if the patient has been adjudicated incompetent to manage his or her personal affairs, or an attorney ad litem appointed for the patient, as authorized by the Texas Mental Health Code Subtitle C, Title 7, Health and Safety Code; the Persons with Mental Retardation Act, Subtitle D, Title 7, Health and Safety Code; Chapter 452, Health and Safety Code, (relating to Treatment of Chemically Dependent Persons); Chapter 5, Texas Probate Code; and Chapter 11, Family Code; or a personal representative if the patient is deceased, provided that the written consent specifies the following:

(1) the information or records to be covered by the release;

(2) the reason or purposes for the release; and

(3) the person to whom the information is to be released.

(e) The patient, or other person authorized to consent, has the right to withdraw his or her consent to the release of any information. Withdrawal of consent does not affect any information disclosed prior to the written notice of the withdrawal.

(f) Any person who receives information made confidential by this act may disclose the information to others only to the extent consistent with the authorized purposes for which consent to release the information was obtained.

(g) An acupuncturist shall furnish legible copies of patient records requested, or a summary or narrative of the records in English, pursuant to a written consent for release of the information as provided by subsection (d) of this section, except if the acupuncturist determines that access to the information would be harmful to the physical, mental, or emotional health of the patient. The acupuncturist may delete confidential information about another person who has not consented to the release. The information shall be furnished by the acupuncturist within 30 days after the date of receipt of the request. Reasonable fees for furnishing the information shall be paid by the patient or someone on his or her behalf. If the acupuncturist denies the request, in whole or in part, the acupuncturist shall furnish the patient a written statement, signed and dated, stating the reason for denial. A copy of the statement denying the request shall be placed in the patient's records. In this subsection, "patient records" means any records pertaining to the history, diagnosis, treatment, or prognosis of the patient.

§ 183.11. Complaint Procedure Notification

Pursuant to § 205.152 of the Act, Chapter 178 of this title (relating to Complaints) shall govern acupuncturists with regard to methods of notification for filing complaints with the agency. If the provisions of Chapter 178 of this title conflict with the Act or rules under this chapter, the Act and provisions of this chapter shall control.

§ 183.12. Medical Board Review and Approval

(a) Pursuant to § 205.202 of the Act, the acupuncture board shall issue a license to practice acupuncture in this state to a person who meets the requirements of the Act and the rules adopted pursuant to the Act without approval of the Medical Board.

(b) Pursuant to § 205.352 of the Act, the acupuncture board shall take disciplinary action against a license holder without approval of the Medical Board.

(c) Pursuant to § 205.101(b) of the Act, a rule adopted by the acupuncture board is subject to Medical board approval, which shall be memorialized in the minutes of the medical board, the minutes of a committee of the medical board, or in a writing signed by the medical board's presiding officer, secretary-treasurer, or authorized committee chairman after consideration of the recommendations of the acupuncture board.

§ 183.13. Construction

The provisions of this chapter shall be construed and interpreted so as to be consistent with the statutory provisions of the Act. In the event of a conflict between this chapter and the provisions of the Act, the provisions of the Act shall control; however, this chapter shall be construed so that all other provisions of this chapter which are not in conflict with the Act shall remain in effect.

§ 183.14. Acudetox Specialist

(a) For purposes of this chapter, an "acudetox specialist" shall be defined as a person who is certified to practice auricular acupuncture for the limited purpose of treating alcoholism, substance abuse, and chemical dependency.

(b) Any person who does not possess a Texas acupuncture license or is not otherwise authorized to practice acupuncture under Tex. Occ. Code Ann. Title 3, Subtitle C, Chapter 205, may practice as an acudetox specialist for the sole purpose of the treatment of alcoholism, substance abuse, or chemical dependency upon obtaining certification as an acudetox specialist only under the following conditions listed in paragraphs (1)–(4) of this subsection:

(1) after issuance of certification by the Medical Board, payment of any required fee and receipt of written confirmation of certification from the Medical Board;

(2) after successful completion of a training program in acupuncture for the treatment of alcoholism, substance abuse, or chemical dependency, which has been approved by the Medical Board with advice from the acupuncture board. Such program in auricular acupuncture shall be 70 hours in length, and shall include a clean needle technique course or equivalent universal infection control precaution procedures course approved by the Medical Board;

(3) if the individual holds an unrestricted and current license, registration, or certification issued by the appropriate Texas regulatory agency authorizing practice as a social worker, a licensed professional counselor, a licensed psychologist, a licensed chemical dependency counselor, a licensed vocational nurse, or a licensed registered nurse; provided, however, that such practice of acudetox is not prohibited by the regulatory agency authorizing such practice as a social worker, professional counselor, psychologist, chemical dependency counselor, licensed vocational nurse, or registered nurse; and,

(4) works under the supervision of a current and active licensed Texas physician or licensed Texas acupuncturist, pursuant to written protocols, who is readily available by telephonic means or other methods of communication. Such protocols shall be agreed upon and signed by the supervising Texas licensee and the acudetox specialist, reviewed and signed at least annually and

maintained on site. The acudetox specialist must submit notification of any changes in, or additions to, the person acting as a supervising physician or acupuncturist for the acudetox specialist not later than the 30th day after the date the change or addition is made.

(c) For purposes of this chapter, auricular acupuncture shall be defined as acupuncture treatment limited to the insertion of needles into five acupuncture points in the ear. These points being the liver, kidney, lung, sympathetic and shen men.

(d) Certification as an acudetox specialist shall be subject to suspension, revocation, or cancellation on any grounds substantially similar to those set forth in the Act, § 205.351 or for practicing acupuncture in violation of this chapter.

(e) Practitioners certified as acudetox specialists shall keep records of patient care which at a minimum shall include the dates of treatment, the purpose for the treatment, the name of the patient, the points used, and the name, signature, and title of the certificate-holder.

(f) The fee for certification as an acudetox specialist for the treatment of alcoholism, substance abuse, or chemical dependency shall be set in such an amount as to cover the reasonable cost of administering and enforcing this chapter without recourse to any other funds generated by the Medical or the Acupuncture Board. The application and renewal fees are defined under § 175.1 and § 175.2 of this title (relating to Application and Administrative Fees and Registration and Renewal Fees).

(g) Certificate-holders under this chapter shall keep a current mailing and practice address on file with the Medical Board and shall notify the Medical Board in writing of any address change within ten days of the change of address.

(h) Individuals practicing as an acudetox specialist under the provisions of this chapter shall ensure that any patient receiving such treatment is notified in writing of the qualifications of the individual providing the acudetox treatment and the process for filing complaints with the Medical Board, and shall ensure that a copy of the notification is retained in the patient's record.

(i) Applications for certification as an acudetox specialist shall be submitted in writing on a form approved by the Medical Board which contains the information set forth in subsection (b) of this section and any supporting documentation necessary to confirm such information.

(j) Each individual who is certified as an acudetox specialist may annually renew certification by completing and submitting to the Medical Board an approved renewal form together with the following as listed in paragraphs (1)–(3) of this subsection:

(1) documentation that the certification or license as required by subsection (b)(3) of this section is still valid;

(2) proof of any Continuing Auricular Acupuncture Education (CAAE) obtained as provided for in § 183.21 of this title (relating to Continuing Auricular Acupuncture Education for Acudetox Specialists); and,

(3) payment of a certification renewal fee as set forth under § 175.2 of this title.

（k）Each individual who obtains certification as an acudetox specialist under this section may only use the titles "Certified Acudetox Specialist" or "C. A. S." to denote his or her specialized training.

§ 183.15.　Use of Professional Titles

（a）A licensee shall use the title "Licensed Acupuncturist," "Lic. Ac.," or "L. Ac.," immediately following his/her name on any advertising or other materials visible to the public which pertain to the licensee's practice of acupuncture, except as provided in subsection（b）of this section. Only persons licensed as an acupuncturist may use these titles. A licensee who is also licensed in Texas as a physician, dentist, chiropractor, optometrist, podiatrist, and /or veterinarian is exempt from the requirement that the licensee's acupuncture title immediately follow his/her name.

（b）If a licensee uses any additional title or designation, it shall be the responsibility of the licensee to comply with the provisions of the Healing Art Identification Act, Texas Occupations Code Annotated, Chapter 104, that require individuals to designate the authority under which the title is used or the college or honorary degree that gives rise to the use of the title. A licensee may use the additional title or designation in materials described in subsection（a）of this section, immediately before or after the title "Licensed Acupuncturist," "Lic. Ac.," or "L. Ac.".

§ 183.16.　Texas Acupuncture Schools

（a）A licensed Texas acupuncturist operating an acupuncture school in Texas which has not yet been accredited by the Accreditation Commission for Acupuncture and Oriental Medicine （ACAOM）or reached candidate status for accreditation by ACAOM, a licensed Texas acupuncturist with any ownership interest in such a school, or a licensed Texas acupuncturist who teaches in or operates such a school, shall ensure that students of the school and applicants to the school are made aware of the provisions of the Medical Practice Act governing acupuncture practice, the rules and regulations adopted by the Texas State Board of Acupuncture Examiners, and the educational requirements for obtaining a Texas acupuncture license to include the rules and regulations establishing the criteria for an approved acupuncture school for purposes of licensure as an acupuncturist by the Texas State Board of Acupuncture Examiners as set forth in subsection （b）of this section.

（b）Compliance with the provisions of subsection（a）of this section shall be accomplished by providing students and applicants with a copy of Subchapter H of the Act, a copy of Chapter 183（Acupuncture）contained in the Rules of the Texas Medical Board, and the following typed statement：

（c）A licensed Texas acupuncturist who operates, teaches at, or owns, in whole or in part, a Texas acupuncture school which is not accredited by ACAOM or is not a candidate for ACAOM accreditation shall not state directly or indirectly, explicitly or by implication, orally or in writing, either personally or through an agent of the acupuncturist or the school, that the school is endorsed, accredited, registered with, affiliated with, or otherwise approved by the Texas State Board of Acupuncture Examiners for any purpose.

(d) Failure to comply with the requirements or abide by the prohibitions of this section shall be grounds for disciplinary action against a licensed Texas acupuncturist who operates, teaches at, or owns, in whole or in part, a Texas acupuncture school which is not accredited by ACAOM or is not a candidate for ACAOM accreditation. Such disciplinary action shall be based on the violation of a rule of the Texas State Board of Acupuncture Examiners as provided for in the Act, § 205.351(a)(6).

(e) For purposes of licensure and regulation of acupuncturists practicing in Texas, ACAOM approved acupuncture schools in Texas meeting the criteria set forth in § 183.2 of this title (relating to Definitions) may issue masters of science in oriental medicine degrees in a manner consistent with the laws of the State of Texas. The Texas State Board of Acupuncture Examiners shall recognize any such lawfully issued degrees. For purposes of licensure and regulation of acupuncturists practicing in Texas, acupuncture schools in Texas which are ACAOM candidates for masters level programs in acupuncture and oriental medicine and who have issued diplomas or degrees during the period of candidacy, may upgrade such degrees to masters degrees upon obtaining full ACAOM accreditation. The Texas State Board of Acupuncture Examiners shall recognize any such lawfully upgraded degrees.

§ 183.17. Compliance

Chapter 189 of this title (relating to Compliance) shall be applied to acupuncturists who are under board orders. If the provisions of Chapter 189 conflict with the Act or rules under this chapter, the Act and provisions of this chapter shall control.

§ 183.18. Administrative Penalties

(a) Pursuant to § 205.352 of the Act and Chapter 165 of the Medical Practice Act, the board by order may impose an administrative penalty, subject to the provisions of the APA, against a person licensed or regulated under the Act who violates the Act or a rule or order adopted under the Act. The imposition of such a penalty shall be consistent with the requirements of the Act and the APA.

(b) The penalty for a violation may be in an amount not to exceed $5,000. Each day a violation continues or occurs is a separate violation for purposes of imposing a penalty.

(c) Prior to the imposition of an administrative penalty by board order, a person must be given notice and opportunity to respond and present evidence and argument on each issue that is the basis for the proposed administrative penalty at a show compliance proceeding.

(d) The amount of the penalty shall be based on the factors set forth under Chapter 190 of this title (relating to Disciplinary Guidelines).

(e) If the board by order determines that a violation has occurred and imposes an administrative penalty on a person licensed or regulated under the Act, the board shall give notice to the person of the board's order which shall include a statement of the right of the person to seek judicial review of the order.

(f) An administrative penalty may be imposed under this section for the following:

(1) failure to timely comply with a board subpoena issued by the board shall be grounds for the imposition of an administrative penalty of no less than $100 and no more than $5,000 for each separate violation;

(2) failure to timely comply with the terms, conditions, or requirements of a board order shall be grounds for imposition of an administrative penalty of no less than $100 and no more than $5,000 for each separate violation;

(3) failure to timely report a change of address to the board shall be grounds for imposition of an administrative penalty of no less than $100 and no more than $5,000 for each separate violation;

(4) failure to timely respond to a patient's communications shall be grounds for imposition of an administrative penalty of no less than $100 and no more than $5,000 for each separate violation;

(5) failure to comply with the complaint procedure notification requirements as set forth in § 183.11 of this chapter (relating to Complaint Procedure Notification) shall be grounds for imposition of an administrative penalty of no less than $100 and no more than $5,000 for each separate violation;

(6) failure to provide show compliance proceeding information in the prescribed time shall be grounds for imposition of an administrative penalty of no less than $100 and no more than $5,000 for each separate violation; and

(7) for any other violation other than quality of care that the board deems appropriate shall be grounds for imposition of an administrative penalty of no less than $100 and no more than $5,000 for each separate violation.

(g) Any order proposed under this section shall be subject to final approval by the board.

(h) Failure to pay an administrative penalty imposed through an order shall be grounds for disciplinary action by the board pursuant to the Act, § 205.351 (a) (10), regarding unprofessional or dishonorable conduct likely to deceive or defraud, or injure the public, and shall also be grounds for the executive director to refer the matter to the attorney general for collection of the amount of the penalty.

(i) A person who becomes financially unable to pay an administrative penalty after entry of an order imposing such a penalty, upon a showing of good cause by a writing executed by the person under oath and at the discretion of the Discipline and Ethics Committee of the board, may be granted an extension of time or deferral of no more than one year from the date the administrative penalty is due. Upon the conclusion of any such extension of time or deferral, if payment has not been made in the manner and in the amount required, action authorized by the terms of the order or subsection (h) of this section.

§ 183.19. Acupuncture Advertising

Acupuncturists shall not authorize or use false, misleading, or deceptive advertising, and, in addition, shall not engage in any of the following:

(1) hold themselves out as a physician or surgeon or any combination or derivative of those terms unless also licensed by the medical board as a physician or surgeon as defined under the Medical Practice Act, Tex. Occ. Code Ann. § 151.002(a)(13) (relating to Definitions);

(2) use the terms "board certified" unless the advertising also discloses the complete name of the board which conferred the referenced certification; or,

(3) use the terms "board certified" or any similar words or phrases calculated to convey the same meaning if the advertised board certification has expired and has not been renewed at the time the advertising in question was published, broadcast, or otherwise promulgated.

§ 183.20. Continuing Acupuncture Education

(a) Purpose. This section is promulgated to promote the health, safety, and welfare of the people of Texas through the establishment of minimum requirements for continuing acupuncture education (CAE) for licensed Texas acupuncturists so as to further enhance their professional skills and knowledge.

(b) Minimum Continuing Acupuncture Education. As a prerequisite to the biennial registration of the license of an acupuncturist, the acupuncturist shall complete 34 hours of CAE every 24 months.

(1) The required hours shall be from courses that meet one of the following criteria at the time the hours are taken:

(A) are designated or otherwise approved for credit by the Texas State Board of Acupuncture Examiners based on a review and recommendation of the course content by the Education Committee of the board as described in subsection (n) of this section;

(B) are offered by providers approved by the Texas State Board of Acupuncture Examiners;

(C) have been approved for CAE credit for a minimum of three years by another state acupuncture board, having first gone through a formal approval process in such state;

(D) approved by the NCCAOM (National Certification Commission for Acupuncture and Oriental Medicine) for professional development activity credit; or

(E) are provided outside of the United States by a provider of continuing acupuncture education that is acceptable to the Board.

(2) The required CAE hours shall include the following core hours:

(A) at least eight hours shall be in general acupuncture therapies;

(B) at least two of the required hours shall be from a course in ethics and safety;

(C) at least six of the required hours shall be in herbology; and

(D) at least four hours of biomedicine.

(3) The remaining CAE hours may be from other courses approved under paragraph (1) of this subsection, subject to the limitations under paragraphs (5) through (7) of this subsection.

(4) Courses may be taught through live lecture, distance learning, or the Internet.

(5) No more than four hours in courses that relate to business practices or office administration may be applied to the total hours required for each registration period.

(6) No more than a total of 16 hours completed under paragraph (1)(D) or (E) of this subsection may be applied to the total hours required each registration period.

(7) At least 18 hours applied to the total hours required each registration period must be approved under paragraph (1)(A) - (C) of this subsection.

(8) The required CAE shall include the completion of a course in human trafficking prevention approved by the executive commissioner of the Texas Health and Human Services Commission. The course may be counted as part of the minimum 18 hours approved under paragraph (1)(A)-(C) of this subsection.

(c) Reporting Continuing Acupuncture Education. An acupuncturist must report on the licensee's registration form whether the licensee has completed the required acupuncture education during the previous two years.

(d) Grounds for Exemption from Continuing Acupuncture Education. An acupuncturist may request in writing and may be exempt from the biennial minimum continuing acupuncture education requirements for one or more of the following reasons:

(1) the licensee's catastrophic illness;

(2) the licensee's military service of longer than one year in duration;

(3) the licensee's acupuncture practice and residence of longer than one year in duration outside the United States; and/or

(4) good cause shown on written application of the licensee which gives satisfactory evidence to the board that the licensee is unable to comply with the requirements of continuing acupuncture education.

(e) Exemption Requests. Exemption requests shall be subject to the approval of the executive director of the board, and shall be submitted in writing at least 30 days prior to the expiration of the license.

(f) Exemption Duration and Renewal. An exemption granted under subsections (d) and (e) of this section may not exceed one year, but may be renewed biennially upon written request submitted at least 30 days prior to the expiration of the current exemption.

(g) Verification of Credits. The board may require written verification of continuing acupuncture education hours from any licensee and the licensee shall provide the requested verification within 30 calendar days of the date of the request. Failure to timely provide the requested verification may result in disciplinary action by the board.

(h) Nonrenewal for Insufficient Continuing Acupuncture Education. Unless exempted under the terms of this section, the apparent failure of an acupuncturist to obtain and timely report the 34 hours of continuing education hours as required and provided for in this section shall result in nonrenewal of the license until such time as the acupuncturist obtains and reports the required hours; however, the executive director of the board may issue to such an acupuncturist a temporary license numbered so as to correspond to the non-renewed license. Such a temporary license issued pursuant to this subsection may be issued to allow the board to verify the accuracy of information related to the continuing acupuncture education hours of the acupuncturist and to allow the acupuncturist who has not obtained or timely reported the required number of hours an opportunity to correct any deficiency so as not to require termination of ongoing patient care.

(i) Fee for Issuance of Temporary License. The fee for issuance of a temporary license pursuant to the provisions of this section shall be in the amount specified under § 175.1 of this title (relating to Application Fees); however, the fee need not be paid prior to the issuance of the temporary license, but shall be paid prior to the renewal of a permanent license.

(j) Application of Additional Hours. Continuing acupuncture education hours that are obtained to comply with the requirements for the preceding registration period, as a prerequisite for licensure renewal, shall first be credited to meet the requirements for that previous registration period. Once the requirements of the previous registration period are satisfied, any additional hours obtained shall be credited to meet the continuing acupuncture education requirements of the current registration period. A licensee may carry forward CAE hours earned prior to a biennial registration report, which are in excess of the 34-hour biennial requirement and such excess hours may be applied to the following registration periods' requirements, except for the required course under subsection (b)(8) of this section. A maximum of 34 total excess hours may be carried forward. Excess CAE hours may not be carried forward or applied to a biennial report of CAE more than two years beyond the date of the registration following the period during which the hours were earned.

(k) False Reports/Statements. An intentionally false report or statement to the board by a licensee regarding continuing acupuncture education hours reportedly obtained shall be a basis for disciplinary action by the board pursuant to the Act, § 205.351(a)(2) and (6).

(l) Monetary Penalty. Failure to obtain and timely report the continuing acupuncture education hours for renewal of a license shall subject the licensee to a monetary penalty for late registration in the amount set forth in § 175.2 and § 175.3 of this title (relating to Registration and Renewal Fees and Penalties).

(m) Disciplinary Action, Conditional Licensure, and Construction. This section shall be construed to allow the board to impose requirements for completion of additional continuing acupuncture education hours for purposes of disciplinary action and conditional licensure.

(n) Required Content for Continuing Acupuncture Education Courses. Continuing Acupuncture

Education courses must meet the following requirements:

(1) the content of the course, program, or activity is related to the practice of acupuncture or oriental medicine, and shall:

(A) be related to the knowledge and/or technical skills required to practice acupuncture; or

(B) be related to direct and/or indirect patient care;

(2) the method of instruction is adequate to teach the content of the course, program, or activity;

(3) the credentials of the instructor (s) indicate competency and sufficient training, education, and experience to teach the specific course, program, or activity;

(4) the education provider maintains an accurate attendance/participation record on individuals completing the course, program, or activity;

(5) each credit hour for the course, program, or activity is equal to no less than 50 minutes of actual instruction or training;

(6) the course, program, or activity is provided by a knowledgeable health care provider or reputable school, state, or professional organization;

(7) the course description provides adequate information so that each participant understands the basis for the program and the goals and objectives to be met; and

(8) the education provider obtains written evaluations at the end of each program, collate the evaluations in a statistical summary, and makes the summary available to the board upon request.

(o) Continuing Acupuncture Education Approval Requests. All requests for approval of courses, programs, or activities for purposes of satisfying CAE credit requirements shall be submitted in writing to the Education Committee of the board on a form approved by the board, along with any required fee, and accompanied by information, documents, and materials accurately describing the course, program, or activity, and necessary for verifying compliance with the requirements set forth in subsection (n) of this section. At the discretion of the board or the Education Committee, supplemental information, documents, and materials may be requested as needed to obtain an adequate description of the course, program, or activity and to verify compliance with the requirements set forth in subsection (n) of this section. At the discretion of the board or the Education Committee, inspection of original supporting documents may be required for a determination on an approval request. The Acupuncture Board shall have the authority to conduct random and periodic checks of courses, programs, or activities to ensure that criteria for education approval as set forth in subsection (n) of this section have been met and continue to be met by the education provider. Upon requesting approval of a course, program, or activity, the education provider shall agree to such checks by the Acupuncture Board or its designees, and shall further agree to provide supplemental information, documents, and material describing the course, program, or activity which, in the discretion of the Acupuncture Board, may be needed for approval or continued approval of the course, program, or activity. Failure of an education provider to provide the necessary information, documents, and materials to show compliance with the standards set forth in subsection (n) of this section shall be grounds for denial of CAE approval or rescission of prior approval in regard to the course, program, or activity.

(p) Reconsideration of Denials of Approval Requests. Determinations to deny approval of a CAE course, program, or activity may be reconsidered by the Education Committee or the board based on additional information concerning the course, program, or activity, or upon a showing of good cause for reconsideration. A decision to reconsider a denial determination shall be a discretionary decision based on consideration of the additional information or the good cause showing. Requests for reconsideration shall be made in writing by the education provider, and may be made orally or in writing by board staff or a committee of the board.

(q) Reconsideration of Approvals. Determinations to approve a CAE course, program, or activity may be reconsidered by the Education Committee or the board based on additional information concerning the course, program, or activity, or upon a showing of good cause. A decision to reconsider an approval determination shall be a discretionary decision based on consideration of the additional information or the good cause showing. Requests for reconsideration may be made in writing by a member of the public or may be made orally or in writing by board staff or a committee of the board.

(r) Criteria for Provider Approval.

(1) In order to be an approved provider, a provider shall submit to the board a provider application on a form approved by the board, along with any required fee. All provider applications and documentation submitted to the board shall be typewritten and in English.

(2) To become an approved provider, a provider shall submit to the board evidence that the provider has three continuous years of previous experience providing at least one different CAE course in Texas in each of those years that were approved by the board. In addition the provider must have no history of complaints or reprimands with the board.

(3) The approval of the provider shall expire three years after it is issued by the board and may be renewed upon the filing of the required application, along with any required fee.

(4) Acupuncture schools and colleges which have been approved by the board, as defined under § 183.2(2) of this title (relating to Definitions), who seek to be approved providers shall be required to submit an application for an approved provider number to the board.

(s) Requirements of Approved Providers.

(1) For the purpose of this chapter, the title "approved provider" can only be used when a person or organization has submitted a provider application form, and has been issued a provider number unless otherwise provided.

(2) A person or organization may be issued only one provider number. When two or more approved providers co-sponsor a course, the course shall be identified by only one provider number and that provider shall assume responsibility for recordkeeping, advertising, issuance of certificates and instructor(s) qualifications.

(3) An approved provider shall offer CAE programs that are presented or instructed by persons who meet the minimum criteria as described in subsection (t) of this section.

(4) An approved provider shall keep the following records for a period of four years in one identified location:

(A) course outlines of each course given;

(B) record of time and places of each course given;

(C) course instructor curriculum vitaes or resumes;

(D) the attendance record for each course; and

(E) participant evaluation forms for each course given.

(5) An approved provider shall submit to the board the following within ten days of the board's request:

(A) a copy of the attendance record showing the name, signature and license number of any licensed acupuncturists who attended the course; and

(B) the participant evaluation forms of the course.

(6) Approved providers shall issue, within 60 days of the conclusion of a course, to each participant who has completed the course, a certificate of completion that contains the following information:

(A) provider's name and number;

(B) course title;

(C) participant's name and, if applicable, his or her acupuncture license number;

(D) date and location of course;

(E) number of continuing education hours completed;

(F) description of hours indicating whether hours completed are in general acupuncture, ethics, herbology, biomedicine, or practice management; and

(G) statement directing the acupuncturist to retain the certificate for at least four years from the date of completion of the course.

(7) Approved providers shall notify the board within 30 days of any changes in organizational structure of a provider and/or the person(s) responsible for the provider's continuing education course, including name, address, or telephone number changes.

(8) Provider approval is non-transferable.

(9) The board may audit during reasonable business hours records, courses, instructors and related activities of an approved provider.

(t) Instructors.

(1) Minimum qualifications of an acupuncturist instructor. The instructor must:

(A) hold a current valid license to practice acupuncture in Texas or other state and be free of any disciplinary order or probation by a state licensing authority; and

(B) be knowledgeable, current and skillful in the subject matter of the course as evidenced through one of the following:

(i) hold a minimum of a master's degree from an accredited college or university or a post-secondary educational institution, with a major in the subject directly related to the content of the program to be presented;

(ii) have experience in teaching similar subject matter content within the last two years in the specialized area in which he or she is teaching;

(iii) have at least one year's experience within the last two years in the specialized area in which he or she is teaching; or

(iv) have graduated from an acceptable acupuncture school, as defined under § 183.2(2) of this title, and have completed 3 years of professional experience in the licensed practice of acupuncture.

(2) Minimum qualifications of a non-acupuncturist instructor. The instructor must:

(A) be currently licensed or certified in his or her area of expertise if appropriate;

(B) show written evidence of specialized training or experience, which may include, but not be limited to, a certificate of training or an advanced degree in a given subject area; and

(C) have at least one year's teaching experience within the last two years in the specialized area in which he or she teaches.

(u) CAE Credit for Course Instruction. Instructors of board-approved CAE courses or courses taught through a program offered by an approved provider for CAE credit may receive three hours of CAE credit for each hour of lecture, not to exceed six hours of continuing education credit per year, regardless of how many hours taught. Participation as a member of a panel presentation for the approved course shall not entitle the participant to earn CAE credit as an instructor. No CAE credit shall be granted to school faculty members as credit for their regular teaching assignments.

(v) Expiration, Denial and Withdrawal of Approval.

(1) Approval of any CAE course shall expire three years after the date of approval.

(2) The board may withdraw its approval of a provider or deny an application for approval if the provider is convicted of a crime substantially related to the activities of a provider.

(3) Any material misrepresentation of fact by a provider or applicant in any information required to be submitted to the board is grounds for withdrawal of approval or denial of an application.

(4) The board may withdraw its approval of a provider after giving the provider written notice setting forth its reasons for withdrawal and after giving the provider a reasonable

opportunity to be heard by the board or its designee.

(5) Should the board deny approval of a provider, the provider may appeal the action by filing a letter stating the reason(s) with the board. The letter of appeal shall be filed with the board within ten days of the mailing of the applicant's notification of the board's denial. The appeal shall be considered by the board.

(w) An acupuncturist, who is a military service member, may request an extension of time, not to exceed two years, to complete any CAE requirements.

§ 183.21. Continuing Auricular Acupuncture Education for Acudetox Specialists

(a) Purpose. This section is promulgated to promote the health, safety, and welfare of the people of Texas through the establishment of minimum requirements for continuing auricular acupuncture education (CAAE) for certified acudetox specialists so as to further enhance their professional skills and knowledge.

(b) Minimum continuing auricular acupuncture education. As a prerequisite to the re-certification of an acudetox specialist, the acudetox specialist shall provide documentation to the Medical Board that the individual has successfully met the continuing education requirements established by the board which includes the following listed in paragraphs (1)-(2) of this subsection:

(1) At least six hours of CAAE each year shall be in the practice of auricular acupuncture;

(2) The required hours shall be from courses that are designated or otherwise approved for credit by the Medical Board at the time the course was taken.

(c) Reporting continuing auricular acupuncture education. An acudetox specialist must report on the certificate-holder's re-certification form the number of hours and type of continuing auricular acupuncture education completed during the previous year.

(d) Grounds for exemption from continuing auricular acupuncture education. An acudetox specialist may request in writing and may be exempt from the annual minimum continuing auricular acupuncture education requirements for one or more of the following reasons listed in paragraphs (1)-(2) of this subsection:

(1) catastrophic illness; and/or

(2) military service of longer than one year in duration;

(e) Exemption requests. Exemption requests shall be subject to the approval of the executive director of the Medical Board, and shall be submitted in writing at least 30 days prior to the expiration of the certificate.

(f) Exemption duration and renewal. An exemption granted under subsections (d) and (e) of this section may not exceed one year, but may be renewed annually upon written request submitted at least 30 days prior to the expiration of the current exemption.

(g) Verification of credits. The board may require written verification of continuing auricular acupuncture education hours from any certified acudetox specialist and the certificate-holder shall provide the requested verification within 30 calendar days of the date of the request. Failure to timely provide the requested verification may result in disciplinary action by the board.

(h) Approval of continuing auricular acupuncture education. Continuing Auricular Acupuncture Education (CAAE) credit hours shall be approved by the Medical Board and shall include education by a ACAOM accredited school or other nationally recognized institution, organization, or training program approved by the Medical Board. Approval of courses shall be by January 1, 1999. The first reporting of CAE shall be required for certification renewal in 2000. Approval shall be based on a showing by the education provider that:

(1) the content of the course, program, or activity is related to the practice of acudetox, and is not a course on practice enhancement, business, or office administration;

(2) the method of instruction is adequate to teach the content of the course, program, or activity;

(3) the credentials of the instructor(s) indicate competency and sufficient training, education, and experience to teach the specific course, program, or activity;

(4) the education provider maintains an accurate attendance/participation record on individuals completing the course, program, or activity; and,

(5) each credit hour for the course, program, or activity is equal to no less than 50 minutes of actual instruction or training.

(i) False Reports/Statements. An intentionally false report or statement to the board by a certificate-holder regarding continuing auricular acupuncture education hours reportedly obtained shall be a basis for disciplinary action by the board pursuant to the Act, § 205.351(a)(2) and (6).

(j) Monetary penalty. Failure to obtain and timely report the continuing auricular acupuncture education hours for renewal of a certificate shall subject the certificate-holder to a monetary penalty for late registration in the amount set forth in § 175.2 of this title (relating to Registration and Renewal Fees) and § 175.3 of this title (relating to Penalties).

(k) Disciplinary action, conditional licensure, and construction. This section shall be construed to allow the board to impose requirements for completion of additional continuing auricular acupuncture education hours for purposes of disciplinary action and conditional licensure.

§ 183.22. Language Requirements

(a) All medical records and prescriptions are to be written in English with the exception of acupuncture terms, including herbs, that are more frequently known by their Chinese or Pinyin translation, if appropriate.

(b) All written instructions to patients must be in English. If the patient does not speak English then the acupuncturist shall make reasonable efforts to translate to the patient's native language.

§ 183.23. Voluntary Surrender of Acupuncture License

Pursuant to Section 205.3522 of the Act, the Board may accept the voluntary surrender of an acupuncture license. Chapter 196 of this title (relating to Voluntary Surrender of a Medical License) shall govern the voluntary surrender of an acupuncture license in a similar manner as that chapter applies to a medical license. Section 183.4 of this title (relating to Licensure) shall govern reapplication after a voluntary surrender.

§ 183.24. Procedure

Chapter 187 of this title (relating to Procedural Rules) shall govern procedures relating to acupuncturists where applicable. If the provisions of Chapter 187 conflict with the Act or rules under this chapter, the Act and provisions of this chapter shall control.

§ 183.25. Inactive Status License

(a) A license holder may have the license holder's license placed on inactive status by applying to the board. A license holder with an inactive status license may not practice as an acupuncturist in Texas.

(b) In order for a license holder to be placed on inactive status, the license holder must have a current registration permit and have a license in good standing.

(c) A license holder who practices as an acupuncturist in Texas while on inactive status is considered to be practicing without a license.

(d) A license holder may return to active status by applying to the board, paying an application fee equal to an application fee for an acupuncture license, complying with the requirements for license renewal under the Act, providing current certifications of good standing from each other state in which the acupuncturist holds an acupuncture license, and complying with subsection (e) of this section.

(e) An inactive status license holder applying to return to active status shall provide sufficient documentation to the board that the applicant has, on a full-time basis as defined in § 183.4(a)(9)(B) of this title (relating to Licensure), actively practiced acupuncture or has been on the active teaching faculty of an acceptable approved acupuncture school, within either of the two years preceding receipt of an application for reactivation. Applicants who do not meet this requirement may, in the discretion of the board, be eligible for the reactivation of a license subject to one or more of the following conditions or restrictions as set forth in paragraphs (1) – (4) of this subsection:

(1) completion of specified continuing acupuncture education hours qualifying under § 183.20 of this title (relating to Continuing Acupuncture Education);

(2) limitation and/or exclusion of the practice of the applicant to specified activities of the practice;

(3) remedial education; and/or

(4) such other remedial or restrictive conditions or requirements which, in the discretion of

the board are necessary to ensure protection of the public and minimal competency of the applicant to safely practice as an acupuncturist.

(f) After five years on inactive status, the license holders license shall be canceled as if by request. The acupuncturist may obtain a new license by complying with the requirements and procedures for obtaining an original license. After such cancellation, the acupuncturist may apply for a new license. The acupuncturist shall be required to follow the standard requirements and procedures for obtaining licensure.

§ 183.26. Retired License

(a) The registration renewal fee shall not apply to retired license holders. To be placed in retired status:

(1) the license holder must not be under an investigation or an active order with the board or otherwise have a restricted license; and

(2) the license holder must request in writing on a form prescribed by the board that his or her license be placed on official retired status.

(b) The following restrictions shall apply to license holders whose licenses are on official retired status:

(1) the license holder must not engage in the practice of acupuncture in any state; and

(2) the license holder's license may not be endorsed to any other state.

(c) A license holder may apply to return to active practice as follows:

(1) A retired status license holder who has been in a retired status for less than two years may apply to return to active status by applying to the board, paying an application fee equal to an application fee for a acupuncture license, complying with the requirements for license renewal under the Act, and complying with paragraph (2)(A)-(D) of this subsection, if applicable.

(2) The request of a retired status license holder seeking a return to active status whose license has been placed on official retired status for two years or longer shall be submitted to the Licensure Committee of the board for consideration and a recommendation to the full board for approval or denial of the request. After consideration of the request and the recommendation of the Licensure Committee, the board shall grant or deny the request. If the request is granted, it may be granted without conditions or subject to such conditions which the board determines are necessary to adequately protect the public including but not limited to:

(A) completion of specified continuing acupuncture education hours qualifying under § 183.20 of this title (relating to Continuing Acupuncture Education);

(B) limitation and/or exclusion of the practice of the applicant to specified activities of practice;

(C) remedial education; and/or

(D) such other remedial or restrictive conditions or requirements which, in the discretion of the board are necessary to ensure protection of the public and minimal competency of the applicant to safely practice as an acupuncturist.

(3) The request of a license holder seeking a return to active status whose license has been placed on official retired status for less than two years may be approved by the executive director of the board or submitted by the executive director to the Licensure Committee for consideration and a recommendation to the full board for approval or denial of the request. In those instances in which the executive director submits the request to the Licensure Committee of the board, the Licensure Committee shall make a recommendation to the full board for approval or denial. After consideration of the request and the recommendation of the Licensure Committee, the board shall grant or deny the request subject to such conditions which the board determines are necessary to adequately protect the public including but not limited to those options provided in paragraph (2)(A)-(D) of this subsection.

(4) In evaluating a request to return to active status, the Licensure Committee or the full board may require a personal appearance by the requesting license holder at the offices of the board, and may also require a physical or mental examination by one or more physicians or other health care providers approved in advance in writing by the executive director, the secretary-treasurer, the Licensure Committee, or other designee(s) determined by majority vote of the board.

§ 183.27. Exemption from Licensure for Certain Military Spouses

(a) The executive director of the Texas Medical Board must authorize a qualified military spouse to engage in the practice of acupuncture in Texas without obtaining a license in accordance with § 55.0041(a), Texas Occupations Code. This authorization to practice is valid during the time the military service member to whom the military spouse is married is stationed at a military installation in Texas, but not to exceed three years.

(b) In order to receive authorization to practice the military spouse must:

(1) hold an active acupuncture license in another state, territory, Canadian province, or country that:

(A) has licensing requirements that are determined by the board to be substantially equivalent to the requirements for licensure in Texas; and

(B) is not subject to any restriction, disciplinary order, probation, or investigation; and

(2) notify the board of the military spouse's intent to practice in Texas on a form prescribed by the board; and

(3) submit proof of the military spouse's residency in this state, a copy of the spouse's military identification card, and proof of the military member's status as an active duty military service member as defined by § 437.001(1), Texas Government Code (relating to Definitions).

(c) While authorized to practice acupuncture in Texas, the military spouse shall comply with all other laws and regulations applicable to the practice of acupuncture in Texas.

(d) Once the board receives the form containing notice of a military spouse's intent to practice in Texas, the board will verify whether the military spouse's license in another state, territory, Canadian province, or country is active and in good standing. Additionally, the board will determine whether the licensing requirements in that jurisdiction are substantially equivalent to the requirements for licensure in Texas.

WEST'S HAWAI'I

§ 436E – 1. Declaration of necessity for regulation and control

The legislature hereby finds and declares that the practice of acupuncture is a theory and method for treatment of illness and disability and for strengthening and invigorating the body and as such affects the public health, safety, and welfare, and therefore there is a necessity that individuals practicing acupuncture be subject to regulation and control.

§ 436E – 2. Definitions

As used in this chapter:

"Acupuncture practitioner" means a person engaged in the practice of acupuncture.

"Board" means the board of acupuncture.

"Department" means the department of commerce and consumer affairs.

"Director" means the director of commerce and consumer affairs.

"Earned degree" means an academically or a clinically obtained degree (not honorary).

"Practice of acupuncture" means stimulation of a certain acupuncture point or points on the human body for the purpose of controlling and regulating the flow and balance of energy in the body. The practice includes the techniques of piercing the skin by inserting needles and point stimulation by the use of acupressure, electrical, mechanical, thermal, or traditional therapeutic means.

§ 436E – 3. License required

Except as otherwise provided by law, no person shall practice acupuncture in this State either gratuitously or for pay, or shall offer to so practice, or shall announce themselves either publicly or privately as prepared or qualified to so practice any method of acupuncture without having a valid unrevoked license or intern permit from the State; provided that the requirement for a permit shall not be enforced until the board has initially adopted rules pursuant to section

436E – 3.6.

§ 436E – 3.5. Physicians and osteopaths not exempt

Persons licensed under chapter 453 who desire to practice acupuncture shall be subject to licensing under this chapter.

§ 436E – 3.6. Acupuncture intern permit required

(a) Except as otherwise provided by law, no person shall practice as an acupuncture intern in this State either gratuitously or for pay, without having first obtained a permit from the board. This permit shall entitle the applicant to engage in the practice of acupuncture for a period of four years under the immediate supervision of a licensed acupuncturist duly licensed under this chapter.

(b) An acupuncture intern permit may be reissued once, for a period not to exceed one year, upon written request to the board and payment of the required fee.

(c) The board shall adopt rules pursuant to chapter 91 defining the functions of an acupuncture intern, establishing the requirements to be met by an applicant for an acupuncture intern permit, and specifying the procedures for the immediate supervision of the acupuncture intern by a licensed acupuncturist.

§ 436E – 4. Exemptions

A licensed acupuncturist of another state or country for demonstrations or lectures to be given at acupuncture or medical society meetings or at acupuncture schools shall be exempt from licensing procedures set forth in this chapter.

§ 436E – 5. Qualifications for examination

(a) No person shall be licensed to practice acupuncture unless the person has passed an examination and has been found to have the necessary qualifications as prescribed in the rules adopted by the board pursuant to chapter 91.

(b) Prior to September 1, 2000, and except as provided in subsection (c), before any applicant shall be eligible for the examination, the applicant shall furnish satisfactory proof to the board that the applicant has received a total of not less than one thousand five hundred hours of education and training consisting of:

(1) A formal program in the science of acupuncture (traditional oriental medicine) at an institute or school approved by the board that:

(A) Shall be for a period of not less than two academic years (not less than six hundred hours); and

(B) Shall result in the award of a certificate or diploma; and

(2) One clinical year in a clinical internship program (not less than twelve months and not less than nine hundred hours) supervised by a licensed acupuncturist; provided that the nine hundred hours of the clinical internship program may be obtained from the institute or school awarding the certificate or diploma or may be obtained under the supervision of a licensed acupuncturist not affiliated with an institute or school.

(c) Students who started training prior to December 31, 1984, in a school approved by the board prior to December 31, 1984, and who complete their training by December 31, 1989, and who file an application with the board before September 1, 2000 shall:

(1) Not lose their rights of continued education, and earned or accumulated credits; and

(2) For the purposes of this chapter, meet requirements for examination and licensure as provided in chapter 436D and rules adopted by the board as they existed on December 31, 1984; provided that the school has not altered its program so as to lower the standards for completion of the program. These students may qualify for examination if they submit evidence of having completed:

(A) At least eighteen months (not less than five hundred seventy-six hours) of academic training; and

(B) At least six months (not less than four hundred eighty hours) of clinical training in the practice of acupuncture on human subjects under the supervision of a licensed acupuncturist.

(d) Notwithstanding subsections (b) and (c), effective September 1, 2000, before any applicant shall be eligible to take the licensing examination, the applicant shall furnish satisfactory proof to the board that the applicant has completed a formal acupuncture program and has received a total of at least two thousand, one hundred seventy-five hours of academic and clinical training consisting of an academic program of at least one thousand, five hundred fifteen hours in the science of acupuncture (traditional oriental medicine) and a clinical training program of at least six hundred sixty hours under the supervision of a licensed acupuncturist, which shall result in the award of a certificate or diploma. For applicants who graduated from an institute, school, or college located in the United States or any territory under the jurisdiction of the United States, the institute, school, or college shall be accredited or recognized as a candidate for accreditation by any acupuncture or oriental medicine accrediting body recognized by the United States Department of Education. For applicants who graduated from a foreign institute, school, or college with a formal program in the science of acupuncture, the applicant, at the applicant's own expense, shall have the applicant's transcripts and curriculum evaluated by a board approved and designated professional evaluator who shall make a determination whether the transcripts and curriculum are at least equivalent to that of the United States accredited acupuncture program, and that the foreign institute is licensed, approved, or accredited by the appropriate governmental authority or an agency recognized by a governmental authority in the respective foreign jurisdiction and whose curriculum is approved by the board.

§ 436E - 6. Board of acupuncture

(a) There shall be a board of acupuncture, the members of which shall be appointed by the governor.

The board shall consist of five persons, two of whom shall be private citizens and three shall be acupuncturists licensed in accordance with this chapter.

(b) Commencing July 1, 1992, and thereafter, each person appointed to the board shall have a four-year term and shall serve not more than two consecutive terms. Members appointed to the board prior to July 1, 1992, shall be permitted to continue to serve on the board until such time when a maximum of eight consecutive years from the date of initial appointment has been attained.

§ 436E – 7. Powers and duties of the board

In addition to any other powers and duties authorized by law, the board shall:

(1) Adopt rules in accordance with chapter 91 to carry out the purposes of this chapter, with special emphasis on the health and safety of the public;

(2) Develop standards for licensure;

(3) Prepare, administer, and grade examinations, provided that the board may contract with a testing agency to provide those services;

(4) Issue, renew, suspend, and revoke licenses;

(5) Register applicants or holders of a license;

(6) Investigate and conduct hearings regarding any violation of this chapter and any rules of the board;

(7) Maintain a record of its proceedings; and

(8) Do all things necessary to carry out the functions, powers, and duties set forth in the chapter.

§ 436E – 8. Repealed by Laws 1992, ch. 202, § 181

§ 436E – 9. Biennial renewal

Every person holding a license under this chapter shall register with the board and pay a biennial fee on or before June 30 of each odd-numbered year. Failure to pay the biennial fee shall constitute a forfeiture of the license as of the date of expiration. Any license so forfeited may be restored within one year after the expiration upon filing of an application and payment of a restoration fee.

§ 436E – 10. Revocation or suspension of licenses

In addition to any other actions authorized by law, any license to practice acupuncture under this chapter may be revoked or suspended by the board of acupuncture at any time in a proceeding before the board for any cause authorized by law, including but not limited to the following:

(1) Obtaining a fee on the assurance that a manifestly incurable ailment can be permanently cured;

(2) The use of false, fraudulent, or deceptive advertising and making untruthful and improbable statements;

(3) Habitually using any habit-forming controlled substance, such as opium or any of its

derivatives, morphine, heroin, or cocaine;

(4) Procuring a license through fraud, misrepresentation, or deceit;

(5) Professional misconduct or gross carelessness or manifest incapacity in the practice of acupuncture; or

(6) Violating any rules adopted under this chapter.

§ 436E – 11.　Repealed by Laws 1992, ch. 202,　§ 182

§ 436E – 12.　Penalty

(a) Any person except a person licensed under this chapter who practices, treats, or instructs in any phase of acupuncture without a license or permit issued by the board, or uses any word or title to induce the belief that they are engaged in the practice of any type of acupuncture, shall be guilty of a misdemeanor and subject to a fine of not less than $50 nor more than $1,000 for each violation.

(b) Any person, except a licensed acupuncturist, who:

(1) Practices or attempts to practice acupuncture;

(2) Buys, sells, or fraudulently obtains any diploma or license to practice acupuncture whether recorded or not;

(3) Uses the title "acupuncturist", "D.Ac." or "D.O.M." or any word or title to induce the belief that the person is engaged in the practice of acupuncture without complying with this chapter; or

(4) Violates this chapter;

shall be penalized as provided in subsection (a). The department may also seek all legal and equitable remedies available to it for the enforcement of the provisions of this chapter, including seeking injunctive relief.

§ 436E – 13.　Use of titles

(a) A licensee who has been awarded a license to practice acupuncture by the board in this State may use the title of "Licensed Acupuncturist" or designation "L.Ac." with the licensee's name in an advertisement for acupuncture or announce or append the designation to the licensee's name.

(b) A licensee who has been awarded an earned doctoral degree may use the designation "Ph.D." in an advertisement for acupuncture or announce or append the designation to the licensee's name if the degree was granted from a university or college recognized by a regional or national accrediting body recognized by the United States Department of Education. A Ph.D. recognized by the board under this subsection shall designate a nonpractitioner as opposed to a practitioner or "doctor" of acupuncture as provided in subsection (c).

(c) A licensee who has been approved by the board to use the doctor of acupuncture title, may use the title "Doctor of Acupuncture" or designation of "D.Ac.", after the licensee's name, or the term "Doctor" or prefix "Dr." provided that the word "Acupuncturist" immediately follows the licensee's name if the term "Doctor", or the prefix "Dr." is used alone.

(d) Before any licensee shall be eligible to use the doctor of acupuncture title, the licensee shall furnish satisfactory proof to the board that the licensee has been awarded an earned doctoral degree in acupuncture (traditional oriental medicine). For licensees who graduated from an institute, school, or college located in the United States or any territory under the jurisdiction of the United States, the institute, school, or college shall be accredited or recognized as a candidate for accreditation by a regional or national accrediting body that is recognized by the United States Department of Education for the accreditation or pre-accreditation ("candidacy") of professional post-graduate doctoral programs in acupuncture and oriental medicine. For licensees who graduated from a foreign institute, school, or college, the licensee, at the licensee's own expense, shall have the licensee's transcripts and curriculum evaluated by a board approved and designated professional evaluator who shall make a determination on whether the transcripts and curriculum are at least equivalent to the United States recognized doctoral program of study in acupuncture and oriental medicine, and that the foreign institute is licensed, approved, or accredited by the appropriate governmental authority or an agency recognized by a governmental authority in the respective foreign jurisdiction and whose curriculum is approved by the board.

(e) Except as provided in this section, use of other titles, prefixes, or designations shall not be permitted.

§ 436E – 14.   Foreign school curricula and standards

The board of acupuncture shall not recognize and approve an earned doctoral degree from a foreign university or college whose curricula and standards are not equivalent to or higher than institutions in the United States which have been recognized and approved by the board in the study or practice of acupuncture.

WEST'S HAWAI'I ADMINISTRATIVE CODE

Subchapter 1.   General Provisions

§ 16 – 72 – 1.   Repealed.
§ 16 – 72 – 2.   Objective.

This chapter is intended to clarify and implement chapter 436E, Hawaii Revised Statutes ("HRS"), to the end that the provisions thereunder may be best effectuated and the public interest most effectively served.

Subchapter 2.   Definitions

§ 16 – 72 – 3.   Definitions.

The definition of terms as appearing in chapter 436E, HRS, shall be adopted by reference.

In addition, as used in this chapter, the following definitions shall be included:

"Acupuncture needle" means a straight, slender rod of various length and diameter, tapered to a sharp point at one end for piercing the skin, with one end for manipulation or maintaining the needle in place, and inserted by an acupuncture practitioner into acupuncture points on the human body. A staple is not an acupuncture needle.

"Acupuncture practitioner" means a person holding a valid license issued by the board of acupuncture in the State.

"Approved post-secondary school" or "post-secondary school" means:

(1) An institute, school, or college accredited by or recognized as a candidate for accreditation by an accrediting body recognized by the United States Department of Education;

(2) An institute, school, or college which, at the time the applicant completed the acupuncture courses, was accredited or a candidate for accreditation by an accrediting body recognized by the United States Department of Education; or

(3) An institute, school or college whose curriculum is approved by the board, but which was not accredited or recognized as a candidate for accreditation because accreditation in acupuncture or another field of medical study was not yet available.

"Approved post-secondary school" in the case of a foreign school means an institute, school or college which is licensed, approved, or accredited by the appropriate governmental authority or an agency recognized by a governmental authority of that country and whose curriculum is approved by the board.

"Approved school", "school approved by the board", or similar words or phrases used in reference to an institute, school, college, or program of acupuncture or traditional Oriental medicine that includes acupuncture means:

(1) For a person who files an application with the board prior to September 1, 2000, an institute, school, college, or program of acupuncture, or traditional Oriental medicine which, at the time of the applicant's graduation, is licensed, approved, a candidate for accreditation, or accredited by the appropriate governmental authority or an agency recognized by a governmental authority in that jurisdiction, state, or country and whose curriculum is approved by the board; or

(2) For a person who files an application with the board on or after September 1, 2000, an institute, school, college, or program of acupuncture or traditional Oriental medicine, which, at the time of the applicant's graduation, is accredited or recognized as a candidate for accreditation by any acupuncture or traditional Oriental medicine accrediting body recognized by the United States Department of Education;

Provided that "approved school" in the case of a foreign school means an institute, school, college, or program with a formal program in the science of acupuncture or traditional Oriental medicine which is licensed, approved, or accredited by the appropriate governmental authority or an agency recognized by a governmental authority in that country and whose curriculum is approved by the board.

"Board" means the board of acupuncture.

"Contact hour" or "hour" means a minimum of fifty minutes of organized classroom instruction or practical clinical training.

"Director" means the director of the department of commerce and consumer affairs.

"Functional disorder" means a condition of the human body in which the symptoms cannot be referred to any organic lesion or change of structure, as opposed to an organic disorder.

"Office" means the physical facilities used for the practice of acupuncture.

"Traditional Oriental medicine" means the system of the healing art which places the chief emphasis on the flow and balance of energy in the human body as being the most important factor in maintaining the well-being of the body in health and disease and includes the practice of acupuncture and herbal medicine.

Subchapter 3. Authorized Practice; Scope of Practice; License

§ 16 – 72 – 4. Authorized practice of acupuncture.

An acupuncture practitioner is authorized to conduct treatment of the human body by means of stimulation of a certain acupuncture point or points for the purpose of controlling and regulating the flow and balance of energy in the body. The practice includes the techniques of piercing the skin by inserting needles and point stimulation by the use of acupressure, electrical, mechanical, thermal therapy, moxibustion, cupping, or traditional therapeutic means.

§ 16 – 72 – 5. Scope of practice of acupuncture.

Acupuncture is used in a wide range of treatment. However, the board recognizes that guidelines on the scope of practice of an acupuncture practitioner should be imposed and establishes the following permissible practices of authorized treatment which consists of pain relief and analgesia; functional and musculoskeletal disorders, including functional components of diseases; and the maintenance of well being, promotion of health, and physiological balance.

§ 16 – 72 – 6. Records.

A licensee shall keep accurate records of each patient the licensee treats. The records shall include the name of the patient, the indication and nature of treatment given, and any other relevant data deemed important by the licensee. Records shall be kept on file for a minimum of seven years and shall be open to inspection at any time by the board or its duly authorized representative.

§ 16 – 72 – 7. Repealed.

§ 16 – 72 – 8. Display of license.

The license certificate shall be conspicuously displayed in the office of practice.

§ 16 – 72 – 9.　Change of address.

A licensee shall notify the board of any change of address within thirty days of the change.

§ 16 – 72 – 10.　Repealed.

§ 16 – 72 – 11.　Supervision and functions of an acupuncture intern in clinical practice.

(a) No licensee shall allow an acupuncture intern to perform acupuncture treatment without the licensee's direct supervision. Direct supervision means that the licensee is physically present prior to, during, and after the intern's treatment of a patient, by instructing and providing active guidance to the intern in the diagnosis and treatment of the patient. In addition, the licensee shall ensure that:

(1) All patients shall be notified and shall consent to treatment by an acupuncture intern; and

(2) Every acupuncture intern under the licensee's supervision shall wear a conspicuously placed name tag stating the person's name and the words "acupuncture intern." The words "acupuncture intern" shall have letters at least one half inch high.

(b) Acupuncture services rendered by an acupuncture intern may include the items delineated in the scope of practice of acupuncture as set forth in section 16 – 72 – 5.

(c) Any violation of this section shall constitute professional misconduct.

Subchapter 4.　Education and Training Requirements

§ 16 – 72 – 14.　Formal education and training requirements.

(a) For applicants applying before September 1, 2000:

(1) An applicant shall submit satisfactory proof of graduation from an approved school, and satisfactory proof of completing a course of study of formal education and clinical training consisting of not less than one thousand five hundred hours.

(2) To satisfy the formal educational requirements, the applicant shall complete a course of study resulting in the award of a certificate or diploma, consisting of not less than two academic years (not less than six hundred hours) of study of acupuncture or traditional Oriental medicine. The course of study shall cover, but shall not be limited to, the following subjects:

(A) History and philosophy of traditional Oriental medicine (Nei-Ching, Taoism, Chi and Hsieh, Yin and Yang, and others);

(B) Traditional human anatomy, including location of acupuncture points;

(C) Traditional physiology, including the five elements organ theory;

(D) Traditional clinical diagnosis, including pulse diagnosis;

(E) Pathology, including the six Yin and seven Chin;

(F) Laws of acupuncture (mother and son, husband and wife, and five elements);

(G) Classification and function of points;

(H) Needle techniques;

(I) Complications;

(J) Forbidden points;

(K) Resuscitation;

(L) Safety and precautions;

(M) Use of electrical devices for diagnosis and treatment;

(N) Public health and welfare;

(O) Hygiene and sanitation;

(P) Oriental herbal studies; and

(Q) Clinical acupuncture practice.

(3) To satisfy the clinical training requirements, the applicant shall complete a course of training consisting of not less than twelve months (not less than nine hundred hours) of clinical internship training under the direct supervision of a licensed acupuncturist. The clinical internship training requirements may be obtained from a licensed acupuncturist at an approved school or from another clinical setting, from a licensed acupuncturist in private practice, or from any combination thereof. The licensed acupuncturist providing direct supervision shall:

(A) Have been licensed and actively practicing for a period of not less than five years prior to the start of the applicant's clinical internship training; and

(B) Have had a current, valid, and unencumbered license during the course of supervision.

(b) Notwithstanding the requirements of subsection (a), an applicant who started training prior to December 31, 1984, in a school approved by the board prior to December 31, 1984, and who completed the required training by December 31, 1989, and who files an application with the board before September 1, 2000, may qualify for licensure, provided that the applicant meets the requirements for examination and licensure as provided in chapter 436D, HRS, and rules adopted by the board as they existed on December 31, 1984, so long as the school has not altered its program so as to lower standards for completion of the program, and provided the applicant submits satisfactory proof of graduation from an approved school, and satisfactory proof of completing a course of study of formal education and clinical training consisting of at least one thousand fifty-six hours.

(1) To satisfy the formal education requirements, the applicant shall have completed a course of study consisting of a minimum duration of eighteen months (at least five hundred seventy-six hours) of acupuncture or traditional Oriental medicine. The course of study shall cover, but not be limited to, the subjects listed in paragraph (a)(2).

(2) To satisfy the clinical training requirements, the applicant shall have completed a course of training consisting of a minimum duration of six months (at least four hundred eighty hours) of clinical training in the practice of acupuncture on human subjects under the direct supervision of a licensed acupuncturist. The clinical training requirements may have been

obtained at an approved school, or from another clinical setting, from a licensed acupuncturist in private practice or from any combination thereof.

(c) An applicant applying on or after September 1, 2000, shall submit satisfactory proof of graduation from an approved school and satisfactory proof of completing a course of study of formal education and clinical training consisting of at least two thousand one hundred seventy five hours.

(1) To satisfy the formal educational requirements, the applicant shall complete an acupuncture and traditional Oriental medicine course of study consisting of not less than one thousand five hundred fifteen hours. The course of study shall cover, but not be limited to, the subjects listed in paragraph (a)(2).

(2) To satisfy the clinical training requirements, the applicant shall complete a course of training consisting of not less than six hundred sixty hours under the supervision of a licensed acupuncturist. The clinical training requirements shall be obtained at an approved school and shall not be obtained from a licensed acupuncturist in private practice or another clinical setting unless it is a part of the clinical training curriculum of an approved school.

§ 16 – 72 – 15.   **Repealed.**

§ 16 – 72 – 16.   **Repealed.**

§ 16 – 72 – 17.   **Academic standards for the use of titles.**

(a) Subject to the provisions herein, a licensee may use an earned degree title if the licensee has completed education in an approved school that includes acupuncture coursework related to the degree.

(b) A licensee who was previously authorized by the board to use a doctoral designation may continue to use that designation until September 1, 2000.

(c) Commencing on September 1, 2000, no licensee shall be allowed to use the doctoral designations "Doctor of Acupuncture", "D. Ac.", or similar title unless that licensee has applied to and received the approval of the board to use the designation. In order for the licensee to receive the board's approval, the licensee shall demonstrate that the licensee has:

(1) An earned doctoral degree in acupuncture or traditional Oriental medicine from an approved school, or shall have completed a program approved by the board in the study or practice of acupuncture or traditional Oriental medicine that consisted of at least five hundred hours in advanced academic education and training that is beyond that required for the L. Ac. entry level. The five hundred hours may include any combination of topics covered in categories I and II listed in "Appendix A" dated April 6, 2000, entitled "Doctoral Program" for determination of credential evaluation; and

(2) At least one thousand five hundred hours of clinical training and practice of acupuncture, traditional Oriental herbal medicine, or traditional Oriental physiotherapy, which may include laboratory work and presentation of scholastic instruction, that was obtained after

the person commenced the doctoral studies.

(d) In determining whether a licensee meets the requirements to use the doctoral designation, the board may require additional information including, but not limited to, the licensee's school catalog course descriptions and documentation of the clinical training and practice of acupuncture.

(e) A licensee who has earned a doctoral title and who wishes to use a doctoral designation after September 1, 2000, shall comply with subsection (c) herein.

(f) A licensee who has been awarded a "Ph.D." in acupuncture or traditional Oriental medicine shall be considered a non-practitioner and shall be permitted to use the designation of "Ph.D." in accordance with subsection 436E – 13(b), HRS.

Subchapter 5. Application for License

§ 16 – 72 – 20. Applications.

(a) Every person seeking a license to practice acupuncture or wishing to use any acupuncture title in the State shall file an application on a form provided by the board. All applications shall be completed in English and shall be accompanied by the following:

(1) The application fee as provided in rules adopted by the director in accordance with chapter 91, HRS, and payable in the form of a personal check, a cashier's check, or a postal money order;

(2) Verification of the required education and training, as applicable;

(3) An affidavit signed by the applicant stating that the applicant has read and shall abide by the board's laws and rules (chapter 436E, HRS, and this chapter) governing the practice of acupuncture; and

(4) Any other documents deemed necessary by the board.

(b) An application for a license may be filed at any time by an applicant who has taken and passed the examination identified in section 16 – 72 – 33 and shall be accompanied by the items required in subsection (a). The applicant shall be responsible for having the testing contractor verify, directly to the board, the passing score of the examination as required in section 16 – 72 – 36.

§ 16 – 72 – 20.1. Application for an acupuncture intern permit.

(a) An application for a permit to work for a period of four years as an acupuncture intern under the direct supervision of a licensed acupuncture practitioner may be filed with the board at any time and shall be accompanied by the required fee. The board may delegate to the board's executive officer the authority to issue an acupuncture intern permit to qualified applicants.

(b) An applicant shall provide verification of the following to the board:

(1) Evidence that the applicant has satisfactorily completed at least three semesters of instruction at an approved school and is currently enrolled in or is a graduate of an approved

school;

(2) A copy of the applicant's diploma or official transcript from an approved school showing the applicant's date of graduation or a letter from the dean or registrar of an approved school stating that the applicant has completed at least three semesters shall be submitted with the application;

(3) The name and license number of the supervising acupuncture practitioner; provided that effective September 1, 2000, the applicant shall also provide the name of the approved school through which the clinical training is being obtained.

(c) An acupuncture intern permit may be reissued for a period not to exceed one year, upon written request to the board and payment of the required fee.

§ 16 – 72 – 21.   **Repealed.**

§ 16 – 72 – 22.   **Repealed.**

§ 16 – 72 – 23.   **Verification of education and training.**

(a) For an applicant applying before September 1, 2000, the following documents shall be submitted as proof of the education and training of the applicant, provided the requirements of subsection 16 – 72 – 14(a) or (b) are met, as applicable:

(1) Verification of academic or educational study and training at an approved school consisting of:

(A) A certified transcript received by the board directly from an approved school and a photostatic copy of the diploma, certificate, or other certified documents from an approved school bearing an official school seal evidencing completion of a program in acupuncture or traditional Oriental medicine which includes acupuncture, and also a copy of the curriculum demonstrating the areas of study taken at an approved school; or

(B) If the school no longer exists or if the school's records have been destroyed for some plausible reason, applicant may submit a sworn affidavit so stating and shall name the school, its address, dates of enrollment and curriculum completed, and the board, in its discretion, may request the applicant also to provide verification from the appropriate governmental authority or an agency recognized by a governmental authority regarding the school's closing or of the unavailability of the school's records, and such other information and documents as the board may deem necessary; and

(C) A statement from the accrediting agency or appropriate governmental authority that the school is accredited or is a candidate for accreditation by an acupuncture accrediting agency recognized by the United States Department of Education, or that the school is licensed, approved, or accredited by the appropriate governmental authority or an agency recognized by a governmental authority in that jurisdiction, state, or country.

(2) Verification of clinical training consisting of:

(A) The name(s) of the licensed acupuncture practitioner(s) under whom the applicant served for the clinical training, the practitioner's license number, a verification of practitioner's dates of licensure, street address of business, the number of hours, dates, and length of training completed by the applicant, and a description of training received by the applicant; and

(B) A certification signed by the acupuncture practitioner under oath that applicant completed a course of clinical training under the practitioner's direction as required in paragraph 16 – 72 – 14(a)(3) or in paragraph 16 – 72 – 14(b)(2), as applicable; or

(C) If the practitioner is deceased or whereabouts not known, the applicant shall so state and shall submit a sworn affidavit certifying to the applicant's completion of clinical training and other documents as the board may deem necessary.

(b) For applicants applying on or after September 1, 2000, the following documents shall be submitted as proof of the education and clinical training of the applicant at an approved school provided they meet the requirements of paragraph 16 – 72 – 14(c):

(1) A certified transcript received directly from an approved school and a photostatic copy of diploma, certificate, or other certified documents from an approved school bearing an official school seal evidencing completion of a program in acupuncture or traditional Oriental medicine, which includes acupuncture, and also a copy of the curriculum demonstrating the areas of study taken at an approved school; or

(2) If the school no longer exists or if the school's records have been destroyed for some plausible reason, the applicant may submit a sworn affidavit so stating and shall name the school, its address, dates of enrollment and curriculum completed and shall also provide verification, from the acupuncture accrediting agency recognized by the United States Department of Education, or in the case of a foreign school, verification from the appropriate governmental authority or an agency recognized by a governmental authority, of the school's closing or of the unavailability of the school's records, and such other information and documents as the board may deem necessary; and

(3) A statement from the accrediting agency or appropriate governmental authority that the school is accredited or is a candidate for accreditation by an acupuncture accrediting agency recognized by the United States Department of Education, or in the case of a foreign school, that the school is licensed, approved, or accredited by the appropriate governmental authority or an agency recognized by a governmental authority in that country.

§ 16 – 72 – 24. Repealed.

§ 16 – 72 – 25. Documents in foreign language.

All documents submitted in a foreign language shall be accompanied by an accurate translation in English. Each translated document shall bear the affidavit of the translator certifying that the translator is competent in both the language of the document and the English language and that the translation is a true and complete translation of the foreign language original, and sworn to before a notary public. Translation of any document relative to a person's application shall be at the expense of the applicant.

§ 16 – 72 – 26. Sufficiency of documents.

In all cases the board's decision as to the sufficiency of documentation shall be final. The board may request further proof of qualification and may also require a personal interview with the applicant to establish the applicant's qualification.

§ 16 – 72 – 27. Deadline for filing application for a license.

The application for a license together with the accompanying documents shall be filed at least seventy-five days before the date of the examination.

§ 16 – 72 – 28. Demand for hearing.

Any person aggrieved by the denial or refusal of the board to issue, renew, restore, or reinstate a license, or by the denial or refusal of the board to permit the use of an academic designation shall submit a request for a contested case hearing pursuant to chapter 91, HRS, and Hawaii Administrative Rules ("HAR"), chapter 16 – 201, the rules of practice and procedure, within sixty days of the date of the refusal or denial. Appeal to the circuit court under section 91 – 14, HRS, or any other applicable statute, may only be taken from the board's final order.

§ 16 – 72 – 29. Repealed.

Subchapter 6. Examinations

§ 16 – 72 – 33. Examination.

(a) Every applicant applying for a license to practice as an acupuncturist shall pass the National Certification Commission for Acupuncture and Oriental Medicine's (NCCAOM) written comprehensive examination or such other written examination as the board may determine.

(b) The examination shall be consistent with the practical and theoretical requirements of acupuncture practice as provided by chapter 436E, HRS, and this chapter. The examination shall stand on its own merits. An applicant shall pass the examination before the applicant can be licensed to practice acupuncture.

(c) The board may contract with an independent testing contractor to provide an examination for the board.

(d) Applicants with disabilities may be afforded special testing arrangements and accommodations provided proper application is made on a form supplied by the board and provided further that they qualify for such arrangements as determined by the board or its designee.

§ 16 – 72 – 34. Frequency.

Examinations shall be conducted at least once a year.

§ 16 – 72 – 35. Language.

The examination shall be given in English; provided that the board may give the written examination in another language upon the applicant's request and subject to the availability of such an examination from the independent testing contractor.

§ 16 – 72 – 36.　Passing score.

The passing score for the written comprehensive examination shall be that minimum score for entry level competency as determined and recommended by the board's testing contractor in accordance with standard psychometric procedures. The passing score for such other written examination required by the board shall be determined by the board.

§ 16 – 72 – 37.　Repealed.

§ 16 – 72 – 38.　Repealed.

§ 16 – 72 – 39.　Repealed.

§ 16 – 72 – 40.　Repealed.

§ 16 – 72 – 41.　Repealed.

§ 16 – 72 – 42.　Repealed.

Subchapter 7.　License Renewal

§ 16 – 72 – 46.　Renewal.

Application for renewal, regardless of the issuance date of the license, shall be made on a form provided by the board on or before June 30 of each odd-numbered year and shall be accompanied by the appropriate renewal fee as provided in rules adopted by the director in accordance with chapter 91, HRS.

§ 16 – 72 – 47.　Renewal due date.

A renewal fee transmitted by mail shall be considered filed when due if the envelope bears a postmark of June 30 of each odd-numbered year or any prior date. Payment of the renewal fee shall be in the form of a personal check, a cashier's check, or a postal money order.

§ 16 – 72 – 48.　Failure to renew; forfeiture; restoration.

Failure to pay the renewal fee when due shall constitute automatic forfeiture of the license. However, a license which has been forfeited for failure to pay the renewal fee may be restored within one year after the date of forfeiture upon compliance with the licensing renewal requirements provided by law and upon written application and payment of the appropriate restoration fees as provided in rules adopted by the director in accordance with chapter 91, HRS. After one year from the date of forfeiture, a license shall not be restored and the person shall be treated as a new applicant and shall meet all the requirements of a new applicant.

Subchapter 8.　Public Health and Sanitation

§ 16 – 72 – 52.　Office.

When acupuncture is conducted in a building used for residential purposes, a room or rooms shall be set apart as an office for the practice and shall be used solely for this purpose. It shall be equipped with a washroom and toilet facilities. An acupuncture office may be inspected at any time during normal business hours by the board or any authorized employee of the department of commerce and consumer affairs.

§ 16 – 72 – 53. Sanitation practices.

Required practices shall include:

(1) A fresh, disposable paper or a fresh sheet shall be used on the examining table for each patient;

(2) Hands shall be washed with soap and water before handling a needle and between treatment of different patients;

(3) A piercing needle shall be previously unused and sterilized;

(4) A piercing needle shall not be used more than once per treatment and shall be disposed of immediately after use in the manner prescribed in paragraph (8) below;

(5) Skin, in the area of any acupuncture procedure, shall be thoroughly swabbed with germicidal solution before using any needles;

(6) If the sterility of an unused needle or instrument has been compromised, it shall be sterilized at a minimum temperature of 250°F (or 121℃) for not less than thirty minutes at fifteen pounds of pressure per square inch before usage;

(7) Prior to its usage on a patient, a reusable instrument or a non-piercing acupuncture needle shall be sterilized at a minimum temperature of 250°F (or 121℃) for not less than thirty minutes at fifteen pounds of pressure per square inch;

(8) All used needles for disposal shall be placed in a hazardous waste container that meets standards set by the department of health. All handling of the container, including but not limited to treating, transporting, and disposing of the container, shall conform with the laws and rules of the department of health; and

(9) Other reasonable sanitation procedures and practices recommended by governmental agencies or manufacturers shall be followed to protect the health and safety of patients and the public.

§ 16 – 72 – 57. Use of titles.

(a) An acupuncturist shall not misrepresent one's academic designation, professional title, qualification, and affiliation in an advertisement.

(b) A licensee who has been awarded an earned doctoral degree from an approved post-secondary school, post-secondary school, approved school, or school approved by the board, and who meets the academic standards set forth in section 16 – 72 – 17 may use the title "Doctor," "Dr.," "Doctor of Acupuncture," "D.Ac.," provided that the word "Acupuncturist" immediately follows the licensee's name.

(c) A licensee who was previously approved by the board to use the doctoral title prior to adoption of this chapter may continue to use the designation until September 1, 2000. In order to continue to use the doctoral title after September 1, 2000, the licensee shall apply for the use of an academic title and shall provide proof to the board of meeting the academic standards of section 16 – 72 – 17. The licensee's failure to apply and to meet the academic standards of section 16 – 72 – 17 by September 1, 2000, shall result in the loss of all rights to the continued usage of the doctoral title and the licensee shall immediately refrain from using the title.

§ 16 – 72 – 58. Repealed.

§ 16 – 72 – 59. Repealed.

§ 16 – 72 – 63. Administrative practice and procedure.

The rules of practice and procedure shall be as provided in HAR, chapter 16 – 201, the rules of practice and procedure of the department of commerce and consumer affairs, which are incorporated by reference and made a part of this chapter.

§ 16 – 72 – 67. Oral testimony.

(a) The board shall accept oral testimony on any item which is on the board's agenda, provided that the testimony shall be subject to the following conditions:

(1) Each person seeking to present oral testimony is requested to notify the board no later than forty-eight hours prior to the meeting, and at that time shall state the item on which testimony is to be presented;

(2) The board may request that any person providing oral testimony submit the remarks, or a summary of the remarks, in writing to the board;

(3) The board may rearrange the items on the agenda for the purpose of providing for the most efficient and convenient presentation of oral testimony;

(4) Persons presenting oral testimony, at the beginning of the testimony, shall identify themselves and the organization, if any, that they represent;

(5) The board may limit oral testimony to a specified time period but in no case shall the period be less than five minutes, and the person testifying shall be informed prior to the commencement of the testimony of the time constraints to be imposed; and

(6) The board may refuse to hear any testimony which is irrelevant, immaterial, or unduly repetitious to the agenda item on which it is presented.

(b) Nothing in this chapter shall require the board to hear or receive any oral or documentary evidence from a person on any matter which is the subject of another proceeding pending subject to the hearing relief, declaratory relief, or rule relief provisions of HAR, chapter 16 – 201.

(c) Nothing in this chapter shall prevent the board from soliciting oral remarks from persons present at the meeting or from inviting persons to make presentations to the board on any particular matter on the board's agenda.

§ 16 – 72 Appendix A. DOCTORAL PROGRAM

Appendix "A"

DOCTORAL PROGRAM

April 6, 2000

CATEGORY I: ORIENTAL MEDICAL SCIENCES
A. ORIENTAL MEDICAL PHILOSOPHY AND CHRONOLOGICAL STUDIES

Study of traditional philosophical literature and cultural perspectives towards Oriental medicine including classical history as related to development of acupuncture and Oriental medicine.

B. ADVANCED DIAGNOSIS AND SYMPTOMATOLOGY

Study of diagnosis techniques, including correlation of necessary data and statistic analysis to evaluate outcomes. Further study of organ system and specific acupuncture procedures to develop accurate diagnostic skills including comparison between classical and modern techniques.

C. ADVANCED MERIDIAN (Channels & Collaterals) SYSTEMS

Study and research of how the systems of the human body integrate with the internal and divergent pathways of the acupuncture meridian system.

D. ADVANCED POINT LOCATION AND FUNCTION

Study of the scientific analysis of acupuncture points based on morphological responses including systems of classical and modern methods of acupuncture point determination. A further study of the new points and scientific review of contraindications.

E. ADVANCED HERBOLOGY

Study of composition and pharmacological analysis of traditional oriental herbal formulas. A further research review of new formulas and pharmacopoeia based on traditional oriental medicine.

F. TRADITIONAL PATHOLOGY AND ETIOLOGY

Advanced studies of traditional oriental and western aspects of pathology and etiology. Study of morphological structure of "Zhang-Fu" and the influence of external, internal, and non-external/non-internal factors and patho-etiological relation with the Chinese bio-clock mechanism.

Study of the biological systemic function of the filtration of body fluids by acupuncture application. Study of the effects of acupuncture on pathological progress, transformations, and molecular metabolism of the organs.

CATEGORY II: ACUPUNCTURE SCIENCES APPLIED IN GENERAL MEDICINE
A. IMMUNOLOGY

Study of the modulation of the body's immunobiological mechanisms and active physiological substance changes with acupuncture and oriental medicine application on anaphylaxis and auto-immune disorders.

B. GYNECOLOGY AND UROLOGY

Study of acupuncture and oriental medicine as applied to gynecology, obstetric problems and female endocrine systems. Study of kidney and genitourinary systems to define clinical implications with acupuncture and oriental medicine applications.

C. NEUROLOGY

Study of neurological effects on the endogenous and vasomotor control with acupuncture application. A neuroanatomy and histological study of the central and peripheral nervous systems to define the significance of acupuncture applications.

D. ORTHOPEDICS

Study of the origin of and acupuncture effect on orthopedic conditions. Study of osteology and analysis of x-rays.

E. GERIATRICS/REHABILITATION/CHRONIC DISEASE

Study of acupuncture and oriental medical aspect applications to aging-related conditions. A study may extend to rehabilitation, chronic disease and pain management.

F. PEDIATRICS

Review of infant and child-related diseases and clinical application of the acupuncture and oriental medicine treatment which may include perinatological care. Study and practice of the pediatric acupuncture therapy instruments.

CATEGORY III: RELATED ADVANCED CLINICAL ACUPUNCTURE AND ORIENTAL MEDICINE

Clinical training practice of acupuncture, and oriental physiotherapy.

Clinical credit may include laboratorial work and presentation of scholastic instruction.

WEST'S NEW MEXICO

WEST'S NEW MEXICO STATUTES ANNOTATED

§ 61 – 14A – 1. Short title

Chapter 61, Article 14A NMSA 1978 may be cited as the "Acupuncture and Oriental Medicine Practice Act".

§ 61 – 14A – 2. Purpose

In the interest of the public health, safety and welfare and to protect the public from the unprofessional, improper, incompetent and unlawful practice of acupuncture and oriental medicine, it is necessary to provide laws and regulations to govern the practice of acupuncture and oriental medicine. The primary responsibility and obligation of the board of acupuncture and oriental medicine is to protect the public.

§ 61 – 14A – 3. Definitions

As used in the Acupuncture and Oriental Medicine Practice Act:

A. "acupuncture" means the surgical use of needles inserted into and removed from the body and the use of other devices, modalities and procedures at specific locations on the body for the prevention, cure or correction of any disease, illness, injury, pain or other condition by controlling and regulating the flow and balance of energy and function to restore and maintain health;

B. "board" means the board of acupuncture and oriental medicine;

C. "doctor of oriental medicine" means a person licensed as a physician to practice acupuncture and oriental medicine with the ability to practice independently, serve as a primary care provider and as necessary collaborate with other health care providers;

D. "moxibustion" means the use of heat on or above specific locations or on acupuncture needles at specific locations on the body for the prevention, cure or correction of any disease, illness, injury, pain or other condition;

E. "oriental medicine" means the distinct system of primary health care that uses all allied techniques of oriental medicine, both traditional and modern, to diagnose, treat and prescribe for the prevention, cure or correction of disease, illness, injury, pain or other physical or mental condition by controlling and regulating the flow and balance of energy, form and function to restore and maintain health;

F. "primary care provider" means a health care practitioner acting within the scope of the health care practitioner's license who provides the first level of basic or general health care for a person's health needs, including diagnostic and treatment services, initiates referrals to other health care practitioners and maintains the continuity of care when appropriate;

G. "techniques of oriental medicine" means:

(1) the diagnostic and treatment techniques used in oriental medicine that include diagnostic procedures; acupuncture; moxibustion; manual therapy, also known as tui na; other physical medicine modalities and therapeutic procedures; breathing and exercise techniques; and dietary, nutritional and lifestyle counseling;

(2) the prescribing, administering, combining and providing of herbal medicines, homeopathic medicines, vitamins, minerals, enzymes, glandular products, natural substances, natural medicines, protomorphogens, live cell products, gerovital, amino acids, dietary and nutritional supplements, cosmetics as they are defined in the New Mexico Drug, Device and Cosmetic Act and nonprescription drugs as they are defined in the Pharmacy Act; and

(3) the prescribing, administering and providing of devices, restricted devices and prescription devices, as those devices are defined in the New Mexico Drug, Device and Cosmetic Act, if the board determines by rule that the devices are necessary in the practice of oriental medicine and if the prescribing doctor of oriental medicine has fulfilled requirements for prescriptive authority in accordance with rules promulgated by the board for the devices enumerated in this paragraph; and

H. "tutor" means a doctor of oriental medicine with at least ten years of clinical experience who is a teacher of acupuncture and oriental medicine.

§ 61 – 14A – 4. License required

Unless licensed as a doctor of oriental medicine pursuant to the Acupuncture and Oriental Medicine Practice Act, no person shall:

A. practice acupuncture or oriental medicine;

B. use the title or represent himself as a licensed doctor of oriental medicine or use any other title, abbreviation, letters, figures, signs or devices that indicate the person is licensed to practice as a doctor of oriental medicine; or

C. advertise, hold out to the public or represent in any manner that he is authorized to practice acupuncture and oriental medicine.

§ 61 – 14A – 4.1. Certified auricular detoxification specialists, supervisors and training programs; fees

A. A person who is not a doctor of oriental medicine or who is not a person certified as an auricular detoxification specialist pursuant to the Acupuncture and Oriental Medicine Practice Act shall not:

(1) practice auricular acupuncture for the treatment of alcoholism, substance abuse or chemical dependency;

(2) use the title of or represent as a certified auricular detoxification specialist or use any other title, abbreviation, letters, figures, signs or devices that indicate that the person is certified to practice as an auricular detoxification specialist; or

(3) advertise, hold out to the public or represent in any manner that the person is authorized to practice auricular detoxification.

B. The board shall issue an auricular detoxification specialist certification to a person who has paid an application fee to the board and has successfully completed all board requirements. The board shall adopt rules that require an applicant to:

(1) successfully complete the national acupuncture detoxification association training or equivalent training approved by the board that shall include clean needle technique training;

(2) demonstrate experience in treatment, disease prevention, harm reduction and counseling of people suffering from alcoholism, substance abuse or chemical dependency or become employed by a substance abuse treatment program;

(3) complete a board-approved training program that will include examinations on clean needle technique, jurisprudence and other skills required by the board; and

(4) demonstrate a record free of convictions for drug- or alcohol-related offenses for at least two consecutive years before the person applied to the board for certification.

C. A certified auricular detoxification specialist is authorized to perform auricular acupuncture and the application to the ear of simple board-approved devices that do not penetrate the skin for the purpose of treating and preventing alcoholism, substance abuse or chemical dependency. The specialist shall use the five auricular point national acupuncture detoxification procedure or auricular procedures approved or established by rule of the board and shall only treat or prevent alcoholism, substance abuse or chemical dependency within a board-approved program that demonstrates experience in disease prevention, harm reduction or the treatment or prevention of alcoholism, substance abuse or chemical dependency.

D. A person certified pursuant to this section shall use the title "certified auricular detoxification specialist" or "C.A.D.S." for the purpose of advertising auricular acupuncture services to the public.

E. A certified auricular detoxification specialist shall apply with the board to renew the certification. The board shall for one year renew the certification of an applicant who pays a renewal fee and completes the requirements established by rule of the board. An applicant who does not apply for renewal before the last date that the certification is valid may be required to pay a late fee pursuant to a rule of the board. The board shall deem a certification for which a renewal has not been applied within sixty days of that date as expired and an applicant that seeks valid certification shall apply with the board for new certification. The board shall by rule require an applicant for renewal of the certification to demonstrate a record free of convictions for drug- or alcohol-related offenses for a minimum of one year prior to application for renewal with the board.

F. A certified auricular detoxification specialist shall practice under the supervision of a licensed doctor of oriental medicine registered with the board as an auricular detoxification specialist supervisor. A supervising doctor of oriental medicine shall be accessible for consultation directly or by telephone to a practicing auricular detoxification specialist. The supervising doctor of oriental medicine shall not supervise more specialists than permitted by board rule. Supervision requirements shall be provided by rule of the board.

G. A doctor of oriental medicine who supervises a certified auricular detoxification specialist shall apply for registration with the board. The board shall issue an auricular detoxification specialist supervisor registration to a doctor of oriental medicine who fulfills board requirements. The board shall by rule require an applicant for registration to list the certified auricular detoxification specialists that will be supervised, pay an application fee for registration and demonstrate clinical experience in treating or counseling people suffering from alcoholism, substance abuse or chemical dependency.

H. A training program that educates auricular detoxification specialists for certification shall apply for approval by the board. The board shall approve a training program that fulfills the board requirements established by rule and that pays an application fee. The approval shall be valid until July 31 following the initial approval.

I. A training program that is approved by the board to provide training for certification of auricular detoxification specialists shall apply to renew the approval with the board. The board shall renew the approval of a program that fulfills board requirements established by rule, and the renewal shall be valid for one year. An applicant who does not renew before the last date that the renewed approval is valid shall pay a late fee. The board shall deem a program approval that is not renewed within sixty days of that date as expired and a program that seeks board approval shall apply with the board for new approval.

J. The board shall impose the following fees:

(1) an application fee not to exceed one hundred fifty dollars ($150) for auricular detoxification specialist certification;

(2) a fee not to exceed seventy-five dollars ($75.00) for renewal of an auricular detoxification specialist certification;

(3) an application fee not to exceed two hundred dollars ($200) for registration of a certified auricular detoxification specialist supervisor;

(4) an application fee not to exceed two hundred dollars ($200) for the approval of an

auricular detoxification specialist training program;

(5) a fee not to exceed one hundred fifty dollars ($150) for the renewal of the approval of an auricular detoxification training specialist training program; and

(6) a late fee not to exceed fifty dollars ($50.00) for applications for renewal filed after the last valid date of a registration, certification, approval or renewal issued pursuant to this section.

K. In accordance with the procedures set forth in the Uniform Licensing Act, the board may deny, revoke or suspend any certification, registration, approval or renewal that a person holds or applies for pursuant to this section upon findings by the board that the person violated any rule established by the board.

§ 61 – 14A – 5. Title

Any person licensed pursuant to provisions of the Acupuncture and Oriental Medicine Practice Act, in advertising his services to the public, shall use the title "doctor of oriental medicine" or "D.O.M.". The title "doctor of oriental medicine" or "D.O.M." shall supersede the use of all other titles that include the words "medical doctor" or the initials "M.D." unless the person is a medical doctor licensed pursuant to provisions of the Medical Practice Act.

§ 61 – 14A – 6. Exemptions

A. Nothing in the Acupuncture and Oriental Medicine Practice Act is intended to limit, interfere with or prevent any other class of licensed health care professionals from practicing within the scope of their licenses, but they shall not hold themselves out to the public or any private group or business by using any title or description of services that includes the term acupuncture, acupuncturist or oriental medicine unless they are licensed under the Acupuncture and Oriental Medicine Practice Act.

B. The Acupuncture and Oriental Medicine Practice Act shall not apply to or affect the following practices if the person does not hold himself out as a doctor of oriental medicine or as practicing acupuncture or oriental medicine:

(1) the administering of gratuitous services in cases of emergency;

(2) the domestic administering of family remedies;

(3) the counseling about or the teaching and demonstration of breathing and exercise techniques;

(4) the counseling or teaching about diet and nutrition;

(5) the spiritual or lifestyle counseling of a person or spiritual group or the practice of the religious tenets of a church;

(6) the providing of information about the general usage of herbal medicines, homeopathic medicines, vitamins, minerals, enzymes or glandular or nutritional supplements; or

(7) the use of needles for diagnostic purposes and the use of needles for the administration of diagnostic or therapeutic substances by licensed health care professionals.

§ 61 – 14A – 7. Board created; appointment; officers; compensation

A. The "board of acupuncture and oriental medicine" is created.

B. The board is administratively attached to the regulation and licensing department.

C. The board shall consist of seven members appointed by the governor for terms of three years each. Four members of the board shall be doctors of oriental medicine who have been residents of and practiced acupuncture and oriental medicine in New Mexico for at least five years immediately preceding the date of their appointment. Three members shall be appointed to represent the public and shall not have practiced acupuncture and oriental medicine in this or any other jurisdiction or have any financial interest in the profession regulated. No board member shall be the owner, principal or director of an institute offering educational programs in acupuncture and oriental medicine. No more than one board member may be from each of the following categories:

(1) a faculty member at an institute offering educational programs in acupuncture and oriental medicine;

(2) a tutor in acupuncture and oriental medicine; or

(3) an officer or director in a professional association of acupuncture and oriental medicine.

D. Members of the board shall be appointed by the governor for staggered terms of three years that shall be made in such a manner that the terms of board members expire on July 1. A board member shall serve until his successor has been appointed and qualified. Vacancies shall be filled for the remainder of the unexpired term in the same manner as the original appointment.

E. A board member shall not serve more than two consecutive full terms, and a board member who fails to attend, after he has received proper notice, three consecutive meetings shall be recommended for removal as a board member unless excused for reasons established by the board.

F. The board shall elect annually from its membership a chairman and other officers as necessary to carry out its duties.

G. The board shall meet at least once each year and at other times deemed necessary. Other meetings may be called by the chairman, a majority of board members or the governor. A simple majority of the board members serving constitutes a quorum of the board.

H. Members of the board shall be reimbursed as provided in the Per Diem and Mileage Act and shall receive no other compensation, perquisite or allowance.

§ 61 – 14A – 8. Board; powers

The board has the power to:

A. enforce the provisions of the Acupuncture and Oriental Medicine Practice Act;

B. promulgate, in accordance with the State Rules Act, all rules necessary for the implementation and enforcement of the provisions of the Acupuncture and Oriental Medicine Practice Act;

C. adopt a code of ethics;

D. adopt and use a seal;

E. inspect facilities of approved educational programs, extern programs and the offices of licensees;

F. promulgate rules implementing continuing education requirements for the purpose of protecting the health and well-being of the citizens of this state and maintaining and continuing informed professional knowledge and awareness; and

G. in accordance with the Uniform Licensing Act:

(1) issue investigative subpoenas for the purpose of investigating complaints against licensees prior to the issuance of a notice of contemplated action;

(2) administer oaths and take testimony on any matters within the board's jurisdiction;

(3) conduct hearings upon charges relating to the discipline of licensees, including the denial, suspension or revocation of a license; and

(4) grant, deny, renew, suspend or revoke licenses to practice acupuncture and oriental medicine or grant, deny, renew, suspend or revoke approvals of educational programs and extern programs for any cause stated in the Acupuncture and Oriental Medicine Practice Act or the rules of the board.

§ 61 – 14A – 8.1. Expanded practice and prescriptive authority; certifications

A. The board shall issue certifications, as determined by rule of the board, for expanded practice and prescriptive authority only for the substances enumerated in Paragraphs (1) and (2) of Subsection C of this section to a doctor of oriental medicine who has submitted completed forms provided by the board, paid the application fee for certification and submitted proof of successful completion of additional training required by rule of the board. The board shall adopt the rules determined by the board of pharmacy for additional training required for the prescribing, administering, compounding or dispensing of caffeine, procaine, oxygen, epinephrine and bioidentical hormones. The board and the board of pharmacy shall consult as appropriate.

B. The board shall issue certifications in the four expanded practices of basic injection therapy, injection therapy, intravenous therapy and bioidentical hormone therapy.

C. The expanded practice and prescriptive authority shall include:

(1) the prescribing, administering, compounding and dispensing of herbal medicines, homeopathic medicines, vitamins, minerals, amino acids, proteins, enzymes, carbohydrates, lipids, glandular products, natural substances, natural medicines, protomorphogens, live cell products, gerovital, dietary and nutritional supplements, cosmetics as they are defined in the New Mexico Drug, Device and Cosmetic Act and nonprescription drugs as they are defined in the Pharmacy Act; and

(2) the prescribing, administering, compounding and dispensing of the following dangerous drugs or controlled substances as they are defined in the New Mexico Drug, Device and Cosmetic

Act, the Controlled Substances Act or the Pharmacy Act, if the prescribing doctor of oriental medicine has fulfilled the requirements for expanded practice and prescriptive authority in accordance with the rules promulgated by the board for the substances enumerated in this paragraph:

(a) sterile water;

(b) sterile saline;

(c) sarapin or its generic;

(d) caffeine;

(e) procaine;

(f) oxygen;

(g) epinephrine;

(h) vapocoolants;

(i) bioidentical hormones;

(j) biological products, including therapeutic serum; and

(k) any of the drugs or substances enumerated in Paragraph (1) of this subsection if at any time those drugs or substances are classified as dangerous drugs or controlled substances.

D. When compounding drugs for their patients, doctors of oriental medicine certified for expanded practice and prescriptive authority shall comply with the compounding requirements for licensed health care professionals in the United States pharmacopeia and national formulary.

§ 61 – 14A – 9. Board; duties

The board shall:

A. establish fees;

B. provide for the examination of applicants for licensing as doctors of oriental medicine as provided in the Acupuncture and Oriental Medicine Practice Act;

C. keep a record of all examinations held, together with the names and addresses of all persons taking the examinations, and the examination results;

D. notify each applicant, in writing, of the results of his examinations within twenty-one days after the results of an examination are available to the board;

E. keep a licensee record in which the names, addresses and license numbers of all licensees shall be recorded together with a record of all license renewals, suspensions and revocations;

F. provide for the granting and renewal of licenses and approval of educational programs; and

G. keep an accurate record of all its meetings, receipts and disbursements.

§ 61 – 14A – 10. Requirements for licensing

The board shall grant a license to practice acupuncture and oriental medicine to a person who has:

A. submitted to the board:

(1) the completed application for licensing on the form provided by the board;

(2) the required documentation as determined by the board;

(3) the required fees;

(4) an affidavit stating that the applicant has not been found guilty of unprofessional conduct or incompetency;

(5) proof, as determined by the board, that the applicant has completed a board-approved educational program in acupuncture and oriental medicine as provided for in the Acupuncture and Oriental Medicine Practice Act and the rules of the board; and

(6) proof that he has passed the examinations approved by the board; and

B. complied with any other requirements of the board.

§ 61 – 14A – 11.　Examinations

A. The board shall establish procedures to ensure that examinations for licensing are offered at least once a year.

B. The board shall establish the deadline for receipt of the application for licensing examination and other rules relating to the taking and retaking of licensing examinations.

C. The board shall establish the passing grades for its approved examinations.

D. The board may approve, and use as a basis for licensure, examinations that are used for national certification or other examinations.

E. The board shall require each qualified applicant to pass a validated, objective written examination that covers areas that are not included in other examinations approved by the board, including, as a minimum, the following subjects:

(1) anatomy and physiology;

(2) pathology;

(3) diagnosis;

(4) pharmacology; and

(5) principles, practices and treatment techniques of acupuncture and oriental medicine.

F. The board may require each qualified applicant to pass a validated, objective practical examination that covers areas that are not included in other examinations approved by the board and that demonstrates his knowledge of and skill in the application of the diagnostic and treatment techniques of acupuncture and oriental medicine.

G. The board shall require each qualified applicant to pass a written or a practical examination or both in the following subjects:

(1) hygiene, sanitation and clean-needle technique; and

(2) needle and instrument sterilization techniques.

H. The board may require each qualified applicant to pass a written examination on the state laws and rules that pertain to the practice of acupuncture and oriental medicine.

I. If English is not the primary language of the applicant, the board may require that the applicant pass an English proficiency examination prescribed by the board.

§ 61 – 14A – 12. Requirements for temporary licensing

A. The board shall establish the criteria for temporary licensing of out-of-state doctors of oriental medicine.

B. The board may grant a temporary license to a person who:

(1) is legally recognized to practice acupuncture and oriental medicine in another state or a foreign country or is legally recognized in another state or foreign country to practice another health care profession and who possesses knowledge and skills that are included in the scope of practice of doctors of oriental medicine;

(2) is under the sponsorship of and in association with a licensed New Mexico doctor of oriental medicine or New Mexico institute offering an educational program approved by the board;

(3) submits the completed application for temporary licensing on the form provided by the board;

(4) submits the required documentation, including proof of adequate education and training, as determined by the board;

(5) submits the required fee for application for temporary licensing;

(6) submits an affidavit stating that the applicant has not been found guilty of unprofessional conduct or incompetency; and

(7) submits an affidavit from the sponsoring and associating New Mexico doctor of oriental medicine or New Mexico institute attesting to the qualifications of the applicant and the activities the applicant will perform.

C. The board may grant a temporary license to allow the temporary licensee to:

(1) teach acupuncture and oriental medicine;

(2) consult, in association with the sponsoring doctor of oriental medicine, regarding the sponsoring doctor's patients;

(3) perform specialized diagnostic or treatment techniques in association with the sponsoring doctor of oriental medicine regarding the sponsoring doctor's patients;

(4) assist in the conducting of research in acupuncture and oriental medicine; and

(5) assist in the implementation of new techniques and technology related to acupuncture and oriental medicine.

D. Temporary licensees may engage in only those activities authorized on the temporary license.

E. The temporary license shall identify the sponsoring and associating New Mexico doctor of oriental medicine or institute.

F. The temporary license shall be issued for a period of time established by rule; provided that temporary licenses may not be issued for a period of time to exceed eighteen months, including renewals.

G. The temporary license may be renewed upon submission of:

（1）the completed application for temporary license renewal on the form provided by the board; and

（2）the required fee for temporary license renewal.

H. In the interim between regular board meetings, whenever a qualified applicant has filed his application and complied with all other requirements of this section, the board's chairman or an authorized representative of the board may grant an interim temporary license that will suffice until the next regular licensing meeting of the board.

§ 61 – 14A – 13. Requirements for expedited licensing

A. The board shall grant a license to practice acupuncture and oriental medicine without examination to a person who has been licensed, certified, registered or legally recognized as a doctor of oriental medicine in another licensing jurisdiction in accordance with Section 61 – 1 – 31.1 NMSA 1978 if the applicant:

（1）submits the completed application for expedited licensing on the form provided by the board;

（2）submits the required documentation as determined by the board;

（3）submits the required fee for application for expedited licensing; and

（4）passes a written examination on the state laws and rules that pertain to the practice of acupuncture and oriental medicine, if the board requires regular applicants for licensure to pass such an examination.

B. The board shall issue the expedited license as soon as practicable but no later than thirty days after the person files an application with the required fees and demonstrates that the person holds a valid, unrestricted license and is in good standing with the licensing board in the other licensing jurisdiction and has practiced for at least two years immediately prior to application in New Mexico. If the board issues an expedited license to a person whose prior licensing jurisdiction did not require examination, the board may require the person to pass an examination before license renewal.

C. The board by rule shall determine the states and territories of the United States and the District of Columbia from which it will not accept an applicant for expedited licensure and determine any foreign countries from which it will accept an applicant for expedited licensure. The board shall post the lists of disapproved and approved licensing jurisdictions on its website. The list of disapproved licensing jurisdictions shall include specific reasons for disapproval. The lists shall be reviewed annually to determine if amendments to the rule are warranted.

§ 61 – 14A – 14. Approval of educational programs

A. The board shall establish by rule the criteria for board approval of educational programs in acupuncture and oriental medicine. For an educational program to meet board approval, proof shall be submitted to the board demonstrating that the educational program as a minimum:

（1）was for a period of not less than four academic years;

(2) included a minimum of nine hundred hours of supervised clinical practice;

(3) was taught by qualified teachers or tutors;

(4) required as a prerequisite to graduation personal attendance in all classes and clinics and, as a minimum, the completion of the following subjects:

(a) anatomy and physiology;

(b) pathology;

(c) diagnosis;

(d) pharmacology;

(e) oriental principles of life therapy, including diet, nutrition and counseling;

(f) theory and techniques of oriental medicine;

(g) precautions and contraindications for acupuncture treatment;

(h) theory and application of meridian pulse evaluation and meridian point location;

(i) traditional and modern methods of qi or life-energy evaluation;

(j) the prescription of herbal medicine and precautions and contraindications for its use;

(k) hygiene, sanitation and clean-needle technique;

(l) care and management of needling devices; and

(m) needle and instrument sterilization techniques; and

(5) resulted in the presentation of a certificate or diploma after completion of all the educational program requirements.

B. All in-state educational programs in acupuncture and oriental medicine with the intent to graduate students qualified to be applicants for licensing examination by the board shall be approved annually by the board. The applicant shall submit the following:

(1) the completed application for approval of an educational program;

(2) the required documentation as determined by the board;

(3) proof, as determined by the board, that the educational requirements provided for in Subsection A of this section are being met; and

(4) the required fee for application for approval of an educational program.

C. Out-of-state educational programs in acupuncture and oriental medicine with the intent to graduate students qualified to be applicants for licensing examination by the board may apply for approval by the board. The applicant shall submit the following:

(1) the completed application for approval of an educational program;

(2) the required documentation as determined by the board;

(3) proof, as determined by the board, that the educational requirements provided for in Subsection A of this section are being met; and

(4) the required fee for application for approval of an educational program.

D. Each in-state approved educational program shall renew its approval annually by submitting prior to the date established by the board:

（1）the completed application for renewal of approval of an educational program on the form provided by the board;

（2）proof, as determined by the board, that the educational requirements provided for in Subsection A of this section are being met; and

（3）the required fee for application for renewal of approval of an educational program.

E. Each out-of-state approved educational program may renew its approval annually by submitting prior to the date established by the board:

（1）the completed application for renewal of approval of an educational program on the form provided by the board;

（2）proof, as determined by the board, that the educational requirements provided for in Subsection A of this section are being met; and

（3）the required fee for application for renewal of approval of an educational program.

F. A sixty-day grace period shall be allowed each educational program after the end of the approval period, during which time the approval may be renewed by submitting:

（1）the completed application for renewal of approval of an educational program on the form provided by the board;

（2）proof, as determined by the board, that the educational requirements provided for in Subsection A of this section are being met;

（3）the required fee for application for renewal of approval of an educational program; and

（4）the required fee for late renewal of approval.

G. An approval that is not renewed by the end of the grace period shall be considered expired, and the educational program must apply as a new applicant.

§ 61 – 14A – 14.1. Students and externs; supervised practice

A. A student enrolled in an approved educational program may practice acupuncture and oriental medicine under the direct supervision of a teacher or tutor as part of the educational program.

B. The board may promulgate rules to govern the practice of acupuncture and oriental medicine by externs. The rules shall include qualifications for externs and supervising doctors of oriental medicine or other supervising health care professionals and the allowable scope of practice for externs. The board may charge a fee for approval and renewal of approval of extern programs. Participation as an extern is optional and not a requirement for licensure.

§ 61 – 14A – 15. License renewal

A. Each licensee shall renew his license annually by submitting prior to the date established by the board:

（1）the completed application for license renewal on the form provided by the board; and

（2）the required fee for annual license renewal.

B. The board may require proof of continuing education or other proof of competency as a requirement for renewal.

C. A sixty-day grace period shall be allowed each licensee after the end of the licensing period, during which time the license may be renewed by submitting:

(1) the completed application for license renewal on the form provided by the board;

(2) the required fee for annual license renewal; and

(3) the required late fee.

D. Any license not renewed at the end of the grace period shall be considered expired and the licensee shall not be eligible to practice within the state. For reinstatement of an expired license within one year of the date of renewal, the board shall establish any requirements or fees that are in addition to the fee for annual license renewal and may require the former licensee to reapply as a new applicant.

§ 61 – 14A – 16.   Fees

Except as provided in Section 61 – 1 – 34 NMSA 1978, the board shall establish a schedule of reasonable nonrefundable fees not to exceed the following amounts:

A. application for licensing $800;

B. application for expedited licensing 750;

C. application for temporary licensing 500;

D. examination, not including the cost of any nationally recognized examination 700;

E. annual license renewal 400;

F. late license renewal 200;

G. expired license renewal 400;

H. temporary license renewal 100;

I. application for approval or renewal of approval of an educational program 600;

J. late renewal of approval of an educational program 200;

K. annual continuing education provider registration 200;

L. application for extended or expanded prescriptive authority 500;

M. application for externship supervisor registration 500;

N. application for extern certification 500; and

O. fees to cover reasonable and necessary administrative expenses.

§ 61 – 14A – 17.   Disciplinary proceedings; judicial review; application of Uniform Licensing Act

A. In accordance with the procedures contained in the Uniform Licensing Act, the board may deny, revoke or suspend any permanent or temporary license held or applied for under the Acupuncture and Oriental Medicine Practice Act, upon findings by the board that the licensee or applicant:

(1) is guilty of fraud or deceit in procuring or attempting to procure a license;

(2) has been convicted of a felony. A certified copy of the record of conviction shall be

conclusive evidence of such conviction;

(3) is guilty of incompetence as defined by board rule;

(4) is habitually intemperate, is addicted to the use of habit-forming drugs or is addicted to any vice to such a degree as to render him unfit to practice as a doctor of oriental medicine;

(5) is guilty of unprofessional conduct, as defined by board rule;

(6) is guilty of any violation of the Controlled Substances Act;

(7) has violated any provision of the Acupuncture and Oriental Medicine Practice Act or rules promulgated by the board;

(8) is guilty of failing to furnish the board, its investigators or representatives with information requested by the board;

(9) is guilty of willfully or negligently practicing beyond the scope of acupuncture and oriental medicine as defined in the Acupuncture and Oriental Medicine Practice Act;

(10) is guilty of failing to adequately supervise a sponsored temporary licensee;

(11) is guilty of aiding or abetting the practice of acupuncture and oriental medicine by a person not licensed by the board;

(12) is guilty of practicing or attempting to practice under an assumed name;

(13) advertises by means of knowingly false statements;

(14) advertises or attempts to attract patronage in any unethical manner prohibited by the Acupuncture and Oriental Medicine Practice Act or the rules of the board;

(15) has been declared mentally incompetent by regularly constituted authorities;

(16) has had a license, certificate or registration to practice as a doctor of oriental medicine revoked, suspended or denied in any jurisdiction of the United States or a foreign country for actions of the licensee similar to acts described in this subsection. A certified copy of the record of the jurisdiction taking such disciplinary action will be conclusive evidence thereof; or

(17) fails, when diagnosing or treating a patient, to possess or apply the knowledge or to use the skill and care ordinarily used by reasonably well-qualified doctors of oriental medicine practicing under similar circumstances, giving due consideration to the locality involved.

B. Disciplinary proceedings may be instituted by any person, shall be by sworn complaint and shall conform with the provisions of the Uniform Licensing Act. Any party to the hearing may obtain a copy of the hearing record upon payment of the costs of the copy.

C. Any person filing a sworn complaint shall be immune from liability arising out of civil action if the complaint is filed in good faith and without actual malice.

D. The licensee shall bear the costs of disciplinary proceedings unless exonerated.

§ 61 – 14A – 18.　Fund created

A. There is created in the state treasury the "board of acupuncture and oriental medicine fund".

B. All money received by the board pursuant to the Acupuncture and Oriental Medicine

Practice Act shall be deposited with the state treasurer for credit to the board of acupuncture and oriental medicine fund. The state treasurer shall invest the fund as other state funds are invested. All balances in the fund shall remain in the fund and shall not revert to the general fund.

C. Money in the board of acupuncture and oriental medicine fund is appropriated to the board and shall be used only for the purpose of meeting the necessary expenses incurred in carrying out the provisions of the Acupuncture and Oriental Medicine Practice Act.

§ 61 – 14A – 19. Penalties

A. A person who violates a provision of the Acupuncture and Oriental Medicine Practice Act is guilty of a misdemeanor and upon conviction shall be punished as provided in Section 31 – 19 – 1 NMSA 1978.

B. In addition to criminal penalties, a person who engages in acupuncture or oriental medicine without a license is subject to disciplinary proceedings by the board. The provisions of Section 61 – 1 – 3.2 NMSA 1978 notwithstanding, the board may impose a civil penalty in an amount not to exceed two thousand dollars ($2,000) against such person and may assess the person for administrative costs, including investigative costs and the cost of conducting a hearing. The fine shall be deposited to the credit of the current school fund

§ 61 – 14A – 20. Criminal Offender Employment Act

The provisions of the Criminal Offender Employment Act shall govern any consideration of criminal records required or permitted by the Acupuncture and Oriental Medicine Practice Act.

§ 61 – 14A – 21. Licensed acupuncture practitioner; license valid under new act

Any person validly licensed as an acupuncture practitioner under prior law of this state shall be deemed licensed under the provisions of the Acupuncture and Oriental Medicine Practice Act.

§ 61 – 14A – 22. Termination of agency life; delayed repeal

The board of acupuncture and oriental medicine is terminated on July 1, 2023 pursuant to the Sunset Act. The board shall continue to operate according to the Acupuncture and Oriental Medicine Practice Act until July 1, 2024. Effective July 1, 2024, Chapter 61, Article 14A NMSA 1978 is repealed.

CODE OF NEW MEXICO RULES

Part 1. General Provisions

16.2.1.1 ISSUING AGENCY

New Mexico Board of Acupuncture and Oriental Medicine.

16.2.1.2 SCOPE

All licensed doctors of oriental medicine, applicants, temporary licensees, applicants for temporary licensure, doctors of oriental medicine certified for expanded practice and applicants for certification, educational courses, externs, auricular detoxification specialists, educational programs and applicants for approval of educational programs.

16.2.1.3 STATUTORY AUTHORITY

This part is promulgated pursuant to the Acupuncture and Oriental Medicine Practice Act, Sections 61 - 14A - 1, 2, 3, 7, 8, 8.1, 14.1 and 9, NMSA 1978.

16.2.1.4 DURATION

Permanent.

16.2.1.5 EFFECTIVE DATE

February 11, 2022 unless a later date is cited at the end of a section or paragraph.

16.2.1.6 OBJECTIVE

This part provides definitions for terms used in the rules in addition to those definitions in the Act, lists the board's duties, clarifies what are not public records, provides for inspection of the board's public records, and provides for telephone conferences.

16.2.1.7 DEFINITIONS

The following definitions apply to the rules and the act.

A. Definitions beginning with "A":

(1) "A4M" is the American academy of anti-aging medicine.

(2) "ACAM" is the American college of alternative medicine.

(3) "ACAOM" is the accreditation commission for acupuncture and oriental medicine.

(4) "Act" is the Acupuncture and Oriental Medicine Practice Act, Sections 61 - 14A - 1 through 61 - 14A - 22 NMSA 1978.

(5) "AMA" is the American medical association.

(6) "Animal acupuncture" is acupuncture performed on any animal other than man. Animal acupuncture is authorized under the supervision of a doctor of veterinary medicine licensed in New Mexico and only under the guidelines of the rules of the New Mexico Veterinary Practice Act 61 - 14 - 1 to 61 - 14 - 20 NMSA 1978 and the rules of the New Mexico board of veterinary medicine 16.25.9.15 NMAC.

(7) "Applicant" is a person who has submitted to the board an application for licensure as a doctor of oriental medicine.

(8) "Applicant for temporary licensure" is a person who has submitted to the board an application for temporary licensure as a doctor of oriental medicine.

(9) "Auricular acupuncture detoxification" is an acupuncture related technique used only in the treatment and prevention of alcoholism, substance abuse and chemical dependency. Auricular acupuncture detoxification may be described or referred to as "auricular detoxification", "acupuncture detoxification", "auricular acupuncture detoxification", or "acudetox".

(10) "Auricular detoxification specialist supervisor" is a doctor of oriental medicine

registered with the board under the provisions of 16.2.16.18 NMAC.

(11) "Auricular detoxification specialist training program" is a training program approved by the board under the provisions of 16.2.16.26 NMAC to train certified auricular detoxification specialists and auricular detoxification supervisors.

(12) "Auricular detoxification specialist training program trainer" is a member of the staff of an auricular detoxification specialist training program who, though not necessarily licensed or certified by the state, shall be deemed to be a certified auricular detoxification specialist only for the purposes of and only for the duration of the auricular detoxification specialist training program.

(13) "Authorized substances" are the specific substances defined in the four certification in 16.2.20 NMAC that are authorized according to Paragraph (1) of Subsection C of Section 61 – 14A – 8 NMSA 1978 of the act for prescription, administration, compounding and dispensing by a doctor of oriental medicine certified for a specific category of expanded practice as defined in 16.2.19 NMAC.

B. Definitions beginning with "B":

(1) "Bioidentical hormones" means compounds, or salt forms of those compounds, that have exactly the same chemical and molecular structure as hormones that are produced in the human body.

(2) "Biomedical diagnosis" is a diagnosis of a person's medical status based on the commonly agreed upon guidelines of conventional biomedicine as classified in the most current edition or revision of the international classification of diseases, ninth revision, clinical modification (ICD – 9 – CM).

(3) "Biomedicine" is the application of the principles of the natural sciences to clinical medicine.

C. Definitions beginning with "C":

(1) "Certified auricular detoxification specialist" is a person certified by the board under the provisions of 16.2.16.10 NMAC to perform auricular detoxification techniques, only on the ears, only in the context of an established treatment program and only under the supervision of an auricular detoxification supervisor registered with the board. A person certified pursuant to Paragraph (1) of Subsection B of 61 – 14A – 4 NMSA 1978 shall use the title of "certified auricular detoxification specialist" or "C.A.D.S."

(2) "Chief officer" is the board's chairperson or his or her designee serving to administer the pre-hearing procedural matters of disciplinary proceedings.

(3) "Clinical experience" is the practice of acupuncture and oriental medicine as defined in the act, after initial licensure, certification, registration or legal recognition in any jurisdiction to practice acupuncture and oriental medicine. A year of clinical experience shall consist of not less than 500 patient hours of licensed acupuncture and oriental medical practice within a calendar year, seeing at least 25 different patients within that year. One patient hour is defined as

one clock hour spent in the practice of oriental medicine with patients.

(4) "Clinical skills examination" is a board approved, validated, objective practical examination that demonstrates the applicants entry level knowledge of and competency and skill in the application of the diagnostic and treatment techniques of acupuncture and oriental medicine and of biomedicine.

(5) "Complainant" is the complaining party.

(6) "Complaint committee" is a board committee composed of the complaint committee chairperson and the complaint manager.

(7) "Complaint committee chairperson" is a member of the board appointed by the board's chairperson.

(8) "Complaint manager" is the board's administrator or any member of the board appointed by the board's chairperson.

D. Definitions beginning with "D":

(1) "Department" is the state of New Mexico regulation and licensing department.

(2) "Detoxification" is a concept in integrative medicine based on the principle that illnesses can be caused by the accumulation of toxic substances (toxins) in the body. Therapeutic support of elimination of these toxins is detoxification.

(3) "Doctor of oriental medicine" is a physician licensed to practice acupuncture and oriental medicine pursuant to the act and as such has responsibility for his or her patient as a primary care physician or independent specialty care physician.

E. Definitions beginning with "E":

(1) "Educational course" is a comprehensive foundation of studies, approved by the board leading to demonstration of entry level competence in the specified knowledge and skills required for the four respective certifications in expanded practice. An educational course is not an educational program as this term is used in the act and the rules and as defined in 16.2.1 NMAC.

(2) "Educational program" is a board approved complete formal program that has the goal of educating a person to be qualified for licensure as a doctor of oriental medicine in New Mexico, is at least four academic years and meets the requirements of Section 61 - 14A - 14 NMSA 1978 of the act and 16.2.7 NMAC.

(3) "Expanded practice" is authorized by of Section 61 - 14 - 8.1 NMSA 1978 of the act and is granted to a doctor of oriental medicine who is certified by the board after fulfilling the requirements, in addition to those necessary for licensure, defined in 16.2.19 NMAC. Expanded practice is in addition to the prescriptive authority granted all licensed doctors of oriental medicine as defined in Paragraph (2) of Subsection G of Section 61 - 14A - 3 NMSA 1978 of the act.

(4) "Extern" is a current applicant undergoing supervised clinical training by an externship supervisor, and who has satisfied the application requirements for extern certification and who

has received an extern certification issued by the board pursuant to 16.2.14 NMAC.

(5) "Externship" is the limited practice of oriental medicine in New Mexico by an extern supervised by an externship supervisor pursuant to 16.2.14 NMAC.

(6) "Externship supervisor" is a doctor of oriental medicine who has at least five clinical experience, maintains a clinical facility and maintains appropriate professional and facility insurance, and who has satisfied the board's application requirements for an externship supervisor and has received an externship supervisor registration issued by the board pursuant to 16.2.14 NMAC.

F. Definitions beginning with "F": [RESERVED]

G. Definitions beginning with "G": "Good cause" is the inability to comply because of serious accident, injury or illness, or the inability to comply because of the existence of an unforeseen, extraordinary circumstance beyond the control of the person asserting good cause that would result in undue hardship. The person asserting good cause shall have the burden to demonstrate that good cause exists.

H. Definitions beginning with "H": [RESERVED]

I. Definitions beginning with "I":

(1) "Inactive licensee" means a licensee in good standing whose license is placed on inactive status by the board and is therefore considered an inactive license in compliance with 16.2.15 NMAC.

(2) "ICE" is the institute for credentialing excellence.

(3) "IFM" is the institute for functional medicine.

J. Definitions beginning with "J": [RESERVED]

K. Definitions beginning with "K": [RESERVED]

L. Definitions beginning with "L":

(1) "Licensee" is a doctor of oriental medicine licensed pursuant to the act.

(2) "License" has the same meaning as defined in Paragraph (1) of Subsection F of Section 61 – 1 – 34 NMSA 1978.

(3) "Licensing candidate" is an applicant whose initial application for licensure as a doctor of oriental medicine has been approved by the board.

(4) "Licensing fee" has the same meaning as defined in Paragraph (2) of Subsection F of Section 61 – 1 – 34 NMSA 1978.

(5) "Licensure by endorsement" is a licensing procedure for the experienced practitioner who completed his initial education in acupuncture and oriental medicine prior to the establishment of current educational standards and who has demonstrated his or her competency through a combination of education, examination, authorized legal practice and clinical experience as defined in 16.2.17 NMAC. Completion of the licensure by endorsement process results in full licensure as a doctor of oriental medicine.

(6) "Limited temporary license" is a license issued under the provisions of 16.2.5.12 NMAC for the exclusive purpose of teaching a single complete course in acupuncture and oriental medicine and assisting in the implementation of new techniques in acupuncture and oriental medicine including the study of such techniques by licensed, registered, certified or legally recognized healthcare practitioners from jurisdictions other than New Mexico. A limited temporary license shall be required for any person who demonstrates, practices or performs diagnostic and treatment techniques on another person as part of teaching or assisting in the implementation of new techniques, if they are not a licensee or temporary licensee. Limited temporary licenses shall not be issued to teachers for the purpose of teaching full semester courses that are part of an approved educational program.

(7) "Live cell products" are living cells from glandular tissues and other tissues.

M. Definitions beginning with "M": "Military service member" has the same meaning as defined in Paragraph (3) of Subsection F of Section 61 - 1 - 34 NMSA 1978.

N. Definitions beginning with "N":

(1) "Natural substances" are substances that exist in or are produced by nature and have not been substantially transformed in character or use.

(2) "NCA" is a notice of contemplated action.

(3) "NCCAOM" is the national certification commission for acupuncture and oriental medicine.

O. Definitions beginning with "O":

(1) "Office" is the physical facility used for the practice of acupuncture and oriental medicine and auricular detoxification.

(2) "Oxidative medicine" is the understanding and evaluation of the oxidation and reduction biochemical functions of the body and the prescription or administration of substances, and the use of devices and therapies to improve the body's oxidation and reduction function and health.

P. Definitions beginning with "P": "Protomorphogens" are extracts of glandular tissues.

Q. Definitions beginning with "Q": [RESERVED]

R. Definitions beginning with "R":

(1) "Respondent" is the subject of the complaint.

(2) "Rules" are the rules, promulgated pursuant to the act, governing the implementation and administration of the act as set forth in 16.2 NMAC.

S. Definitions beginning with "S":

(1) "Substantial equivalent" means the determination by the board that the education, examination, and experience requirements contained in the statutes and rules of another jurisdiction are comparable to, or exceed the education, examination, and experience requirements of the Acupuncture and Oriental Medicine Practice Act, Sections 61 - 14A - 1 NMSA 1978 et. seq.

(2) "Supervised clinical observation" is the observation of acupuncture and oriental medical

practice, in actual treatment situations under appropriate supervision.

(3) "Supervised clinical practice" is the application of acupuncture and oriental medical practice, in actual treatment situations under appropriate supervision.

(4) "Supervision" is the coordination, direction and continued evaluation at first hand of the student in training or engaged in obtaining clinical practice and shall be provided by a qualified instructor or tutor as set forth in 16.2.7 NMAC. No more than four students shall be under supervision for supervised clinical practice and no more than four students shall be under supervision for supervised clinical observation by a qualified instructor at any time.

T. Definitions beginning with "T":

(1) "Temporary licensee" is a doctor of oriental medicine who holds a temporary license pursuant to the act, 61 – 14 – 12 NMSA 1978 and 16.2.5 NMAC.

(2) "Therapeutic serum" is a product obtained from blood by removing the clot or clot components and the blood cells.

(3) "Treatment program" is an integrated program that may include medical and counseling services for disease prevention, harm reduction or the treatment or prevention of alcoholism, substance abuse or chemical dependency that is located at a fixed location or in a mobile unit and approved by the board under the provisions of 16.2.16.28 NMAC.

U. Definitions beginning with "U": "USP 797" is the United States pharmacopeia Chapter 797 pharmaceutical compounding.

V. Definitions beginning with "V": "Veteran" has the same meaning as defined in Paragraph (4) of Subsection F of Section 61 – 1 – 34 NMSA 1978.

W. Definitions beginning with "W": [RESERVED]

X. Definitions beginning with "X": [RESERVED]

Y. Definitions beginning with "Y": [RESERVED]

Z. Definitions beginning with "Z": [RESERVED]

16.2.1.8 BOARD DUTIES

In addition to its duties described in the act, the board shall:

A. Keep a file of all approved educational programs.

B. Issue certificates of approval of educational programs.

C. Delegate its ministerial duties if it so chooses.

D. Notify the governor when any board member has missed three consecutive meetings.

E. Elect a chairperson and a vice-chairperson at the first board meeting after January first each year.

F. The board shall perform such other duties and shall exercise such other powers as may be conferred upon it by statute, or as may be reasonably implied from such statutory powers and duties and as may be reasonably necessary in the performance of its responsibilities under the act.

16.2.1.9　PUBLIC RECORDS

All records kept by the board shall be available for public inspection pursuant to the New Mexico Inspection of Public Records Act, Section 14 - 2 - 1, NMSA 1978, et seq., except as provided herein.

A. During the course of the processing and investigation of a complaint, and before the vote of the board as to whether to dismiss the complaint or to issue a notice of contemplated action as provided in the Uniform Licensing Act, Section 61 - 1 - 1, NMSA 1978, et seq., and in order to preserve the integrity of the investigation of the complaint, records and documents that reveal confidential sources, methods, information or licensees accused, but not charged yet with a violation of the act, shall be confidential and shall not be subject to public inspection. Such records shall include evidence in any form received or compiled in connection with any such investigation of the complaint or of the licensee by or on behalf of the board by any investigating agent or agency.

B. Upon the completion of the processing and investigation of the complaint, and upon the decision of the board to dismiss the complaint or to issue a notice of contemplated action, the confidentiality privilege conferred by Subsection A of 16.2.1.9 NMAC shall dissolve, and the records, documents or other evidence pertaining to the complaint and to the investigation of the complaint shall be available for public inspection.

C. All tests and test questions by which applicants are tested shall not be available to public inspection, as there is a countervailing public policy requiring that such records remain confidential in order to ensure the integrity of a licensing exam intended to protect the public health, safety and welfare from incompetent practitioners.

D. The board or its administrator may charge a fee not to exceed one dollar per page for documents 11 inches by 17 inches or smaller in size for copying public records.

16.2.1.10　TELEPHONE CONFERENCES

Pursuant to the provisions of the Open Meetings Act, Section 10 - 15 - 1.C, NMSA 1978, as amended, board members may participate in a meeting of the board by means of a conference telephone or similar communications equipment when it is otherwise difficult or impossible for the member to attend the meeting in person, provided that each board member participating by conference telephone can be identified when speaking, all participants are able to hear each other at the same time and members of the public attending the meeting must be able to hear any member of the board who speaks during the meeting. Participation of a board member by such means shall constitute presence in person at the meeting.

16.2.1.11　DISASTER OR EMERGENCY PROVISION

Doctors of oriental medicine, educational programs and auricular detoxification specialists currently licensed and in good standing or otherwise meeting the requirements for New Mexico licensure in a state which a federal disaster has been declared may apply for licensure in New

Mexico under 16.2.1.11 NMAC during the four months following the declared disaster. The application for emergency provisional licensure shall be made to the board and shall include:

A. an application under this provision shall be made to the board that is complete and in English on a form provided by the board that shall include the applicant's name, address, date of birth and social security number accompanied by proof of identity, which may include a copy of drivers license, passport or other photo identification issued by a governmental entity; and the applicants signature on the affidavit made part of the application form;

B. an affidavit attesting to the consequences suffered by the applicant as a result of the federal disaster;

C. evidence of completion of requirements specified in 16.2.3, 16.2.4, 16.2.7, 16.2.10, and 16.2.16 NMAC; if the applicant is unable to obtain documentation from the federal declared disaster area or as a result of the declared federal disaster the board may accept other documentation in lieu of the forms required under 16.2.3, 16.2.4, 16.2.7, 16.2.10, and 16.2.16 NMAC; the board reserves the right to request additional documentation, including but not limited to, recommendation forms and work experience verification forms prior to approving licensure;

D. exceptions may be made for good cause;

E. an affidavit certifying that all the documents submitted with the application are true and accurate or are faithful copies of the original;

F. nothing in this section shall constitute a waiver of the requirements for licensure contained in 16.2.3, 16.2.4, 16.2.7, 16.2.10, and 16.2.16 NMAC; and

G. the applicant is responsible for reading, understanding and complying with the state of New Mexico laws and rules regarding this application as well as the practice of acupuncture and oriental medicine.

Part 2.   Scope of Practice

16.2.2.1   ISSUING AGENCY

New Mexico Board of Acupuncture and Oriental Medicine.

16.2.2.2   SCOPE

All licensed doctors of oriental medicine, all licensed doctors of oriental medicine certified for expanded practice as defined in 16.2.19 NMAC, temporary licensees engaging in only those activities authorized on the temporary license, externs engaging in only those activities authorized by the externship and students enrolled in an educational program in acupuncture and oriental medicine approved by the board working under the direct supervision of a teacher at the approved educational program as part of the educational program in which they are enrolled.

16.2.2.3   STATUTORY AUTHORITY

This part is promulgated pursuant to the Acupuncture and Oriental Medicine Practice Act,

Sections 61 – 14A – 3, 4, 6, 8 and 8.1 NMSA 1978.

16.2.2.4 DURATION

Permanent.

16.2.2.5 EFFECTIVE DATE

02 – 15 – 05, unless a later date is cited at the end of a section.

16.2.2.6 OBJECTIVE

This part clarifies the scope of practice of doctors of oriental medicine, temporary licensees, externs and students and doctors of oriental medicine certified for expanded practice.

16.2.2.7 DEFINITIONS

Refer to definitions in 16.2.1.7 NMAC (Section 7 of Part 1 of the rules).

16.2.2.8 SCOPE OF PRACTICE

Pursuant to Section 61 – 14A – 3 NMSA 1978, the practice of oriental medicine in New Mexico is a distinct system of primary health care with the goal of prevention, cure, or correction of any disease, illness, injury, pain or other physical or mental condition by controlling and regulating the flow and balance of energy, form and function to restore and maintain health. Oriental medicine includes all traditional and modern diagnostic, prescriptive and therapeutic methods utilized by practitioners of acupuncture and oriental medicine. The scope of practice of doctors of oriental medicine shall include but is not limited to:

A. evaluation, management and treatment services;

B. diagnostic examination, testing and procedures;

C. the ordering of diagnostic imaging procedures and laboratory or other diagnostic tests;

D. the surgical procedures of acupuncture and other related procedures;

E. the stimulation of points, areas of the body or substances in the body using qi, needles, heat, cold, color, light, infrared and ultraviolet, lasers, sound, vibration, pressure, magnetism, electricity, electromagnetic energy, bleeding, suction, or other devices or means;

F. physical medicine modalities, procedures and devices;

G. therapeutic exercises, qi exercises, breathing techniques, meditation, and the use of biofeedback devices and other devices that utilize heat, cold, color, light, infrared and ultraviolet, lasers, sound, vibration, pressure, magnetism, electricity, electromagnetic energy and other means therapeutically;

H. dietary and nutritional counseling and the prescription or administration of food, beverages and dietary supplements therapeutically;

I. counseling and education regarding physical, emotional and spiritual balance in lifestyle;

J. prescribing, administering, combining, providing, compounding and dispensing any non-injectable herbal medicine, homeopathic medicines, vitamins, minerals, enzymes, glandular products, natural substances, protomorphogens, live cell products, amino acids, dietary and nutritional supplements; cosmetics as they are defined in the New Mexico Drug, Device and

Cosmetic Act and nonprescription drugs as they are defined in the Pharmacy Act;

K. the prescription or administration of devices, restricted devices and prescription devices as defined in the New Mexico Drug, Device and Cosmetic Act (Section 26 – 1 – 1 NMSA 1978) by a doctor of oriental medicine who meets the requirements of 16.2.2.9 NMAC.

16.2.2.9   DEVICES, RESTRICTED DEVICES AND PRESCRIPTION DEVICES

The board determines that devices, restricted devices and prescription devices as defined in the New Mexico Drug, Device and Cosmetic Act (Section 26 – 1 – 1 NMSA 1978) are necessary in the practice of oriental medicine. Doctors of oriental medicine who have the training recommended by the manufacturer of the device shall be authorized to prescribe, administer or dispense the device.

16.2.2.10   SCOPE OF PRACTICE FOR EXPANDED PRACTICE

A. In addition to the scope of practice for a licensed New Mexico doctor of oriental medicine, the scope of practice for those certified in expanded practice shall include certification in any or all of the following modules: basic injection therapy, injection therapy, intravenous therapy and bioidentical hormone therapy. practitioners previously certified as Rx1 extended prescriptive authority, will be certified for basic injection therapy and practitioners previously certified as Rx2 expanded prescriptive authority, will be certified for injection therapy, intravenous therapy and bioidentical hormone therapy.

B. The expanded practice shall include:

(1) the prescribing, administering, compounding and dispensing of herbal medicines, homeopathic medicines, vitamins, minerals, amino acids, proteins, enzymes, carbohydrates, lipids, glandular products, natural substances, natural medicines, protomorphogens, live cell products, gerovital, dietary and nutritional supplements, cosmetics as they are defined in the New Mexico Drug, Device and Cosmetic Act (26 – 1 – 1 NMSA 1978) and nonprescription drugs as they are defined in the Pharmacy Act (61 – 11 – 1 NMSA 1978); and

(2) the prescribing, administering, compounding and dispensing of the following dangerous drugs or controlled substances as they are defined in the New Mexico Drug, Device and Cosmetic Act, the Controlled Substances Act (30 – 31 – 1 NMSA 1978) or the Pharmacy Act:

(a) sterile water;

(b) sterile saline;

(c) sarapin or its generic;

(d) caffeine;

(e) procaine;

(f) oxygen;

(g) epinephrine;

(h) vapocoolants;

(i) bioidentical hormones; and

(j) biological products, including therapeutic serum.

C. When compounding drugs for their patients, doctors of oriental medicine certified for expanded practice and prescriptive authority shall comply with the compounding requirements for licensed health care professionals in the United States pharmacopeia and national formulary.

16.2.2.11 [RESERVED]

16.2.2.12 PRESCRIPTION PADS

A doctor of oriental medicine, when prescribing, shall use prescription pads imprinted with his name, address, telephone number and license number. If a doctor of oriental medicine is using a prescription pad printed with the names of more than one doctor of oriental medicine, each doctor of oriental medicine shall have a separate signature line indicating the name and license number. Each specific prescription shall indicate the name of the doctor of oriental medicine for that prescription.

16.2.2.13 [RESERVED]

16.2.2.14 [RESERVED]

Part 3. Application for Licensure (Refs & Annos)

16.2.3.1 ISSUING AGENCY

New Mexico Board of Acupuncture and Oriental Medicine.

16.2.3.2 SCOPE

All applicants for licensure as doctors of oriental medicine.

16.2.3.3 STATUTORY AUTHORITY

This part is promulgated pursuant to the Acupuncture and Oriental Medicine Practice Act, Sections 61 − 14A − 4, 6, 8, 9 and 10, NMSA 1978

16.2.3.4 DURATION

Permanent.

16.2.3.5 EFFECTIVE DATE

February 11, 2022, unless a later date is cited at the end of a section.

16.2.3.6 OBJECTIVE

This part lists the requirements that an applicant must fulfill in order to apply for licensure as a doctor of oriental medicine.

16.2.3.7 DEFINITIONS

Refer to definitions in 16.2.1.7 NMAC.

16.2.3.8 GENERAL REQUIREMENTS

A. Any applicant who has been subject to any action or proceeding comprehended by Subsection A of 16.2.3.8 NMAC may be subject to disciplinary action, including denial, suspension or revocation of licensure, pursuant to the provisions of Section 61 − 14A − 17 NMSA 1978; and subject to the Uniform Licensing Act, Section 61 − 1 − 1 NMSA 1978, et seq., and subject to the Criminal Offender Employment Act, Section 28 – 2 – 1 NMSA 1978, et seq.

B. Any applicant who provides the board with false information or makes a false statement to the board may be subject to disciplinary action, including denial, suspension or revocation of licensure, pursuant to the provisions of Section 61 – 14A – 17 NMSA 1978, and to the Uniform Licensing Act, Section 61 – 1 – 1 NMSA 1978, et seq.

16.2.3.9   EDUCATIONAL PROGRAM REQUIREMENTS

Every applicant shall provide satisfactory proof that he completed a board approved educational program as defined in 61 – 14A – 14 NMSA 1978 of the act and 16.2.7 NMAC. If the educational program is no longer in existence, or if the applicant's records are not available 2 for good cause, the applicant shall submit an affidavit so stating and shall identify the educational program, and shall provide the address, dates of enrollment, and curriculum completed, along with such other information and documents as the board shall deem necessary. The board, in its sole and sound discretion, may accept or reject as adequate and sufficient such evidence presented in lieu of the records otherwise required.

16.2.3.10   CRIMINAL CONVICTIONS

A. Convictions for any of the following offenses, or their equivalents in any other jurisdiction, are disqualifying criminal convictions that may disqualify an applicant from receiving or retaining a license, including temporary licenses and auricular detoxification specialist certificates, issued by the board:

(1) homicide;

(2) aggravated assault, aggravated battery, kidnapping, false imprisonment, human trafficking, or other crimes of violence against persons;

(3) robbery, larceny, burglary, extortion, receiving stolen property, possession of burglary tools, unlawful taking of a motor vehicle, or other crimes involving theft or appropriation of personal property or funds;

(4) rape, criminal sexual penetration, criminal sexual contact, incest, indecent exposure, child solicitation, or other crimes constituting sexual offenses;

(5) driving under the influence of intoxicating liquor or drugs within the five years prior to the date of application;

(6) trafficking controlled substances, specifically excluding cannabis or cannabis-derived products, within the five years prior to the date of application;

(7) crimes involving child abuse or neglect;

(8) fraud, forgery, money laundering, embezzlement, credit card fraud, counterfeiting, financial exploitation, or other crimes of altering any instrument affecting the rights or obligations of another;

(9) making a false statement under oath or in any official document;

(10) an attempt, solicitation or conspiracy involving any of the felonies in this subsection.

16.2.3.11 INITIAL LICENSURE APPLICATION

Upon approval of an application for licensure that fulfills the requirements listed below, the board shall issue a license that will be valid until July 31 following the initial licensure, except that licenses initially issued after May 1 will not expire until July 31 of the next renewal period as defined in 16.2.8.9 NMAC; the application requirements for a license shall be receipt of the following by the board:

A. the fee for application for licensure specified in 16.2.10 NMAC;

B. an application for licensure that is complete and in English on a form provided by the board that shall include the applicant's name, address, date of birth and social security number, if available;

C. two passport-type photographs of the applicant taken not more than six months prior to the submission of the application;

D. an affidavit as provided on the "initial licensure application" as to whether the applicant:

(1) has been subject to any disciplinary action in any jurisdiction related to the practice of acupuncture and oriental medicine, or related to any other profession including other health care professions for which the applicant is licensed, certified, registered or legally recognized to practice including resignation from practice, withdrawal or surrender of applicants license, certificate or registration during the pendency of disciplinary proceedings or investigation for potential disciplinary proceedings;

(2) has been a party to litigation in any jurisdiction related to the applicants practice of acupuncture and oriental medicine, or related to any other profession including other health care professions for which the applicant is licensed, certified, registered or legally recognized to practice;

(3) is in arrears on a court-ordered child support payment; or

(4) has violated any provision of the act or the rules;

E. an official license history, which is a certificate from each jurisdiction stating the disciplinary record of the applicant, from each jurisdiction where the applicant has been licensed, certified, registered or legally recognized to practice any profession, including health care professions, in any jurisdiction, pursuant to any authority other than the New Mexico Acupuncture and Oriental Medicine Practice Act;

F. an affidavit as provided on the "initial licensure application" stating that the applicant understands that:

(1) an applicant who has been subject to any action or proceeding comprehended by Subsection D of 16.2.3.10 NMAC may be subject to disciplinary action at any time, including denial, suspension or revocation of licensure, pursuant to the provisions of the act, Section 61 - 14A - 17 NMSA 1978; and subject to the Uniform Licensing Act, Section 61 - 1 - 1 NMSA 1978, and subject to the Criminal Offender Employment Act, Section 28 - 2 - 1 NMSA

1978; and

(2) an applicant who provides the board with false information or makes a false statement to the board may be subject to disciplinary action, including denial, suspension or revocation of licensure, pursuant to the provisions of the act, Section 61 – 14A – 17 NMSA 1978, and the Uniform Licensing Act, Section 61 – 1 – 1 NMSA 1978;

G. an affidavit as provided on the "initial licensure application" stating that the applicant understands that:

(1) the applicant is responsible for reading, understanding and complying with the state of New Mexico laws and rules regarding this application as well as the practice of acupuncture and oriental medicine;

(2) the license must be renewed annually by July 31; and

(3) the applicant must notify the board within ten days if the applicant's address changes;

H. a copy of the applicant's certificate or diploma from an educational program evidencing completion of the required program; this copy shall include on it an affidavit certifying that it is a true copy of the original;

I. an official copy of the applicant's transcript that shall be sent directly to the board in a sealed envelope by the educational program from which the applicant received the certificate or diploma, and that shall verify the applicant's satisfactory completion of the required academic and clinical education and that shall designate the completed subjects and the hours of study completed in each subject; or this copy of the transcript shall remain in the closed envelope secured with the official seal of the educational program and shall be sent by the applicant to the board along with the applicant's application for licensure; and

J. an accurate translation in English of all documents submitted in a foreign language; each translated document shall bear the affidavit of the translator certifying that he or she is competent in both the language of the document and the English language and that the translation is a true and faithful translation of the foreign language original; each translated document shall also bear the affidavit of the applicant certifying that the translation is a true and faithful translation of the original; each affidavit shall be signed before a notary public; the translation of any document relevant to an application shall be at the expense of the applicant.

16.2.3.12 EXAMINATION REQUIREMENTS

The examination requirements specified in 16.2.4 NMAC shall be received at the board office within 12 months of the receipt of the initial application at the board office, with the exception of the national certification commission for acupuncture and oriental medicine (NCCAOM) score requirements which need to be submitted to the board office within 24 months of the initial application.

16.2.3.13 DOCUMENTS IN A FOREIGN LANGUAGE

All documents submitted in a foreign language must be accompanied by an accurate translation in English. Each translated document shall bear the affidavit of the translator certifying that he or she is competent in both the language of the document and the English language and that the translation is a true and faithful translation of the foreign language original. Each translated document shall also bear the affidavit of the applicant certifying that the translation is a true and faithful translation of the original. Each affidavit shall be signed before a notary public. The translation of any document relevant to an applicant's application shall be at the expense of the applicant.

16.2.3.14   SUFFICIENCY OF DOCUMENT

The board shall determine the sufficiency of the documentation that supports the application for licensure. The board may, at its discretion, request further proof of qualifications or require a personal interview with any applicant to establish his or her qualifications. If requested by the board, all further proof of qualifications shall be received at the board office at least 45 days before the clinical skills examination date. Any required personal interview will be scheduled as determined by the board.

16.2.3.15   DEADLINE FOR COMPLETING ALL REQUIREMENTS FOR LICENSURE

Documentation required for licensure shall be received at the board office no later than 12 months after the initial application is received at the board office, with the exception of the national certification commission for acupuncture and oriental medicine (NCCAOM) score requirements which need to be submitted to the board office within 24 months of the initial application.

16.2.3.16   NOTIFICATION OF LICENSURE

The applicant shall be notified of approval or denial of his completed application requirements including examination requirements by mail postmarked no more than 21 days from the board's receipt of all required documentation. The board shall issue a license to all applicants who have met the requirements of 16.2.3 NMAC and 16.2.4 NMAC.

16.2.3.17   EXPIRATION AND ABANDONMENT OF APPLICATION

If all application requirements have not been met within 24 months of the initial application, the application will expire and will be deemed abandoned. Exceptions may be made, at the board's discretion, for good cause. If the application is abandoned and the applicant wants to reapply for licensure, the applicant shall be required to submit the completed current application form, pay the current application fee and satisfy the requirements for licensure then in effect at the time of the new application.

Part 4.   Examinations

16.2.4.1   ISSUING AGENCY

New Mexico Board of Acupuncture and Oriental Medicine.

16.2.4.2   SCOPE

All applicants for licensure as doctors of oriental medicine.

16.2.4.3 STATUTORY AUTHORITY

This part is promulgated pursuant to the Acupuncture and Oriental Medicine Practice Act, Sections 61 – 14A – 8, 9, 10(F) and 11, NMSA 1978.

16.2.4.4 DURATION

Permanent.

16.2.4.5 EFFECTIVE DATE

July 1, 1996, unless a later date is cited at the end of a section.

16.2.4.6 OBJECTIVE

This part clarifies the contents, language, number and type of the examinations for licensure, the requirements for issuance of a license, the frequency of examination administration and re-examination requirements in the event of a failing score.

16.2.4.7 DEFINITIONS

Refer to definitions in 16.2.1.7 NMAC (Section 7 of Part 1 of the rules).

16.2.4.8 APPROVED EXAMINATIONS

The board approved examinations shall consist of a written examination portion and a practical examination portion. All required NCCAOM examinations must be completed prior to taking the clinical skills examination.

A. The written examinations approved by the board shall be:

(1) the national certification commission for acupuncture and oriental medicine foundations of oriental medicine module;

(2) the national certification commission for acupuncture and oriental medicine acupuncture module;

(3) the national certification commission for acupuncture and oriental medicine Chinese herbology module;

(4) the national certification commission for acupuncture and oriental medicine biomedicine module;

(5) the national certification commission for acupuncture and oriental medicine approved clean needle technique course; and

(6) the board approved and board administered jurisprudence examination covering the act and the rules.

B. The practical examinations approved by the board shall be:

(1) the national certification commission for acupuncture and oriental medicine point location module; and

(2) the clinical skills examination; the clinical skills examination includes examination in acupuncture, herbal medicine and biomedicine competencies.

C. The board may adopt such other examinations as may be necessary for psychometric evaluation of its approved examinations.

16.2.4.9　EXAMINATION LANGUAGE

All examinations required by the board shall be given in English.

16.2.4.10　EXAMINATION REQUIREMENTS FOR LICENSURE

The following shall be the examination requirements for licensure. All fees for nationally recognized examinations shall be paid by the applicant and are not included in fees charged by the board.

A. Achievement of a passing score as determined by the national certification commission for acupuncture and oriental medicine (NCCAOM) on each of the following prior to taking the clinical skills exam:

(1) the NCCAOM foundations of oriental medicine module;

(2) the NCCAOM acupuncture module;

(3) the NCCAOM Chinese herbology module;

(4) the NCCAOM biomedicine module; and

(5) the NCCAOM point location module.

B. Achievement of a passing score of at least 75 percent on the clinical skills examination. To determine a passing score when the applicant is examined by more than one examiner, if the applicant is examined by two examiners, the applicant must receive a score of at least 75 percent after both scores are averaged and if the applicant is examined by three examiners, the applicant must receive a score of at least 75 percent from a majority of the examiners.

C. Successful completion of the national certification commission for acupuncture and oriental medicine approved clean needle technique course.

D. Achievement of a passing score of not less than 90 percent on the board approved and board administered jurisprudence examination covering the act and the rules.

E. Applicants who completed the national certification commission for acupuncture and oriental medicine (NCCAOM) examinations in acupuncture and Chinese herbology prior to June 2004 are not required to pass the NCCAOM foundations of oriental medicine module.

16.2.4.11　CLINICAL SKILLS EXAMINATION FREQUENCY AND DEADLINES

The board shall hold a clinical skills examination at least once each year provided that applications for licensure are pending. The initial application specified in 16.2.3.11 NMAC shall be received at the board office at least 60 calendar days before the next scheduled clinical skills examination date. The board shall send a written response to the applicant informing the applicant of the application's completeness or needed documentation postmarked at least 45 calendar days before the next scheduled clinical skills examination date. All documentation required to complete the initial application for licensure shall be received at the board office at least 35 calendar days before the next scheduled clinical skills examination date. If the application requirements are received at the board office after a deadline, the application will be held and not processed until the deadline schedule for the next subsequent clinical skills examination. The applicant shall be notified of approval or denial of his or her completed initial application for licensure specified in 16.2.3.11, by mail or electronic means at least 25 calendar days prior to the next scheduled clinical skills examination date.

16.2.4.12 CLINICAL SKILLS EXAMINATION CONFIRMATION

The board approved confirmation card, provided to the applicant, shall be sent to the applicant within fifteen days of receipt of the clinical skills examination fee specified in 16.2.10 NMAC. Confirmation of clinical exam passage will be valid for 24 months from the date of initial application. After 24 months have passed, the applicant will have to retake the clinical exam and reapply as a new applicant and pay required fees specified in 16.2.10 NMAC.

16.2.4.13 PAYMENT OF CLINICAL SKILLS EXAMINATION FEE

The non refundable clinical skills examination fee specified in 16.2.10 NMAC shall be paid by check or money order in U.S. funds and received in the board's office at least 31 calendar days prior to the next scheduled clinical skills examination.

16.2.4.14 CLINICAL SKILLS EXAMINATION COMMITMENT

Upon receipt of the clinical skills examination fee for the next scheduled clinical skills examination, the applicant shall sit for the exam or forfeit the fee. The non-refundable clinical skills examination fee may be applied to a subsequent exam only as provided in Section 15 of 16.2.4 NMAC.

16.2.4.15 FORFEITURE OF CLINICAL SKILLS EXAMINATION FEE

Once the clinical skills examination fee is received in the board office, the applicant shall take the next scheduled clinical skills examination or forfeit the clinical skills examination fee. Under special circumstances the applicant may be allowed to take the next subsequent scheduled clinical skills examination without paying an additional examination fee.

16.2.4.16 FAILING SCORE

In the event that an applicant fails to achieve a passing score on the clinical skills examination, he may apply as provided in 16.2.4.17 NMAC, and must pay the required fees.

16.2.4.17 RE – EXAMINATION

Applicants who have failed the clinical skills examination may apply to take the next subsequent clinical skills examination. The applicant shall notify the board of his commitment to take the next subsequent clinical skills examination with a written and signed letter received at the board office at least 60 days before the next clinical skills examination date. The applicant shall then be notified by the board of his acceptance to take the next clinical skills examination by mail or electronic means at least 45 days prior to the next scheduled clinical skills examination date. The applicant shall pay the clinical skills examination fee in accordance with the provisions of 16.2.4.13 NMAC. If the applicant does not pass the next scheduled clinical skills examination, the applicant shall file a new application on the current form provided by the board, pay all the required fees, and satisfy all current requirements in effect at the time the application is made. If the applicant passes the exam, but does not complete license application within 24 months, the applicant will have to reapply as an initial applicant.

16.2.4.18 EXAMINERS

The board shall select a group of doctors of oriental medicine to act as examiners for the clinical skills examination. These examiners shall have had five years of clinical experience at the time they are selected. The board or its designated agent shall train these examiners to judge applicants taking the board approved clinical skills examination in the application of the diagnostic and treatment techniques of acupuncture and oriental medicine.

16.2.4.19 REVIEW OF CLINICAL SKILLS EXAMINATION SCORE

Applicants may request review of their clinical skills examination results by the board or its examination committee for significant procedural or computational error if such review request is received in writing at the board office within 25 calendar days of notification to the applicant of the clinical skills examination results.

Part 5. Temporary Licensing

16.2.5.1 ISSUING AGENCY

New Mexico Board of Acupuncture and Oriental Medicine.

16.2.5.2 SCOPE

All licensees, applicants, temporary licensees, applicants for temporary licensure, externs, educational programs and applicants for approval of educational programs.

16.2.5.3 STATUTORY AUTHORITY

This part is promulgated pursuant to the Acupuncture and Oriental Medicine Practice Act, Sections 61 - 14A - 8, 9 and 12, NMSA 1978.

16.2.5.4 DURATION

Permanent.

16.2.5.5 EFFECTIVE DATE

February 11, 2022, unless a later date is cited at the end of a section.

16.2.5.6 OBJECTIVE

This part establishes requirements for temporary licensure and limited temporary licensure, prior disciplinary action relating to other licenses, prior litigation and prior felonies, the educational requirements for temporary licensure, the renewal period for temporary licensure and the requirements for renewal of temporary licenses.

16.2.5.7 DEFINITIONS

Refer to definitions in 16.2.1.7 NMAC.

16.2.5.8 GENERAL REQUIREMENTS

A. Any applicant for temporary licensure or applicant for a limited temporary license who has been subject to any action or proceeding comprehended by Subsection E of 16.2.5.10 NMAC and Subsection D of 16.2.5.12 NMAC, may be subject to disciplinary action at any time, including denial, suspension or revocation of licensure, pursuant to the provisions of the act, Section 61 – 14A – 17 NMSA 1978; and subject to the Uniform Licensing Act, Section 61 – 1 – 1 NMSA 1978, et seq., and subject to the Criminal Offender Employment Act, Section 28 – 2 – 1 NMSA 1978, et seq.

B. Any applicant for temporary licensure or an applicant for a limited temporary license who provides the board with false information or makes a false statement to the board may be subject to disciplinary action, including denial, suspension or revocation of licensure, pursuant to the provisions of the act, Section 61 – 14A – 17 NMSA 1978, and the Uniform Licensing Act, Section 61 – 1 – 1 NMSA 1978, et seq.

16.2.5.9 TEMPORARY LICENSE EDUCATIONAL REQUIREMENTS

A. An applicant for temporary licensure shall provide satisfactory proof that he or she has completed an approved educational program. An applicant for temporary licensure who is legally recognized in any state or foreign country to practice another health care profession and who possesses knowledge and skills that are included in the scope of practice of doctors of oriental medicine shall provide satisfactory proof that he or she has completed the education required for legal recognition in that state or foreign country.

B. The board, by a vote of the majority of the members of the board acting at a duly convened meeting of the board, may determine not to require the applicant for temporary licensure to complete the requirements of Subsection A of 16.2.5.9 NMAC, if the board determines that there is good cause and the health and safety of the citizens of New Mexico will not be jeopardized.

16.2.5.10 TEMPORARY LICENSE APPLICATION

Upon approval of an application for a temporary license that fulfills the requirements listed below, the board shall issue a temporary license that will be valid for the dates specified on the license but shall not exceed six months. The temporary license shall include the name of the temporary licensee, the effective dates of the license, the name of the sponsoring New Mexico doctor of oriental medicine or New Mexico educational program, and a statement that the license shall be for the exclusive purpose of one or more of the following: teaching acupuncture and oriental medicine; consulting, in association with the sponsoring doctor of oriental medicine, regarding the sponsoring doctor's patients; performing specialized diagnostic or treatment techniques in association with the sponsoring doctor of oriental medicine regarding the sponsoring doctor's patients; assisting in the conducting of research in acupuncture and oriental medicine; or assisting in the implementation of new techniques and technology related to acupuncture and oriental medicine. The application requirements for a limited temporary license shall be receipt of the following by the board.

A. The fee for application for temporary license specified in 16.2.10 NMAC.

B. An application for temporary license that is complete and in English on a form provided by the board that shall include the applicant's name, address, date of birth, social security number, if available, and the name of the sponsoring and associating New Mexico doctor of oriental medicine or New Mexico educational program.

C. One passport-type photograph of the applicant taken not more than six months prior to the submission of the application.

D. An affidavit as provided on the "temporary license application" from the sponsoring and associating New Mexico doctor of oriental medicine or New Mexico educational program attesting to the qualifications of the applicant and the activities the applicant will perform.

E. An affidavit as provided on the "temporary license application" as to whether the applicant:

(1) has been subject to any disciplinary action in any jurisdiction related to the practice of acupuncture and oriental medicine, or related to any other profession including other health care professions for which the applicant is licensed, certified, registered or legally recognized to practice including resignation from practice, withdrawal or surrender of applicants license, certificate or registration during the pendency of disciplinary proceedings or investigation for potential disciplinary proceedings; or

(2) has been a party to litigation in any jurisdiction related to the applicants practice of acupuncture and oriental medicine, or related to any other profession including other health care professions for which the applicant is licensed, certified, registered or legally recognized to practice; or

(3) is in arrears on a court-ordered child support payment.

F. An official license history, which is a certificate from each jurisdiction stating the disciplinary record of the applicant, from each jurisdiction where the applicant has been licensed, certified, registered or legally recognized to practice any other profession, including other health care professions, in any jurisdiction, pursuant to any authority other than the New Mexico Acupuncture and Oriental Medicine Practice Act.

G. An affidavit as provided on the "temporary license application" stating that the applicant understands that:

(1) an applicant who has been subject to any action or proceeding comprehended by Subsection E of 16.2.5.10 NMAC may be subject to disciplinary action at any time, including denial, suspension or revocation of licensure, pursuant to the provisions of the act, Section 61 - 14A - 17 NMSA 1978; and subject to the Uniform Licensing Act, Section 61 - 1 - 1 NMSA 1978, and subject to the Criminal Offender Employment Act, Section 28 - 2 - 1 NMSA 1978; and

(2) an applicant who provides the board with false information or makes a false statement to the board may be subject to disciplinary action, including denial, suspension or revocation of

licensure, pursuant to the provisions of the act, Section 61 – 14A – 17 NMSA 1978, and the Uniform Licensing Act, Section 61 – 1 – 1 NMSA 1978.

H. An affidavit as provided on the "temporary license application" stating that the applicant understands that:

(1) the applicant is responsible for reading, understanding and complying with the state of New Mexico laws and rules regarding this application as well as the practice of acupuncture and oriental medicine; and

(2) the applicant must notify the board within ten days if the applicant's address changes or the circumstances of the applicant's relationship to the sponsoring and associating New Mexico doctor of oriental medicine or New Mexico educational program change; and

(3) the applicant may only engage in those activities authorized on the temporary license and only in association with the sponsoring and associating New Mexico doctor of oriental medicine or New Mexico educational program for the limited time specified on the temporary license.

I. A copy of the applicant's license, certification or registration or other document proving that the applicant is legally recognized in another state or country to practice acupuncture and oriental medicine or another health care profession and who possesses knowledge and skill that are included in the scope of practice of doctors of oriental medicine. The copy shall include on it an affidavit by the applicant certifying that it is a true copy of the original. For applicants in the United States who practice in a state in which there is no legal recognition, a copy of the certification document in acupuncture, Chinese herbal medicine or Asian body work, whichever is appropriate for the type of material they will be teaching or studying, by the national certification commission for acupuncture and oriental medicine (NCCAOM) shall be sufficient. The copy shall include on it an affidavit by the applicant certifying that it is a true copy of the original. For applicants outside the United States who practice in a country in which there is no specific legal recognition document but where graduation from an appropriate educational program is the legal requirement for practice, the above provisions in this paragraph shall not apply.

J. A copy of the applicant's diploma for graduation from the educational program that is required to be licensed, certified, registered or legally recognized to practice in the state or country where the applicant practices. This copy shall include on it an affidavit by the applicant certifying that it is a true copy of the original.

K. An official copy of the applicant's transcript that shall be sent directly to the board in a sealed envelope by the educational program from which the applicant received the certificate or diploma, and that shall verify the applicant's satisfactory completion of the required academic and clinical education and that shall designate the completed subjects and the hours of study completed in each subject. This copy of the transcript shall remain in the closed envelope secured with the official seal of the educational program and shall be sent by the applicant to the board along with the applicant's application for licensure.

L. An affidavit stating that the applicant has been officially informed by the board in writing that either of the following two requirements has been fulfilled:

(1) the educational program in acupuncture and oriental medicine from which the applicant graduated has been approved by the board as an educational program; or

(2) the board, by a vote of the majority of the members of the board acting at a duly convened meeting of the board, has determined not to require the applicant for temporary licensure to have graduated from an approved educational program as provided for in Subsection B of 16.2.5.9 NMAC.

M. An accurate translation in English of all documents submitted in a foreign language. Each translated document shall bear the affidavit of the translator certifying that they are competent in both the language of the document and the English language and that the translation is a true and faithful translation of the foreign language original. Each translated document shall also bear the affidavit of the applicant certifying that the translation is a true and faithful translation of the original. Each affidavit shall be signed before a notary public. The translation of any document relevant to an application shall be at the expense of the applicant.

16.2.5.11 TEMPORARY LICENSE RENEWAL

A temporary license issued by the board may be renewed a maximum of two times only, for a period of six months for each renewal. Renewals shall run sequentially so that a renewal shall begin immediately when the previous temporary license period expires. Upon approval of an application for renewal of a temporary license that fulfills the requirements listed below, the board shall issue a temporary license. The application requirements for renewal of a temporary license shall be receipt of the following by the board:

A. The fee for renewal of a temporary license specified in 16.2.10 NMAC.

B. An application for renewal of a temporary license that is complete and in English on a form provided by the board that shall include the applicant's name, address, date of birth, social security number, if available, and the name of the sponsoring and associating New Mexico doctor of oriental medicine or New Mexico educational program.

C. An affidavit from the sponsoring and associating New Mexico doctor of oriental medicine or New Mexico educational program attesting to the qualifications of the applicant and the activities the applicant will perform.

16.2.5.12 LIMITED TEMPORARY LICENSE APPLICATION

Upon approval of an application for a limited temporary license that fulfills the requirements listed below, the board shall issue a limited temporary license that will be valid for the dates specified on the license but shall not exceed 12 consecutive months from the date of issuance and is not renewable. A limited temporary license shall be for the exclusive purpose of teaching a single complete course in acupuncture and oriental medicine and assisting in the implementation of new techniques in acupuncture and oriental medicine including the study of such techniques by licensed, registered, certified or legally recognized health care practitioners from jurisdictions other than New Mexico. A limited temporary license shall be required for any person who demonstrates, practices or performs diagnostic and treatment techniques on another person as part of teaching or assisting in the implementation of new techniques, if they are not a licensee or temporary licensee. Limited temporary licenses shall not be issued to teachers for the purpose of teaching full semester courses that are part of an approved educational program. The limited temporary license shall include the name of the limited temporary license holder, the effective dates of the license, the name of the sponsoring New Mexico doctor of oriental medicine or New Mexico educational program, and a statement that the license shall be for the exclusive purpose of teaching acupuncture and oriental medicine, and assisting in the implementation of new techniques in acupuncture and oriental medicine including the study of such techniques by licensed, registered, certified or legally recognized health care practitioners from jurisdictions other than New Mexico. The requirements for a limited temporary license shall be:

A. the fee for application for a limited temporary license specified in 16.2.10 NMAC;

B. an application for limited temporary license that is complete and in English on a form provided by the board that shall include the applicant's name, address, date of birth, social security number, if available, and the name of the sponsoring and associating New Mexico doctor of oriental medicine or New Mexico educational program;

C. an affidavit as provided on the "temporary license application" from the sponsoring and associating New Mexico doctor of oriental medicine or New Mexico educational program attesting to the qualifications of the applicant and the activities the applicant will perform; and

D. an affidavit as to whether the applicant:

(1) has been subject to any disciplinary action in any jurisdiction related to the practice of acupuncture and oriental medicine, or related to any other profession including other health care professions for which the applicant is licensed, certified, registered or legally recognized to practice including resignation from practice, withdrawal or surrender of applicants license, certificate or registration during the pendency of disciplinary proceedings or investigation for potential disciplinary proceedings; or

(2) has been a party to litigation in any jurisdiction related to the applicants practice of acupuncture and oriental medicine, or related to any other profession including other health care professions for which the applicant is licensed, certified, registered or legally recognized to practice; or

(3) is in arrears on a court-ordered child support payment; and

E. an affidavit as provided on the "temporary license application" stating that the applicant understands that:

(1) an applicant who has been subject to any action or proceeding comprehended by Subsection D of 16.2.5.12 NMAC, may be subject to disciplinary action at any time, including denial, suspension or revocation of licensure, pursuant to the provisions of the act, Section 61 - 14A - 17 NMSA 1978; and subject to the Uniform Licensing Act, Section 61 - 1 - 1 NMSA 1978, and subject to the Criminal Offender Employment Act, Section 28 - 2 - 1 NMSA 1978; and

(2) an applicant who provides the board with false information or makes a false statement to the board may be subject to disciplinary action, including denial, suspension or revocation of licensure, pursuant to the provisions of the act, Section 61 - 14A - 17 NMSA 1978, and the Uniform Licensing Act, Section 61 - 1 - 1 NMSA 1978; and

F. an affidavit as provided on the "temporary license application" stating that the applicant understands that:

(1) the applicant is responsible for reading, understanding and complying with the state of New Mexico laws and rules regarding this application as well as the practice of acupuncture and oriental medicine; and

(2) the applicant must notify the board within ten days if the applicant's address changes or the circumstances of the applicant's relationship to the sponsoring and associating New Mexico doctor of oriental medicine or New Mexico educational program change; and

(3) the applicant may only engage in those activities authorized on the temporary license and only in association with the sponsoring and associating New Mexico doctor of oriental medicine or New Mexico educational program for the limited time specified on the temporary license; and

G. a copy of the applicant's license, certification or registration or other document proving that the applicant is legally recognized in another state or country to practice acupuncture and oriental medicine or another health care profession and who possesses knowledge and skill that are included in the scope of practice of doctors of oriental medicine; the copy shall include on it an affidavit by the applicant certifying that it is a true copy of the original; for applicants in the United States who practice in a state in which there is no legal recognition, a copy of the certification document in acupuncture, Chinese herbal medicine or Asian body work, whichever is appropriate for the type of material they will be teaching or studying, by the national certification commission for acupuncture and oriental medicine (NCCAOM) shall be sufficient; the copy shall include on it an affidavit by the applicant certifying that it is a true copy of the original; for applicants outside the United States who practice in a country in which there is no specific legal recognition document but where graduation from an appropriate educational program is the legal requirement for practice, the above provisions in this paragraph shall not apply; and

H. a copy of the applicant's diploma for graduation from the educational program that is required to be licensed, certified, registered or legally recognized to practice in the state or country where the applicant practices; this copy shall include on it an affidavit by the applicant certifying that it is a true copy of the original; and

I. an accurate translation in English of all documents submitted in a foreign language; each translated document shall bear the affidavit of the translator certifying that they are competent in both the language of the document and the English language and that the translation is a true and faithful translation of the foreign language original; each translated document shall also bear the affidavit of the applicant certifying that the translation is a true and faithful translation of the original; each affidavit shall be signed before a notary public; the translation of any document relevant to an application shall be at the expense of the applicant.

Part 6.   Reciprocal Licensing

16.2.6.1   ISSUING AGENCY
New Mexico Board of Acupuncture and Oriental Medicine.

16.2.6.2   SCOPE
All licensees and applicants.

16.2.6.3   STATUTARY AUTHORITY
This part is promulgated pursuant to the Acupuncture and Oriental Medicine Practice Act, Sections 61 – 14A – 8, 9 and 13, NMSA 1978.

16.2.6.4   DURATION
Permanent

16.2.6.5   EFFECTIVE DATE
December 1, 2001 unless a later date is cited at the end of a section.

16.2.6.6   OBJECTIVE
This part establishes that there are currently no reciprocal licensing agreements between the board and other states or countries.

16.2.6.7   DEFINITIONS
Refer to definitions in 16.2.1.7 NMAC (Section 7 of Part 1 of the rules).

16.2.6.8   RECIPROCAL LICENSING
Currently there are no states or countries with which the board has reciprocal licensing agreements.

Part 7.   Educational Programs

16.2.7.1   ISSUING AGENCY
New Mexico Board of Acupuncture and Oriental Medicine

16.2.7.2   SCOPE
All licensed doctors of oriental medicine, temporarily licensed doctors of oriental medicine,

approved educational programs and all applicants for licensure as a doctor of oriental medicine, temporary licensure and for approval of an educational program.

16.2.7.3　STATUTORY AUTHORITY

This part is promulgated pursuant to the Acupuncture and Oriental Medicine Practice Act, Sections 61 – 14A – 8, 9 and 14, NMSA 1978.

16.2.7.4　DURATION

Permanent.

16.2.7.5　EFFECTIVE DATE

October 22, 2003, unless a later date is cited at the end of a section.

16.2.7.6　OBJECTIVE

This part establishes the requirements for approval of educational programs, the requirements for making an application for approval of an educational program, the renewal of the approval of the educational program and the requirement of notification of changes.

16.2.7.7　DEFINITIONS

Refer to definitions in 16.2.1.7 NMAC (Section 7 of Part 1 of the rules).

16.2.7.8　EDUCATIONAL PROGRAM REQUIREMENTS

All educational programs shall be approved by the board. Using the requirements of 16.2.7.8 NMAC and 16.2.7.9 NMAC (Sections 8 and 9 of Part 7 of the rules), the board will evaluate whether or not an educational program shall be approved. If a visit is necessary to evaluate the educational program, the cost of the visit, including any administrative costs, shall be paid in advance by the educational program.

A. The foundation educational program requirement shall be the four academic year masters of oriental medicine program that meets the national certification commission for acupuncture and oriental medicine (NCCAOM) accreditation/equivalent education policy as defined here. Graduation/education must be obtained from a formal education program that has met the standards of the accreditation commission for acupuncture and oriental medicine (ACAOM) or an equivalent educational body. A program may be established as having satisfied this requirement by demonstration of one of the following:

(1) accreditation or candidacy for accreditation by ACAOM; or

(2) approval by a foreign government's ministry of education, ministry of health, or equivalent foreign government agency; each candidate must submit their documents for approval by a foreign credential equivalency service approved by the NCCAOM for that purpose; programs attempting to meet the eligibility requirement under this method must also meet the curricular requirements of ACAOM in effect at the time of application; or

(3) approval by a foreign private accreditation agency that has an accreditation process and standards substantially equivalent to that of ACAOM, and that is recognized for that purpose by the appropriate government entity in that foreign country; each candidate must submit their

documents for approval by a foreign credential equivalency service approved by the NCCAOM for that purpose; programs attempting to meet the eligibility requirement under this method must also meet the curricular requirements of ACAOM in effect at the time of application.

B. The educational program shall provide a program that shall be at least four academic years and shall include in-class education that comprises a minimum of 2,400 clock hours of classes including a minimum of 1,100 hours of didactic education in acupuncture and oriental medicine and a minimum of 900 hours of supervised clinical practice, instruction and observation in acupuncture and oriental medicine. The curriculum shall provide the knowledge and skills required to maintain appropriate standards of acupuncture and oriental medical care.

C. The educational program shall include a didactic curriculum that educates and graduates physicians who are competent to practice acupuncture and oriental medicine and who are able to diagnose, prescribe, and treat accurately and that specifically includes, in addition to the requirements of the act, oriental principles of life therapy, including the prescription of herbal medicine, diet and nutrition, manual therapy/physical medicine and counseling, not to exceed 900 hours of the required 2,400 hours specified in Subsection B of 16.2.7.8 NMAC (Subsection 8.B. of Part 7 of the rules) and that includes a minimum of 450 hours of education in herbal medicine.

D. The educational program shall include a clinical curriculum that includes clinical instruction and direct patient contact. This clinical part of the educational program shall include at least 900 hours of supervised clinical practice, instruction and observation in the following areas:

(1) the observation of and assistance in the application of principles and techniques of oriental medicine including diagnosis, acupuncture, moxibustion, manual therapy/physical medicine, diet and nutrition, counseling and the prescription of herbal medicine; and

(2) a minimum of 400 hours of actual treatment in which the student is required to perform complete treatment as the primary student practitioner.

E. The educational program shall include a curriculum that educates and graduates physicians who are competent to demonstrate a clinically relevant, complementary and integrative knowledge of biomedicine and biomedical diagnosis sufficient to treat and refer patients when appropriate.

F. The educational program may honor credit from other educational programs.

G. The names and educational qualifications of all teaching supervisors, resident teachers, and visiting teachers of acupuncture and oriental medicine shall be submitted to the board and shall meet the following:

(1) all teachers of acupuncture and oriental medicine in New Mexico shall have a license or temporary license to practice acupuncture and oriental medicine in New Mexico issued by the board; any educational program in violation of this provision shall be subject to suspension or revocation of the educational program approval or subject to disciplinary proceedings, including

fines as defined in 16.2.12 NMAC（Part 12 of the rules）；

（2）all teachers of acupuncture and oriental medicine at educational programs outside New Mexico shall be licensed, certified, registered or legally recognized to practice acupuncture and oriental medicine in the state or country in which he or she practices and teaches; any educational program in violation of this provision shall be subject to suspension or revocation of the educational program approval or subject to disciplinary proceedings, including fines as defined in 16.2.12 NMAC（Part 12 of the rules）；

（3）exceptions may be made at the board's discretion and for good cause.

H. Educational programs may employ or contract with tutors to teach components of the educational program. Educational programs may honor credit from tutors. A tutor is defined in the act as "a doctor of oriental medicine with at least ten years of clinical experience who is a teacher of acupuncture and oriental medicine."

I. The educational program may be subject to inspection by the board.

16.2.7.9 EDUCATIONAL PROGRAM CERTIFICATE OR DIPLOMA AND TRANSCRIPT REQUIREMENTS

Educational programs shall provide the following：

A. A transcript of grades, as part of the student's record, that includes the following：

（1）Name of the student；

（2）Address of the student；

（3）Date of birth；

（4）Course titles；

（5）Grade received in each course; and

（6）Number of clock hours per course.

B. A certificate or diploma stating that the student has satisfactorily completed the educational program only after personal attendance in all required classes, and satisfactory completion of the educational program requirements.

16.2.7.10 APPLICATION FOR ANNUAL APPROVAL OF AN EDUCATIONAL PROGRAM

All educational programs in New Mexico are required to be annually approved by the board. Any educational program outside New Mexico, that so chooses, may apply to receive annual approval status. These educational programs shall be granted approval after submitting to the board：

A. The initial application fee for annual approval of an educational program specified in 16.2.10 NMAC（Part 10 of the rules）and paid by certified check or money order in U. S. funds; and

B. An application that is complete and in English on a form prescribed by the board that contains the matriculation date for the educational program and the information necessary to verify that the standards of professional education required by 16.2.7.8 and 16.2.7.9 NMAC (Sections 8 and 9 of Part 7 of the rules) are being met including an official copy of the curriculum. The board shall act upon the application within sixty (60) days of the receipt of the application and shall inform the educational program of the status of the application in writing by mail postmarked within seven (7) days of acting on it.

16.2.7.11 APPLICATION FOR SINGLE INSTANCE APPROVAL OF AN EDUCATIONAL PROGRAM

An educational program that does not have annual approval status from the board shall receive a single instance approval of the educational program for use by a single applicant after the educational program that graduated the applicant has submitted to the board:

A. The application fee for a single instance approval of an educational program, specified in 16.2.10 NMAC (Part 10 of the rules), paid by certified check or money order in U.S. funds; and

B. An application that is complete and in English on a form prescribed by the board that contains the matriculation date for the educational program and the information necessary to verify that the standards of professional education required by 16.2.7.8 and 16.2.7.9 NMAC (Sections 8 and 9 of Part 7 of the rules) are being met including an official copy of the curriculum. The application and the application fee shall be received at the board's office at least ninety (90) days prior to the next scheduled clinical skills examination. The board shall send a written response to the applicant for approval of an educational program informing the applicant of the application's completeness or needed documentation postmarked at least eighty-five (85) days before the next scheduled clinical skills examination date. All documentation requested to complete the application shall be received at the board's office at least seventy (70) days before the next scheduled clinical skills examination date. The applicant shall be notified of approval or denial of the application in writing by mail postmarked at least sixty (60) days prior to the next scheduled clinical skills examination date. Note that the above deadlines exist to synchronize with the deadlines for applicants regarding the clinical skills exam as defined in 16.2.4.11 NMAC (Section 11 of Part 4 of the rules).

16.2.7.12 ANNUAL RENEWAL, LATE RENEWAL AND EXPIRED APPROVAL

To maintain annual approval status, an educational program shall submit by May 1st an annual renewal application that is complete and in English on a form prescribed by the board and the required fee for renewal of approval of an educational program, specified in 16.2.10 NMAC (Part 10 of the rules), paid by certified check or money order in U.S. funds. The approval period is defined as August 1st to July 31st of the subsequent year. The approval expires at 12:00 midnight on July 31st. Renewal applications received after September 30th of any year must be submitted with the late fee specified in 16.2.10 NMAC (Part 10 of the rules) and paid by certified check or money order in U.S. funds. If the annual renewal application and fee are not received within sixty (60) days after expiration, following the approval period, the annual approval is expired and the educational program shall submit the initial application and initial application fee to become approved.

16.2.7.13 NOTIFICATION OF CHANGES

If ownership of the educational program changes or the educational program is substantially changed the educational program shall notify the board within ten (10) days of such change. The educational program may then be subject to inspection. The educational program shall be on a probationary approval status until final approval is given under the changed circumstances.

ARIZONA

Article 1.   Acupuncture Board of Examiners
(Refs & Annos)

§ 32 – 3901.   Definitions

In this chapter, unless the context otherwise requires:

1. "Acupuncture":

(a) Means a system of medicine based in traditional practices and informed by contemporary science.

(b) Includes the following:

(i) Puncturing the skin by thin, solid needles to reach subcutaneous structures.

(ii) Stimulating the needles to effect a positive therapeutic response.

(iii) Removing needles.

(iv) Using and prescribing adjunctive therapies.

(v) Using and prescribing herbal therapies commensurate with the acupuncturist's education and training.

(vi) Using decision-support tools, including physical and clinical examinations.

(vii) ordering diagnostic imaging and clinical laboratory procedures to determine the nature of care or to form a basis for referral to other licensed health care professionals, or both.

2. "Acupuncture assistant" means an unlicensed person who has completed a training program approved by the board, who assists in basic health care duties in the practice of acupuncture under the supervision of a licensed acupuncturist and who performs delegated duties commensurate with the acupuncture assistant's education and training, but who does not evaluate, interpret, design or modify established treatment programs of acupuncture care.

3. "Adjunctive therapies" means the manual, mechanical, magnetic, thermal, electrical or

285

electromagnetic stimulation of acupuncture points and energy pathways, auricular and detoxification therapy, the use of ion cord devices, electroacupuncture, nutritional counseling, therapeutic exercise, the use of nonionizing lasers and acupressure.

4. "Board" means the acupuncture board of examiners.

5. "Herbal therapies" means prescribing, administering, injecting, compounding and dispensing herbal medicines and plant, animal, mineral and natural substances.

6. "Supervision" means that the supervising licensed acupuncturist is present in the facility where the acupuncture assistant is performing services and is available for consultation regarding procedures that the licensed acupuncturist has authorized and for which the licensed acupuncturist remains responsible.

7. "Trauma" means the experience of significant psychological distress following any terrible or life-threatening event.

8. "Unprofessional conduct" includes the following, whether occurring in this state or elsewhere:

(a) Wilfully disclosing a professional secret or wilfully violating a privileged communication except as either of these may otherwise be required by law.

(b) Committing a felony as evidenced by conviction by a court of competent jurisdiction.

(c) Being habitually intemperate in the use of alcohol or any substance abuse that interferes with the ability to safely practice acupuncture.

(d) Committing conduct that the board determines is gross malpractice, repeated malpractice or any malpractice resulting in the death of a patient.

(e) Impersonating another acupuncturist or any other practitioner of the healing arts.

(f) Falsely acting or assuming to act as a member, an employee or an authorized agent of the board.

(g) Procuring or attempting to procure a license pursuant to this chapter by fraud or misrepresentation.

(h) Refusing to divulge to the board on demand the acupuncture method used in the treatment of a patient.

(i) Giving or receiving or aiding or abetting the giving or receiving of rebates, either directly or indirectly.

(j) Knowingly making any false or fraudulent statement, written or oral, in connection with the practice of acupuncture.

(k) Having a license refused, revoked or suspended by any other state, district or territory of the United States or any other country, unless the action was not taken for reasons relating to the person's ability to safely and skillfully practice acupuncture or relating to an act of unprofessional conduct.

(1) Committing conduct that is contrary to the recognized standards or ethics of the

acupuncture profession or that may constitute a danger to the health, welfare or safety of the patient or the public.

(m) Committing any conduct or having any condition that may impair the ability to safely and skillfully practice acupuncture.

(n) Violating or attempting to violate, directly or indirectly, assisting in or abetting the violation of or conspiring to violate this chapter or board rules.

(o) Advertising in a false, deceptive or misleading manner.

(p) Failing or refusing to maintain adequate patient health records or failing or refusing to make health records promptly available to the patient or to another health practitioner or provider on request and receipt of proper authorization.

(q) Deriving direct or indirect compensation from referring a patient without disclosing to the patient in writing the extent of the compensation.

(r) Deriving a financial interest in products the acupuncturist endorses or recommends to the patient without disclosing to the patient in writing the extent of the financial interest.

(s) Having sexual intimacies with a patient in the practice of acupuncture.

(t) Failing to appropriately exercise control over or supervise an acupuncture student employed by or assigned to the practitioner in the practice of acupuncture.

(u) Failing to furnish information in a timely manner to the board or its investigators or representatives if the information is legally requested by the board.

(v) Supervising or engaging in a clinical training program in acupuncture without being approved and registered by the board for that program.

(w) Knowingly making a false, fraudulent or misleading statement, written or oral, to the board.

(x) Failing to exercise proper care for a patient by abandoning or neglecting a patient in need of immediate care without making reasonable arrangements for the continuation of care or by failing to refer the patient to another appropriate health care provider when necessary.

(y) Failing to use needles that have been sterilized according to clean needle technique principles approved by the board.

(z) Failing to demonstrate professional standards of care and training and education qualifications, as established by the board in rule, for performing a therapeutic modality.

(aa) Prescribing or administering medicine or drugs, except as allowed pursuant to this chapter.

§ 32 – 3902. Acupuncture board of examiners; members; qualifications; terms; removal; compensation

A. The acupuncture board of examiners is established consisting of the following members who are appointed by the governor:

1. Through January 16, 2022, four members who are licensed to practice acupuncture pursuant

to this chapter and who have practiced acupuncture in this state or any other state for at least one year. Not more than two of these members may be graduates of the same school or college of acupuncture. The governor may make these appointments from a list of names submitted by a statewide acupuncture society.

2. Through January 17, 2022, three consumers who：

（a）Are not employed in a health profession.

（b）Do not have any pecuniary interest in a school of medicine or health care institution.

（c）Demonstrate an interest in health issues in this state.

3. Through January 17, 2022, two members who are licensed pursuant to chapter 8, 13, 14, 17 or 29 of this title. These members shall not be licensed pursuant to the same chapter.

4. Beginning January 17, 2022, one member who is certified or licensed to practice auricular acupuncture or acupuncture pursuant to this chapter.

5. Beginning January 20, 2022, three members who are licensed to practice acupuncture pursuant to this chapter and who have practiced acupuncture in this or any other state for at least one year. Not more than two of these members may be graduates of the same school or college of acupuncture. The governor may make these appointments from a list of names submitted by a statewide acupuncture society.

6. For appointments made on or after January 18, 2022, two consumers who meet all of the following：

（a）Are not employed in a health profession.

（b）Do not have any pecuniary interest in a school of medicine or health care institution.

（c）Demonstrate an interest in health issues in this state.

7. For appointments made on or after January 18, 2022, one member who is licensed pursuant to chapter 8, 13, 14, 17 or 29 of this title.1

B. Before appointment by the governor, a prospective member of the board shall submit a full set of fingerprints to the governor for the purpose of obtaining a state and federal criminal records check pursuant to § 41－1750 and Public Law 92－544. The department of public safety may exchange this fingerprint data with the federal bureau of investigation.

C. Board members shall be residents of this state for at least one year immediately preceding their appointment.

D. Board members serve three-year terms to begin and end on the third Monday in January. A member shall not serve more than two consecutive terms.

E. The board shall meet in January of each year to elect a chairperson and vice chairperson.

F. The board shall meet quarterly and at the call of the chairperson or a majority of board members.

G. Board members are eligible to receive compensation in an amount not to exceed $50 per day for each day of actual service in the business of the board and are eligible for reimbursement of expenses necessarily and properly incurred in attending board meetings.

H. The governor may remove a board member from office for malfeasance, dishonorable conduct or unprofessional management of board duties.

I. The term of any member automatically ends on resignation or absence from this state for a period of at least six months. The governor shall fill vacancies for an unexpired portion of a term in the same manner as regular appointments.

J. Board members and board employees are not subject to civil liability for any act done or proceeding undertaken or performed in good faith and in furtherance of the purposes of this chapter.

§ 32 – 3903.　Powers and duties of the board

A. The board shall:

1. Adopt rules necessary to enforce this chapter.

2. Initiate investigations and take disciplinary actions to enforce this chapter.

3. Evaluate the qualifications of applicants and issue licenses to qualified applicants.

4. Adopt and use a seal to authenticate official board documents.

5. Establish fees pursuant to § 32 – 3927.

6. Adopt rules for clinical training.

B. The board may:

1. Subject to title 41, chapter 4, article 4, 1 employ personnel needed to carry out board functions.

2. Purchase, lease, rent, sell or otherwise dispose of personal and real property for the operations of the board.

3. Approve examinations for licensure.

§ 32 – 3904.　Executive director; personnel; duties; compensation

A. Subject to title 41, chapter 4, article 4, 1 the board may appoint an executive director who serves at the pleasure of the board. The executive director shall not be a board member.

B. The executive director is eligible to receive compensation set by the board within the range determined pursuant to § 38 – 611.

C. The executive director shall:

1. Perform the administrative duties of the board.

2. Subject to title 41, chapter 4, article 4, employ personnel needed to carry out board functions.

3. Perform other duties as directed by the board.

§ 32 – 3905.　Acupuncture board of examiners fund

A. The acupuncture board of examiners fund is established consisting of fees collected pursuant to § 32 – 3927. The board shall administer the fund. Pursuant to §§ 35 – 146 and 35 – 147, the board shall deposit ten per cent of all monies collected under this chapter in the state general fund and deposit the remaining ninety per cent in the acupuncture board of examiners fund.

B. Monies deposited in the acupuncture board of examiners fund are subject to § 35 – 143.01.

§ 32 – 3906.　Third party reimbursements

This chapter does not require direct third party reimbursement to persons who are licensed pursuant to this chapter.

Article 2.　Licensure

§ 32 – 3921.　Licensure; acts and persons not affected

A. A person shall not practice acupuncture without a license issued pursuant to this chapter.

B. This chapter does not apply to:

1. Health care professionals licensed pursuant to this title practicing within the scope of their license.

2. A student enrolled in a school of acupuncture approved by the board practicing acupuncture under the direct supervision of an acupuncturist licensed pursuant to this chapter as a part of a course of study approved by the board.

3. The practice of acupuncture in this state by a person licensed or certified to perform acupuncture by any other jurisdiction if the person is doing so in the course of regular instruction of a school of acupuncture approved by the board or in an educational seminar by a professional organization of acupuncture, if in the case of an educational seminar the practice is supervised directly by a person licensed pursuant to this chapter or by a health professional licensed pursuant to this title whose scope of practice includes acupuncture.

4. An acupuncturist who resides outside the state and who is authorized to practice acupuncture in that jurisdiction, if the person engages in a single or infrequent consultation with an acupuncturist licensed in this state and the consultation regards a specific patient or patients.

5. A person who self-administers acupuncture.

§ 32 – 3922.　Acupuncture detoxification specialist for chemical dependency or trauma; certificate; requirements; fingerprints; informed consent; definition

A. The board may issue an acupuncture detoxification specialist certificate to a person who practices auricular acupuncture for the purpose of treating alcoholism, substance abuse, trauma or chemical dependency if the person does all of the following:

1. Provides documentation of successfully completing a board-approved training program in acupuncture for treating alcoholism, substance abuse, trauma or chemical dependency that meets or exceeds standards of training established by the national acupuncture detoxification association or a board-approved group.

2. Provides documentation satisfactory to the board of successfully completing a board-approved clean needle technique course.

3. Submits an application as prescribed by the board and a fee prescribed by § 32 – 3927.

4. Submits a full set of fingerprints to the board for the purpose of obtaining a state and federal criminal records check pursuant to § 41 – 1750 and Public Law 92 – 544. The department of public safety may exchange this fingerprint data with the federal bureau of investigation.

5. Discloses in an application for initial certification or recertification all other active and past professional health care licenses and certificates issued to the applicant in this state or by another state, district or territory of the United States.

B. A certificate issued pursuant to this section allows the certificate holder to practice auricular acupuncture under the supervision of a person who is licensed pursuant to this chapter.

C. A certificate issued pursuant to this section is valid for one year. The certificate may be renewed by the board if the certificate holder submits an application as prescribed by the board and a fee prescribed by § 32 – 3927 before the certificate expires.

D. Before treating a patient, an auricular acupuncturist shall obtain from the patient a signed informed consent that has been approved by the board.

E. For the purposes of this section, "auricular acupuncture" means applying acupuncture needles to the pinna, lobe or auditory meatus to treat alcoholism, substance abuse, trauma or chemical dependency.

§ 32 – 3923.   Use of title or abbreviation by licensee; prohibited acts; posting of license

A. A person who is licensed pursuant to this chapter may use the title "licensed acupuncturist" and the abbreviation "L.Ac.".

B. A person who is not licensed pursuant to this chapter shall not use any title, abbreviation, words, letters, signs or figures to indicate that the person is licensed pursuant to this chapter.

C. Possession of a license pursuant to this chapter does not by itself entitle a person to use the title "doctor" or "physician".

D. A person who is licensed pursuant to this chapter shall post the license or an official duplicate of the license in a conspicuous location in the reception area of each office facility of that licensee.

E. A person who is licensed pursuant to this chapter shall not represent to any member of the public that, by virtue of that license, the person is licensed to practice any modality other than acupuncture.

§ 32 – 3924.   Qualifications for licensure

To receive a license to practice acupuncture pursuant to this chapter, a person shall submit an application as prescribed by the board. The applicant shall disclose in an application for initial licensure all other active and past professional health care licenses and certificates issued to the applicant in this state or by another state, district or territory of the United States. The application shall document to the board's satisfaction that the applicant has successfully completed a clean needle technique course approved by the board and meets all of the following:

1. Has either:

(a) Been certified in acupuncture by the national certification commission for acupuncture and oriental medicine, or its successor organization, or another certifying body or examination that is recognized by the board.

(b) Passed the point location module, foundations of oriental medicine module, biomedicine module and acupuncture module offered by the national certification commission for acupuncture and oriental medicine.

(c) Been licensed by another state with substantially similar standards, and has not had certification or licensure revoked.

2. Has graduated from or completed training in a board-approved program of acupuncture with a minimum of one thousand eight hundred fifty hours of training that includes at least eight hundred hours of board-approved clinical training.

3. Beginning July 1, 2016, has submitted a full set of fingerprints to the board for the purpose of obtaining a state and federal criminal records check pursuant to § 41 – 1750 and Public Law 92 – 544. The department of public safety may exchange this fingerprint data with the federal bureau of investigation.

§ 32 – 3925. Renewal of license; continuing education

A. Except as provided in § 32 – 4301, a license issued pursuant to this chapter is subject to renewal each year and expires unless renewed.

B. The executive director shall send a renewal application to each licensee at least sixty days before expiration of the license.

C. A licensee shall submit to the board on request documentation satisfactory to the board that the licensee has successfully completed at least fifteen hours of board-approved continuing education each year.

D. On compliance with board requirements for the renewal of licenses, the board may reinstate a license canceled for failure to renew.

§ 32 – 3926. Visiting professor certificate

A. The board may issue a visiting professor certificate to an acupuncturist who has received a teaching position in a school of acupuncture in this state if that person demonstrates to the satisfaction of the board that the person has at least five years' experience in the practice of acupuncture and has adequate skill and training. The acupuncturist shall submit an application as prescribed by the board and shall submit the fee prescribed pursuant to § 32 – 3927.

B. A certificate issued pursuant to this section allows the certificate holder to practice acupuncture only in relation to the certificate holder's faculty position duties.

C. A certificate issued pursuant to this section is valid for one year. The board may grant a one year extension if the certificate holder submits an application at least thirty days before the certificate expires. The board may grant a total of two one-year extensions.

§ 32 – 3927. Fees

A. By a formal vote at its annual meeting the board shall establish nonrefundable fees that do not exceed the following:

1. For issuance of an initial license, six hundred dollars.

2. For an application for a license or certificate, one hundred fifty dollars.

3. For renewal of a license, six hundred dollars.

4. For late renewal of a license, an additional one hundred dollars.

5. For issuance of a duplicate license or certificate, fifty dollars.

6. For issuance of an initial visiting professor certificate, six hundred dollars.

7. For renewal of a visiting professor certificate, six hundred dollars.

8. For issuance of an initial auricular acupuncture certificate, two hundred fifty dollars.

9. For renewal of an auricular acupuncture certificate, two hundred fifty dollars.

10. For copying records, documents, letters, minutes, applications and files, twenty-five cents a page.

11. For a copy of the minutes to board meetings during the current calendar year, twenty-five dollars for each set of minutes.

B. The board shall charge additional fees for services not required to be provided by this chapter but that the board determines are necessary and appropriate to carry out this chapter. The fees shall not exceed the actual cost of providing these services.

Article 3. Regulation

§ 32 – 3951. Denial, revocation or suspension of license; hearings; alternative sanctions

A. The board may deny, revoke or suspend a license issued under this chapter for any of the following reasons:

1. Conviction of a felony or a misdemeanor involving moral turpitude. The record of the conviction or a certified copy from the clerk of the court where the conviction occurred or from the judge of that court is sufficient evidence of conviction.

2. Securing a license under this chapter through fraud or deceit.

3. Unprofessional conduct or incompetence in the conduct of the licensee's practice.

4. Using a false name or alias in the practice of the licensee's profession.

5. Violating this chapter or board rules.

B. If the board determines pursuant to a hearing that grounds exist to revoke or suspend a license, the board may do so permanently or for a fixed period of time and may impose conditions prescribed by the board. The board may also impose a civil penalty of not more than ten thousand dollars for each violation of this chapter. The board shall deposit, pursuant to §§ 35 – 146 and 35 – 147, civil penalties collected pursuant to this subsection in the state general fund.

C. The board may deny a license without holding a hearing. After receiving notification of the denial, the applicant may request a hearing to review the denial.

D. The board shall conduct any hearing to revoke or suspend a license pursuant to title 41, chapter 6, article 10.1 Any person appearing before the board may be represented by an attorney.

E. Instead of denying, revoking or suspending a license the board may file a letter of concern, issue a decree of censure, prescribe a period of probation or restrict or limit the practice of a licensee. The board may also issue a nondisciplinary order requiring the licensee to complete a prescribed number of hours of continuing education in an area or areas prescribed by the board to provide the licensee with the necessary understanding of current developments, skills, procedures or treatment.

F. The board shall promptly notify a licensee's employer if the director initiates a disciplinary action against the licensee.

G. The board may appoint an investigator to provide information to the board concerning an alleged violation of this chapter.

H. The board on its own initiative or on application of any person involved in an investigation or proceeding conducted by the board may issue subpoenas compelling the attendance and testimony of witnesses or demanding the production for examination or copying of documents, reports, records or any other evidence relating to a board investigation or proceeding.

§ 32 – 3952.　Right to examine and copy evidence

In connection with a board investigation conducted pursuant to 32 – 3951, the board at all reasonable times has the right to examine and copy any documents, reports, records or other physical evidence of any person being investigated or reports, records and any other documents maintained by and in the possession of any clinic, licensee's office or other public or private agency and any health care institution as defined in § 36 – 401 if the board believes this information is related to unprofessional conduct or the mental or physical ability of a licensee to practice acupuncture.

§ 32 – 3953.　Injunctive relief; bond; service of process

A. In addition to all other available remedies, if the board has any reason to believe that a person has violated this chapter or a board rule, the board through the attorney general or the county attorney of the county in which the violation is alleged to have occurred may apply to the superior court in that county for an injunction restraining that person from engaging in the violation.

B. The court shall issue a temporary restraining order, a preliminary injunction or a permanent injunction without requiring the board to post a bond.

C. Service of process may be on the defendant in any county of this state where the defendant is found.

§ 32 – 3954.　Violation; classification

A person who violates this chapter is guilty of a class 1 misdemeanor.

§ 32 – 3955. Acupuncture assistants; scope of duties; registration required; use of title

A. This chapter does not prohibit an acupuncture assistant from assisting a licensed acupuncturist pursuant to rules adopted by the board, consistent with the following:

1. An acupuncture assistant may:

(a) Remove acupuncture needles.

(b) Monitor acupuncture procedures such as the application of heat or moxibustion.

(c) Perform noncritical functions such as gathering basic patient information, taking blood pressure and attending to patient treatment rooms.

2. An acupuncture assistant may not insert acupuncture needles or evaluate, interpret, design or modify established treatment programs of acupuncture care.

3. An acupuncture assistant shall register with the board on a form prescribed by the board. The board may suspend or revoke the registration of an acupuncture assistant who violates any provision of this chapter related to the practice of acupuncture or who indulges in conduct or a practice that is detrimental to the health or safety of the public.

B. It is unlawful for a person to do either of the following:

1. Work as an acupuncture assistant except under the supervision of a licensed acupuncturist pursuant to this chapter and the rules adopted by the board.

2. Use the abbreviation "a. a." or the term "acupuncture assistant" unless the person is working under the supervision of a licensed acupuncturist pursuant to this chapter and the rules adopted by the board.

ARIZONA ADMINISTRATIVE CODE

Article 1.   General Provisions (Refs & Annos)

R4 – 8 – 101. Definitions

The definitions in A.R.S. § 32 – 3901 apply to this Chapter. Additionally, in this Chapter:

"ACAOM" means the Accreditation Commission for Acupuncture and Oriental Medicine.

"Acupuncture program" means a Board-approved training designed to prepare a student for the NCCAOM examination and licensure.

"Acupuncture student" means an individual enrolled in an acupuncture or auricular acupuncture training program.

"Acupuncturist" means an individual licensed or certified by the Board to practice acupuncture in this state.

"Administrative completeness review" means the Board's process for determining whether an applicant provided a complete application packet.

"Applicant" means an individual who applies to the Board for an initial or renewal license or certificate.

"Application packet" means the fees, forms, documents, and additional information the Board requires to be submitted by an applicant or on an applicant's behalf.

"Approved continuing education" means a planned educational experience the Board determines meets the criteria in R4 − 8 − 408.

"Auricular acupuncture" means a therapy in which the five-needle protocol is used to treat alcoholism, substance abuse, or chemical dependency.

"Clean needle technique" means a manner of needle sterilization and use that avoids the spread of disease and infection, protects the public and the patient, and complies with state and federal law.

"Clinical hours" means actual clock hours that a student spends providing patient care under the supervision of an individual licensed under R4 − 8 − 203 or R4 − 8 − 208.

"Course" means a systematic learning experience that assists a participant to acquire knowledge, skills, and information relevant to the practice of acupuncture.

"Day" means calendar day.

"Five-needle protocol" means a therapy, developed by NADA to treat alcoholism, substance abuse, or chemical dependency, which involves inserting five needles into specific points on the outer ear.

"Hour" means at least 50 minutes of course participation.

"Letter of concern" means an alternative sanction that informs a licensee or certificate holder that, while the evidence does not warrant disciplinary action, the Board believes the licensee or certificate holder should change certain practices and failure to change the practices may result in disciplinary action. A letter of concern is a public document that may be used in future disciplinary proceedings.

"NADA" means the National Acupuncture Detoxification Association.

"NCCAOM" means the National Certification Commission for Acupuncture and Oriental Medicine.

"Respondent" means an individual accused of violating A.R.S. Title 32, Chapter 39 or this Chapter.

"Successful completion of a clean needle technique course" means a course participant: Attended the course, and received a passing score on an examination or other confirmation from the course provider that evidences the participant mastered the course content.

"Supervisor" means an acupuncturist licensed by the Board who is responsible for the oversight and direction of an acupuncture student or a certificate holder.

R4 − 8 − 102.   Authentication of Documentation; Translation; Verification

A. An applicant shall ensure that a document submitted to the Board by or on behalf of the applicant has an official or government seal or written verification authenticating the document. If the Board determines that an applicant cannot obtain the seal or verification through the exercise of due diligence, the Board shall waive this requirement.

B. An applicant shall ensure that an official copy of any diploma, transcript, license, certificate, examination score, or other document required for application is forwarded directly to the Board by the issuing entity.

C. An applicant shall ensure that a document submitted in a language other than English is accompanied by an original English translation, performed by a qualified translator who is not the applicant. The applicant shall ensure that the translation is accompanied by an Affidavit of Accuracy in which the translator who performed or verified the translation affirms, under oath and penalty of perjury, that the entire document has been translated, nothing has been omitted or added, and the translation is true and correct. The Board shall return an original translation to the applicant only if the applicant provides a photocopy of the entire translation, including the Affidavit of Accuracy.

D. The following persons are regarded as qualified translators:

1. An officer or employee of an official translation bureau or governmental agency;

2. A professor or instructor who teaches the translated language at an accredited college or university in the United States. The professor or instructor shall ensure that the Affidavit of Accuracy includes the name of the course taught, is on official letterhead of the college or university, and is notarized;

3. An American consul in the country where the translated document was issued. If a private translator translated the document, the American consul shall verify the translation as required under subsection (C) and the identity of the translator; and

4. A consul general or diplomatic representative accredited in the United States, or other representative of a foreign government agency. If a private translator translated the document, the representative shall verify the translation as required under subsection (C) and the identity of the translator.

R4 – 8 – 103.   Change of Mailing Address, E-mail Address, or Telephone Numbers

The Board shall communicate with a licensee, certificate holder, or a person holding an approval from the Board using the contact information provided to the Board. To ensure timely communication from the Board, a licensee, certificate holder, or person holding an approval from the Board shall notify the Board, in writing, within 30 days of any change of mailing address (giving both the old and the new address), e-mail address, or residential, business, or mobile telephone number.

R4 – 8 – 104.   Expired

R4 – 8 – 105.   Time-frames for Licensure, Certification, and Approval

A. For the purpose of A.R.S. § 41 – 1073, the Board establishes the time-frames listed in

Table 1. An applicant or a person requesting an approval from the Board and the Executive Director of the Board may agree in writing to extend the substantive review and overall time-frames by no more than 25% of the overall time-frame.

B. The administrative completeness review time-frame begins when the Board receives an application packet or a request for approval. During the administrative completeness review time-frame, the Board shall notify the applicant or person requesting approval that the application packet or request for approval is either complete or incomplete. If the application packet or request for approval is incomplete, the Board shall specify in the notice what information is missing.

C. An applicant or person requesting approval whose application packet or request for approval is incomplete, shall submit the missing information to the Board within the time to complete listed in Table 1. Both the administrative completeness review and overall time-frames are suspended from the date of the Board's notice under subsection (B) until the Board receives all of the missing information.

D. Upon receipt of all missing information, the Board shall notify the applicant or person requesting approval that the application packet or request for approval is complete. The Board shall not send a separate notice of completeness if the Board grants or denies a license, certificate, or approval within the administrative completeness time-frame listed in Table 1.

E. The substantive review time-frame listed in Table 1 begins on the date of the Board's notice of administrative completeness.

F. If the Board determines during the substantive review that additional information is needed, the Board shall send the applicant or person requesting approval a comprehensive written request for additional information.

G. An applicant or person requesting approval who receives a request under subsection (F), shall submit the additional information to the Board within the time for response listed in Table 1. Both the substantive review and overall time-frames are suspended from the date of the Board's request until the Board receives the additional information.

H. An applicant or person requesting approval may receive a 30-day extension of the time provided under subsection (C) or (G) by providing written notice to the Board before the time expires. If an applicant or person requesting approval fails to submit to the Board the missing or additional information within the time provided under Table 1 or the time as extended, the Board shall close the applicant's or person's file. To receive further consideration, an applicant or person requesting approval whose file is closed shall re-apply.

I. Within the overall time-frame listed in Table 1, the Board shall:

1. Grant a license, certificate, or approval if the Board determines that the applicant or person requesting approval meets all criteria required by statute and this Chapter; or

2. Deny a license, certificate, or approval if the Board determines that the applicant or person requesting approval does not meet all criteria required by statute and this Chapter.

J. If the Board denies a license, certificate, or approval, the Board shall send the applicant or person requesting approval a written notice explaining:

1. The reason for denial, with citations to supporting statutes or rules;

2. The applicant's or person's right to appeal the denial by filing an appeal under A.R.S. Title 41, Chapter 6, Article 10;

3. The time for appealing the denial; and

4. The applicant's or person's right to request an informal settlement conference.

K. If a time-frame's last day falls on a Saturday, Sunday, or official state holiday, the next business day is the time-frame's last day.

R4 – 8 – 105 Tbl. 1. Time-frames (in days)

Type of license, certificate, or approval	Authority	Administrative Completeness Time-frame	Time to Complete	Substantive Review Time-frame	Time to Respond	Overall Time-frame
Acupuncture License	ARS 32 – 3924; R4 – 8 – 203	20	30	40	30	60
Visiting Professor Certificate	ARS 32 – 3926; R4 – 8 – 208	20	30	40	30	60
Auricular Acupuncture Certificate	ARS 32 – 3922; R4 – 8 – 301	20	30	40	30	60
Auricular Acupuncture Training Program	ARS 32 – 3922; R4 – 8 – 401	20	30	40	30	60
Acupuncture Program	ARS 32 – 3924 (2); R4 – 8 – 403	20	30	40	30	60
Clinical Training Program	ARS 32 – 3924 (2); R4 – 8 – 403	20	30	40	30	60
Clean Needle Technique Course	ARS 32 – 3924; R4 – 8 – 402	20	30	40	30	60
Continuing Education Approval	ARS 32 – 3925; R4 – 8 – 409	20	30	40	30	60
Renewal of License or Certificate	ARS 32 – 3925; R4 – 8 – 204 or R4 – 8 – 303	20	30	40	30	60
Extension of Visiting Professor Certificate	ARS 32 – 3926 (C); R4 – 8 – 208	20	30	40	30	60
Reinstatement of License	ARS 32 – 3925 (D); R4 – 8 – 205	20	30	40	30	60

R4 - 8 - 106.　Fees

A. Under the authority provided at A.R.S.　§ 32 - 3927, the Board establishes and shall collect the following fees:

1. Application for an acupuncture license: $150;

2. Issuance of an initial acupuncture license: $275;

3. Renewal of an acupuncture license: $275;

4. Additional fee for late renewal of an acupuncture license: $100;

5. Application for an auricular acupuncture certificate: $75;

6. Issuance of an initial auricular acupuncture certificate: $75;

7. Renewal of an auricular acupuncture certificate: $75;

8. Visiting professor certificate: $600;

9. Extension of a visiting professor certificate: $600; and

10. Duplicate license or certificate: $50.

B. Except as provided in subsections (B)(1) through (B)(3) or as required under A.R.S. § 41 - 1077, all fees are nonrefundable. The Board shall refund the fee paid under subsection (A)(2) or (A)(6) if:

1. The Board denies a license or certificate to an applicant,

2. The Board closes the file of an applicant under R4 - 8 - 105, or

3. An applicant withdraws an application.

R4 - 8 - 107.　Materials Incorporated by Reference

A. The Board incorporates the following material by reference:

1. "NADA Registered Trainer Resource Manual," 1999, published by the National Acupuncture Detoxification Association, 3220 N Street NW #275, Washington, D.C. 20007;

2. "Clean Needle Technique Manual for Acupuncturists," 5th edition, 2004, published by the National Acupuncture Foundation, P.O. Box 137, Chaplin, CT 06235; and

3. "Accreditation Handbook," Part One, 2005, published by the Accreditation Commission for Acupuncture and Oriental Medicine, Maryland Trade Center #3, 7501 Greenway Center Drive, Suite 260, Greenbelt, MD 20770.

B. The materials incorporated by reference under subsection (A) contain no later editions or amendments and are on file with the Board.

Article 2.　Acupuncture Licensing; Visiting Professor Certificate

R4 - 8 - 201.　Renumbered

R4 - 8 - 202.　Renumbered

R4 - 8 - 203.　Application for Acupuncture License

A. To be licensed to practice acupuncture, an applicant shall submit an application packet to the Board that includes:

1. An application, on a form provided by the Board, that provides the following information about the applicant:

a. Name;

b. Other names by which the applicant has been known;

c. Date of birth;

d. Social Security number;

e. Home, business, and e-mail addresses;

f. Home, business, and mobile telephone numbers;

g. A statement of whether the applicant has ever been permitted by law to practice a health-care profession in this or another state, territory, or district of the United States, or another country or subdivision of another country, and if so:

(i) A list of the jurisdictions in which the applicant has been permitted by law to practice a health-care profession;

(ii) The number of each license;

(iii) The date each license was issued;

(iv) The date each license expired or expires;

(v) Limitations, if any, for each license;

(vi) Whether each license was granted by endorsement, examination, or another means;

h. A statement of whether the applicant is certified by the NCCAOM, and if so, whether the certification is active and current, and the dates of issuance and expiration;

i. If not certified by the NCCAOM, a statement of whether the applicant:

(i) Has passed all the following NCCAOM modules: Point Location; Foundations of Oriental Medicine; Biomedicine; and Acupuncture; or

(ii) Has passed the State of California Acupuncture Licensing Examination;

j. A statement of whether the applicant has completed an acupuncture program accredited within the United States or another country or subdivision of another country, and if so, the date of program completion;

k. A statement of whether the applicant has ever had a licensing authority of another state, district, or territory of the United States, or another country or subdivision of another country, deny the applicant a license or certificate to practice acupuncture, and if so, the name of the jurisdiction denying a license or certificate, date of the denial, and an explanation of the circumstances;

l. A statement of whether the applicant has ever had a licensing authority of another state, district, or territory of the United States, or another country or subdivision of another country, revoke, suspend, limit, restrict, or take any other action regarding the applicant's license or certificate to practice acupuncture, and if so, the name of the jurisdiction taking the action, the action taken, date of the action, and an explanation of the circumstances;

m. A statement of whether the applicant has ever been convicted of a crime, including driving under the influence of drugs or alcohol, other than a minor traffic offense, and if so, the name of the jurisdiction in which convicted, the nature of the crime, date of the conviction, and current status;

n. A statement of whether the applicant has ever had a claim for malpractice or a lawsuit filed against the applicant alleging professional malpractice or negligence in the practice of acupuncture, and if so, the claim or case number, date of the claim or lawsuit, the matters alleged, and whether the claim or lawsuit is still pending or the manner in which it was resolved;

o. A statement of whether the applicant has any condition that may impair the applicant's ability to practice acupuncture safely and skillfully, and if so, the nature of the condition and any accommodations necessary;

p. A statement of whether the applicant has ever resigned, voluntarily or involuntarily, from a healthcare facility while under investigation, and if so, the name of the health-care facility, the date of the resignation, and an explanation of the circumstances; and

q. A statement of whether the applicant has ever had a health-care facility terminate, restrict, or take any other action regarding the applicant's employment, professional training, or privileges, and if so, the name of the health-care facility, the date of the action, and an explanation of the circumstances;

2. An official record or document that relates to the applicant's explanation of an item under subsections (A)(1)(k) through (A)(1)(q);

3. Documentation of one of the following:

a. Certification from the NCCAOM or its successor;

b. Certification by another certifying body recognized by the Board;

c. Certification as a result of passing a licensing or certifying examination in acupuncture; or

d. Authorization by law to practice acupuncture in another state, district, or territory of the United States, or another country or subdivision of another country with licensing standards substantially similar to those in this Chapter that has not been revoked;

4. Documentation of successfully completing a Board-approved clean needle technique course. A copy of the certificate of completion showing the name of the course and the date on and location at which the course was completed is acceptable documentation;

5. A 2″ × 2″ photograph, taken within the last year, that shows the front of the applicant's face;

6. A completed Arizona Statement of Citizenship and Alien Status for State Public Benefits, which is a form available from the Board; and

7. A complete set of fingerprints that meet the criteria of the Federal Bureau of Investigation and are taken by a law enforcement agency or other qualified entity;

8. The amount charged by the Department of Public Safety to process fingerprints for a state and federal criminal records check; and

9. The application and initial licensing fees prescribed by the Board under R4 − 8 − 106(A) (1) and (A)(2).

B. In addition to the materials required under subsection (A), an applicant shall provide evidence that the applicant completed at least 1,850 hours of training in acupuncture, including at least 800 clinical hours, by having submitted directly to the Board an official transcript from each school at which the applicant attended a Board-approved acupuncture program showing:

1. The name and address of the school,

2. The dates on which the applicant attended the school,

3. The courses and clinical training completed by the applicant,

4. The number of hours in each course or clinical training,

5. The grade or score obtained by the applicant in each course or clinical training, and

6. Whether the applicant received a diploma or degree from the school.

C. In addition to complying with subsections (A) and (B), an applicant shall sign, date, and have notarized an affidavit that indicates all information provided in the application packet, including any accompanying documents submitted by or on behalf of the applicant, are true, complete, and correct.

R4 − 8 − 204. Renewal of an Acupuncture License

A. An acupuncture license expires 12 months after the date issued.

B. The Board shall provide a licensee with 60-days notice of the need to renew. It is the responsibility of the licensee to renew timely. Failure to receive notice of the need to renew does not excuse failure to renew timely.

C. If a licensee fails to submit a renewal application packet as described in subsection (D) on or before the expiration date, the licensee shall cease the practice of acupuncture.

D. To renew an acupuncture license, a licensee shall submit to the Board:

1. A renewal application that provides the following information about the licensee:

a. Name;

b. License number;

c. Business name;

d. Home, business, and e-mail addresses;

e. Home, business, and mobile telephone numbers;

f. A statement of whether during the last 12 months a licensing authority of another state, district, or territory of the United States or another country or subdivision of another country denied the licensee a license or certificate to practice acupuncture and if so, the name of the jurisdiction denying a license or certificate, date of the denial, and an explanation of the circumstances;

g. A statement of whether during the last 12 months a licensing authority of another state, district, or territory of the United States or another country or subdivision of another country revoked, suspended, limited, restricted, or took other action regarding the license of the licensee and if so, the name of the jurisdiction taking action against the license, the action taken, date of the action, and an explanation of the circumstances;

h. A statement of whether during the last 12 months the licensee has been convicted of a crime, including driving under the influence of drugs or alcohol, other than a minor traffic offense, and if so, the name of the jurisdiction in which convicted, the nature of the crime, date of the conviction, and current status;

i. A statement of whether during the last 12 months a claim for malpractice or a lawsuit was filed against the licensee alleging professional malpractice or negligence in the practice of acupuncture, and if so, the claim or case number, date of the claim or lawsuit, the matters alleged, and whether the claim or lawsuit is still pending or the manner in which it was resolved;

j. A statement of whether during the last 12 months the licensee has any condition that may impair the licensee's ability to practice acupuncture safely and skillfully, and if so, the nature of the condition and any accommodations necessary;

k. A statement of whether during the last 12 months the licensee resigned, voluntarily or involuntarily, from a health-care facility while under investigation, and if so, the name of the health-care facility, the date of the resignation, and an explanation of the circumstances; and

l. A statement of whether during the last 12 months the licensee had a health-care facility terminate, restrict, or take any other action regarding the licensee's employment, professional training, or privileges, and if so, the name of the health-care facility, the date of the action, and an explanation of the circumstances;

2. An affirmation that the licensee completed the continuing education required under R4 - 8 - 206;

3. An affirmation that the licensee is in compliance with the requirements at A.R.S. § 32 - 3211;

4. A completed Arizona Statement of Citizenship and Alien Status for State Public Benefits, which is a form available from the Board;

5. The renewal fee required under R4 - 8 - 106(A)(3); and

6. The licensee's dated signature affirming that the information provided is accurate, true, and complete.

R4 - 8 - 205.　Reinstatement of an Acupuncture License

A. An individual whose acupuncture license expires because of failure to renew timely under R4 - 8 - 204(D) may apply to the Board for reinstatement of the acupuncture license by submitting, within 60 days after expiration of the license;

1. The application packet described under R4 - 8 - 204(D);

2. A sworn affidavit that the individual has not practiced acupuncture since the license expired; and

3. The fee prescribed under R4 − 8 − 106 (A) (4) for late renewal of an acupuncture license.

B. The Board shall not reinstate an acupuncture license that expires more than 60 days before the former licensee complies with subsection (A). If an acupuncture license is expired for more than 60 days, the former licensee may apply for licensure by complying with R4 − 8 − 203.

R4 − 8 − 206.   Continuing Education Requirement

A. A licensee shall complete at least 15 hours of approved continuing education per year.

B. The Board shall award hours in an approved continuing education as follows:

1. Seminar or workshop: One hour of continuing education for each contact hour;

2. Course at an accredited educational institution: 15 hours of continuing education for each semester hour;

3. Self-study, online, or correspondence course: Hours of continuing education determined by the course provider;

4. Teaching an approved continuing education: One hour of continuing education for each hour taught;

5. Having an article on the practice of acupuncture or traditional East-Asian medicine published in a peer-reviewed professional journal or in a text book: 15 hours of continuing education;

6. Attending a Board meeting: One hour for attending one meeting during a year; and

7. Having a text book published relating to the practice of acupuncture or traditional East-Asian medicine: 15 hours of continuing education.

C. The Board shall limit the number of hours of approved continuing education awarded as follows:

1. No more than 30 percent of the required hours may be obtained from teaching an approved continuing education. Hours may be obtained from teaching a particular approved continuing education only once during each year. No hours may be obtained from participating as a member of a panel at an approved continuing education; and

2. Hours that exceed the maximum required during a year may not be carried over to a subsequent year.

D. A licensee shall obtain a certificate or other evidence of attendance from the provider of each approved continuing education attended that includes the following:

1. Name of the licensee;

2. License number of the licensee;

3. Name of the approved continuing education;

4. Name of the continuing education provider;

5. Name of the entity that approved the continuing education;

6. Date, time, and location of the approved continuing education; and

7. Number of hours of approved continuing education.

E. A licensee shall maintain the evidence of attendance described in subsection (D) for two years and make the evidence available to the Board under R4 - 8 - 207 and as otherwise required under this Chapter.

R4 - 8 - 207. Audit of Compliance and Sanction for Noncompliance with Continuing Education Requirement

When notice of the need to renew a license is provided, the Board shall also provide notice of an audit of continuing education records to a random sample of licensees. A licensee subject to a continuing education audit shall submit the documentation required under R4 - 8 - 206(D) at the same time that the licensee submits the renewal application packet required under R4 - 8 - 204(D). If a licensee fails to submit the required documentation with the renewal application packet before the date of expiration, the license expires.

R4 - 8 - 208. Application for Visiting Professor Certificate; Extension of Visiting Professor Certificate

A. To obtain a visiting professor certificate, an applicant shall submit to the Board:

1. The application form required under R4 - 8 - 203(A) and a signed verification that the information provided is accurate, true, and complete;

2. The fee required under R4 - 8 - 106(A)(8);

3. Documentation of at least five years of experience in the practice of acupuncture;

4. Evidence of skill and training in the subject that the applicant will be teaching, including one of the following:

a. Documentation from a college or university of experience, education, or other training in the subject the applicant will be teaching;

b. Documentation of experience in teaching the same or similar subject matter content within the two years before the application; or

c. Documentation of one year of experience within the last two years in the specialized area in which the applicant is teaching; and

5. A detailed plan outlining the duties of the visiting professor.

B. A visiting professor certificate is valid for one year from the date issued. To extend a visiting professor certificate for another year, the certificate holder shall, at least 30 days before the certificate expires, submit to the Board an application for extension. An application for extension includes:

1. The renewal application form described in R4 - 8 - 204(D)(1) including a signed verification that the information provided is accurate, true, and complete;

2. A letter on official letterhead from an official of the school of acupuncture at which the

visiting professor will be teaching requesting that the extension be granted; and

3. The fee required under R4 – 8 – 106(A) (9).

C. The Board shall not extend a visiting professor certificate more than twice.

R4 – 8 – 209.   Repealed

R4 – 8 – 210.   Repealed

Article 3.   Auricular Acupuncture Certification (Refs & Annos)

R4 – 8 – 301.   Application for Auricular Acupuncture Certificate

To be certified as an auricular acupuncturist to provide auricular acupuncture services in a Board-approved alcoholism, substance abuse, or chemical dependency program, an applicant shall submit an application packet to the Board that includes:

1. An application, on a form provided by the Board, that provides the following information about the applicant:

a. Name;

b. Other names by which the applicant has been known;

c. Date of birth;

d. Social Security number;

e. Home, business, and e-mail addresses;

f. Home, business, and mobile telephone numbers;

g. A statement of whether the applicant has ever been permitted by law to practice auricular acupuncture in another state, territory, or district of the United States, or another country or subdivision of another country, and if so:

i. A list of the jurisdictions in which the applicant has been permitted by law to practice auricular acupuncture;

ii. The number of each license or certificate;

iii. The date each license or certificate was issued;

iv. The date each license or certificate expired or expires;

v. Limitations, if any, for each license or certificate;

vi. Current status of each license or certificate; and

vii. Whether each license or certificate was granted by endorsement, examination, or another means;

h. A statement of whether the applicant has ever had a licensing authority of another state, district, or territory of the United States, or another country or subdivision of another country, deny the applicant a license or certificate to practice auricular acupuncture, and if so, the name of the jurisdiction denying a license or certificate, date of the denial, and an explanation of the circumstances;

i. A statement of whether the applicant has ever had a licensing authority of another state, district, or territory of the United States, or another country or subdivision of another country, revoke, suspend, limit, restrict, or take any other action regarding the applicant's license or certificate to practice auricular acupuncture, and if so, the name of the jurisdiction taking the action, the action taken, date of the action, and an explanation of the circumstances;

j. A statement of whether the applicant has ever been convicted of a crime, including driving under the influence of drugs or alcohol, other than a minor traffic offense, and if so, the name of the jurisdiction in which convicted, the nature of the crime, date of the conviction, and current status;

k. A statement of whether the applicant has ever had a claim for malpractice or a lawsuit filed against the applicant alleging professional malpractice or negligence in the practice of auricular acupuncture, and if so, the claim or case number, date of the claim or lawsuit, the matters alleged, and whether the claim or lawsuit is still pending or the manner in which it was resolved;

l. A statement of whether the applicant has any condition that may impair the applicant's ability to practice auricular acupuncture safely and skillfully, and if so, the nature of the condition and any accommodations necessary;

m. A statement of whether the applicant has ever resigned, voluntarily or involuntarily, from a healthcare facility while under investigation, and if so, the name of the health-care facility, the date of the resignation, and an explanation of the circumstances; and

n. A statement of whether the applicant has ever had a health-care facility terminate, restrict, or take any other action regarding the applicant's employment, professional training, or privileges, and if so, the name of the health-care facility, the date of the action, and an explanation of the circumstances;

2. An official record or document that relates to the applicant's explanation of an item under subsections (1)(h) through (1)(n);

3. The application and initial certification fees prescribed by the Board under R4 – 8 – 106 (A)(5) and (A)(6);

4. Documentation of successfully completing a Board-approved:

a. Training program in auricular acupuncture for the treatment of alcoholism, substance abuse, or chemical dependency. A copy of the certificate of completion showing the name, date, and location of the course is acceptable documentation; and

b. Clean needle technique course. A copy of the certificate of completion showing the name, date, and location of the course is acceptable documentation;

5. The name, license number, and telephone number of the Arizona licensed acupuncturist who will supervise the applicant if the applicant is certified;

6. A 2″ × 2″ photograph, taken within the last year, that shows the front of the applicant's

face and that the applicant signs on the back or the white frame around the photograph;

7. A completed Arizona Statement of Citizenship and Alien Status for State Public Benefits, which is a form available from the Board; and

8. The applicant's dated and notarized signature affirming that the information provided in the application, including any accompanying documents submitted by or on behalf of the applicant, are true and complete.

R4 - 8 - 302.   Requirements for the Practice of Auricular Acupuncture

A. A holder of an auricular acupuncture certificate shall provide auricular acupuncture services only in an alcoholism, substance abuse, or chemical dependency program approved by the Board or the state or federal government.

B. A holder of an auricular acupuncture certificate shall provide auricular acupuncture services only under the supervision of an individual licensed under A.R.S. § 32 - 3924 and R4 - 8 - 203.

C. The Board approves an alcoholism, substance abuse, or chemical dependency program that provides services and is licensed by the Arizona Department of Health Services as a behavioral health agency under A.R.S. Title 36, Chapter 4.

R4 - 8 - 303.   Renewal of an Auricular Acupuncture Certificate

A. An auricular acupuncture certificate expires 12 months after the date issued.

B. The Board shall provide a certificate holder with 60-days notice of the need to renew. It is the responsibility of the certificate holder to renew timely. Failure to receive notice of the need to renew does not excuse failure to renew timely.

C. If a certificate holder fails to submit a renewal application packet as described in subsection (D) on or before the expiration date, the certificate holder shall cease the practice of auricular acupuncture.

D. To renew an auricular acupuncture certificate, a certificate holder shall submit to the Board:

1. A renewal application that provides the following information listed about the certificate holder:

a. Name;

b. Certificate number;

c. Renewal date;

d. The name, address, and telephone number of the alcoholism, substance abuse, or chemical dependency facility at which the certificate holder works;

e. Residential and e-mail addresses;

f. Residential and mobile telephone numbers;

g. A statement of whether during the last 12 months a licensing authority of another state, district, or territory of the United States or another country or subdivision of another country denied the certificate holder a license or certificate to practice auricular acupuncture and if so, the name of the jurisdiction denying a license or certificate, date of the denial, and an explanation of the circumstances;

h. A statement of whether during the last 12 months a licensing authority of another state, district, or territory of the United States or another country or subdivision of another country revoked, suspended, limited, restricted, or took other action regarding the license or certificate of the certificate holder and if so, the name of the jurisdiction taking action, the action taken, date of the action, and an explanation of the circumstances;

i. A statement of whether during the last 12 months the certificate holder has been convicted of a crime, including driving under the influence of drugs or alcohol, other than a minor traffic offense, and if so, the name of the jurisdiction in which convicted, the nature of the crime, date of the conviction, and current status;

j. A statement of whether during the last 12 months a claim for malpractice or a lawsuit was filed against the certificate holder alleging professional malpractice or negligence in the practice of auricular acupuncture, and if so, the claim or case number, date of the claim or lawsuit, the matters alleged, and whether the claim or lawsuit is still pending or the manner in which it was resolved;

k. A statement of whether during the last 12 months the certificate holder has any condition that may impair the certificate holder's ability to practice auricular acupuncture safely and skillfully, and if so, the nature of the condition and any accommodations necessary;

l. A statement of whether during the last 12 months the certificate holder resigned, voluntarily or involuntarily, from a health-care facility while under investigation, and if so, the name of the health-care facility, the date of the resignation, and an explanation of the circumstances;

m. A statement of whether during the last 12 months the certificate holder had a health-care facility terminate, restrict, or take any other action regarding the certificate holder's employment, professional training, or privileges, and if so, the name of the health-care facility, the date of the action, and an explanation of the circumstances; and

n. The name, license number, and telephone number of the licensed acupuncturist who supervises the certificate holder;

2. A completed Arizona Statement of Citizenship and Alien Status for State Public Benefits, which is a form available from the Board;

3. The renewal fee required under R4 − 8 − 106(A)(7); and

4. The certificate holder's dated signature affirming that the information provided is accurate, true, and complete.

E. The Board does not have authority to reinstate an expired auricular acupuncture certificate. An individual whose auricular acupuncture certificate expires because of failure to renew timely under subsection (D) may apply for certification by complying with R4 − 8 − 301.

R4 – 8 – 304. Notice of Change in Supervisor

A. A certificate holder shall provide written notice to the Board within 10 days after one of the following occurs:

1. The certificate holder changes employment from one approved alcoholism, substance abuse, and chemical dependency program to another;

2. The certificate holder ceases to practice as an auricular acupuncturist; or

3. The licensed acupuncturist supervising the certificate holder changes.

B. A certificate holder required to provide notice under subsection (A), shall include the following information in the notice:

1. Name and certificate number of the certificate holder;

2. Name and address of the approved alcoholism, substance abuse, and chemical dependency program at which the certificate holder is employed; and

3. Name, license number, and telephone number of the licensed acupuncturist supervising the certificate holder; or

4. A statement that the certificate holder is not practicing as an auricular acupuncturist.

R4 – 8 – 305. Recodified

R4 – 8 – 306. Recodified

R4 – 8 – 307. Recodified

R4 – 8 – 308. Recodified

R4 – 8 – 309. Recodified

R4 – 8 – 310. Recodified

R4 – 8 – 311. Recodified

R4 – 8 – 312. Recodified

Article 4. Training Programs and Continuing Education

R4 – 8 – 401. Auricular Acupuncture Training Program Approval

A. The Board approves an auricular acupuncture training program that is recognized by NADA.

B. To obtain Board approval of an auricular acupuncture training program that is not approved under subsection (A), the provider of the training program shall submit to the Board evidence that the program is:

1. Conducted in accordance with the "NADA Registered Trainer Resource Manual," which is incorporated by reference in R4 – 8 – 107; and

2. Approved by another board-approved certifying entity for acupuncture.

R4 – 8 – 402. Clean Needle Technique Course Approval

To be approved by the Board, a person that proposes to conduct a clean needle technique course shall submit to the Board evidence that the course is conducted in accordance with "Clean Needle Technique Manual for Acupuncturists," which is incorporated by reference in R4 – 8 – 107.

R4 – 8 – 403.　Approval of an Acupuncture or Clinical Training Program

A. To be approved by the Board, the provider of an acupuncture program shall submit to the Board either：

1. Documentation that the acupuncture program is a candidate for accreditation or has accreditation through the ACAOM and provides at least 1,850 hours of training, including at least 800 hours of clinical training; or

2. Documentation that the acupuncture program meets the standards at R4 – 8 – 404(A).

B. To be approved by the Board, the provider of an acupuncture clinical training program shall submit to the Board either：

1. Documentation that the clinical training program is part of an acupuncture program that is a candidate for accreditation or has accreditation through the ACAOM, or is itself a candidate for accreditation or has accreditation through ACAOM; or

2. Documentation that the clinical program meets the standards at R4 – 8 – 404(B).

R4 – 8 – 404.　Standards for an Acupuncture or Clinical Training Program

A. The Board shall approve an acupuncture program that does not meet the standard at R4 – 8 – 403(A)(1) only if the program：

1. Is for at least three years;

2. Complies with the essential requirements and attendant criteria in Part One of the "Accreditation Handbook", which is incorporated by reference in R4 – 8 – 107; and

3. Provides the following course content and minimum hours：

a. Traditional East – Asian medical theory, diagnosis, treatment techniques in acupuncture, and related studies：690 hours;

b. Clinical training：800 hours; and

c. Biomedical clinical sciences：360 hours.

B. The Board shall approve an acupuncture clinical training program that does not meet the standard of R4 – 8 – 403(B)(1) only if the clinical training program：

1. Is operated by a person who owns and operates an acupuncture clinic,

2. Provides at least 75% of clinical instruction in the acupuncture clinic, and

3. Provides direct patient contact in the following：

a. Supervised observation of the clinical practice of acupuncture with case presentations and discussions;

b. Application of Eastern and Western diagnostic procedures in evaluating a patient; and

c. Clinical treatment of a patient with acupuncture techniques.

R4 – 8 – 405.　Documentation Required for Approval

To obtain Board approval of an acupuncture or clinical training program under R4 – 8 – 404, the provider of the program shall submit or have the custodian of program records submit to the Board documents and other evidence that demonstrates that the program meets the standards in R4 − 8 − 404. These documents and other evidence may include catalogues, course descriptions, curricula plans, and study bulletins.

R4 − 8 − 406.   Repealed

R4 − 8 − 407.   Program Monitoring; Records; Reporting

A. The provider of an approved acupuncture or clinical training program shall submit to the Board, within 60 days after the close of the program's fiscal year, a letter attesting that the acupuncture or clinical training program continues to meet the standards of R4 − 8 − 403 or R4 − 8 − 404, and a course catalog that includes:

1. A description of the courses in the next year's proposed curriculum;

2. A list of members of the program faculty, administration, and governing body; and

3. A description of the program facility.

B. A representative of the Board may conduct an onsite visit of an approved acupuncture or clinical training program to review and evaluate the status of the program. The provider of the approved program shall reimburse the Board for direct costs incurred in conducting this review and evaluation.

C. The provider of an approved acupuncture or clinical training program shall ensure that all student records are maintained in English.

D. The provider of an approved acupuncture or clinical training program shall, within 30 days, report to the Board any failure to meet the standards at R4 − 8 − 403 or R4 − 8 − 404.

R4 − 8 − 408.   Approval of Continuing Education

A. The Board shall approve a continuing education only if the continuing education:

1. Is related to the knowledge or technical skills used to practice acupuncture safely and competently; or

2. Is related to direct or indirect acupuncture patient care, including practice management, medical ethics, or Chinese language; and

3. Includes a method by which the continuing education participants evaluate:

a. The extent to which the continuing education met its stated objectives,

b. The adequacy of the instructor's knowledge of the subject taught,

c. The use of appropriate teaching methods, and

d. The applicability or usefulness of the information provided; and

4. Provides continuing education participants with a certificate of attendance that meets the requirements at R4 − 8 − 206(D).

B. The Board shall approve a continuing education, without application under R4 − 8 − 409, if the continuing education is:

1. Approved by a licensing board of acupuncture in another state,

2. Provided by the Continuing Education Council of NCCAOM, or

3. Provided by a board-approved acupuncture or clinical training program.

R4 − 8 − 409.　Application for Continuing Education Approval

A. To obtain the Board's approval for a continuing education, the provider of the continuing education shall submit to the Board at least 45 days before teaching the continuing education:

1. A form, which is available from the Board, containing the following information:

a. Title of the continuing education;

b. Name and address of the continuing education provider;

c. Name, telephone and fax numbers of a contact person for the continuing education provider;

d. Date, time, and place at which the continuing education will be taught, if known;

e. Subject matter of the continuing education;

f. Method of instruction; and

g. Number of continuing education hours requested; and

2. The following documents:

a. Curriculum vitae of the continuing education instructor,

b. Objective of the continuing education,

c. Detailed outline of the continuing education,

d. Agenda for the continuing education showing the hours of instruction and the subject matter taught during each hour,

e. Method by which participants evaluate the continuing education, and

f. Certificate of attendance that meets the requirements at R4 − 8 − 206(D).

B. The provider of a continuing education that is not approved under R4 − 8 − 408(B) shall not advertise that the continuing education is approved by the Board until the Board acts on an application submitted under subsection (A).

C. The Board's approval of a continuing education is valid for one year unless there is a change in subject matter, instructor, or hours of instruction. At the end of one year or when there is a change in subject matter, instructor, or hours of instruction, the continuing education provider shall apply again for approval.

R4 − 8 − 410.　Repealed

R4 − 8 − 411.　Preceptorship Training Standards—Expired

R4 − 8 − 412.　Approval of Preceptorship Training Program Supervisor — Expired

Article 5.　Supervision; Recordkeeping

R4 − 8 − 501.　Treatment of Patients by Acupuncture Students; Supervision

A. Before a supervising acupuncturist allows an acupuncture student to treat a patient, the supervising acupuncturist shall:

1. Consult with the acupuncture student regarding the treatment to be provided;

2. Ensure that the acupuncture student has the level of training required to provide the treatment safely and effectively;

3. Ensure that written evidence of informed consent is obtained from the patient indicating that the patient knows a student will be treating the patient; and

4. Ensure that the supervisor is physically present in the clinic during any patient treatment performed by the acupuncture student.

B. If an acupuncture student treats a patient, the supervising acupuncturist shall ensure that records of the treatment:

1. Are maintained as required under R4 − 8 − 502;

2. Include the written evidence of informed consent required under subsection (A)(3), and

3. Indicate the names of both the supervising acupuncturist and the acupuncture student.

R4 − 8 − 502.   Recordkeeping

A. An acupuncturist shall:

1. Make a complete, legible, and accurate record of each patient to whom an acupuncture treatment is given. The acupuncturist shall ensure that a patient record is in English and includes:

a. Name of the patient,

b. Patient history,

c. Dates of treatment,

d. Treatment given, and

e. Progress made during acupuncture treatments; and

2. Maintain a patient record for six years after the last treatment of the patient or as prescribed at A.R.S. § 12 − 2297, whichever date occurs later.

B. The provider of an acupuncture, auricular acupuncture, or clinical training program shall:

1. Make accurate and complete records of:

a. Compliance with the program standards in Article 4, and

b. Students enrolled in the program. The provider shall ensure that a student record indicates:

i. Name of the student;

ii. Date enrolled;

iii. Courses taken;

iv. Grade obtained in each course;

v. Date on which the program was completed or the student ceased to participate; and

vi. Whether the student was awarded a diploma, degree, or certificate of completion.

2. Maintain the records required under subsection (B)(1)(a) for six years, and

3. Maintain the records required under subsection (B)(1)(b) for 25 years after the student completes or is last enrolled in the program or as required by A.R.S. § 32 − 3001 et seq. and the rules of the Board of Private Postsecondary Education, whichever is longer.

C. The provider of an approved continuing education shall:

1. Make accurate and complete records of:

a. The Board's approval of the continuing education;

b. The date, time, and location of each presentation of the continuing education; and

c. Participants at each presentation of the continuing education.

2. Maintain the records required under subsection (C)(1) for two years.

R4 - 8 - 503.　Supervision of an Auricular Acupuncturist

A licensed acupuncturist supervising an auricular acupuncture certificate holder shall:

1. Be available promptly to consult with the auricular acupuncture certificate holder in person, by telephone, or electronically during normal working hours; and

2. Ensure that the auricular acupuncture certificate holder performs auricular acupuncture safely and effectively and complies with the law regarding auricular acupuncture.

R4 - 8 - 504.　Recodified

R4 - 8 - 505.　Recodified

R4 - 8 - 506.　Recodified

Article 6.　Complaints; Hearing Procedures; Discipline

R4 - 8 - 601.　Making a Complaint

A. Anyone, including the Board, may file a complaint that alleges a violation of A.R.S. Title 32, Chapter 39 or this Chapter.

B. A complaint may be filed against:

1. An individual licensed under A.R.S. § 32 - 3921 and R4 - 8 - 203;

2. An individual certified under A.R.S. § 32 - 3922 and R4 - 8 - 301;

3. An individual certified under A.R.S. § 32 - 3926 and R4 - 8 - 208; or

4. An individual who is not exempt under A.R.S. § 32 - 3921(B) and believed to be practicing acupuncture without a license or certificate issued under A.R.S. Title 32, Chapter 39 and this Chapter.

C. To file a complaint, an individual shall provide the following information, either orally or in writing, to the Board:

1. Date;

2. Name, address, and telephone number of the individual complained against;

3. Name, address, and telephone number of the complainant;

4. If the complaint is filed on behalf of a third party, the name and address of the third party;

5. The date on which the complaint was last discussed with the individual complained against or a representative of an involved business:

a. A statement of whether the last discussion of the complaint was by telephone or in person, and

b. The name of the individual with whom the complaint was last discussed; and

6. A detailed description, including dates, of the events alleged to constitute a violation of A.R.S. Title 32, Chapter 39 or this Chapter.

D. A complainant shall file a complaint within 90 days of the events alleged to constitute a violation of A.R.S. Title 32, Chapter 39 or this Chapter.

E. A complainant may withdraw a complaint at any time by providing notice to the Board.

R4 – 8 – 602. Complaint Procedures

A. The Board shall review a complaint to determine whether it meets the requirements under R4 – 8 – 601. If a complaint does not meet the requirements under R4 – 8 – 601, the Board shall provide written notice to the complainant that the complaint is dismissed without further action.

B. If the Board determines that a complaint meets the requirements under R4 – 8 – 601, the Board shall assess whether the complaint alleges a violation of A.R.S. Title 32, Chapter 39 or this Chapter and:

1. Dismiss the complaint if the Board determines that the allegation, if true, does not amount to a violation of A.R.S. Title 32, Chapter 39 or this Chapter and provide written notice of the dismissal to the complainant; or

2. Serve a copy of the complaint on the respondent if the Board determines that the allegation, if true, amounts to a violation of A.R.S. Title 32, Chapter 39 or this Chapter and provide the respondent with 20 days to submit:

a. A response in which the individual admits, denies, or further explains each allegation in the complaint; and

b. Records relevant to the complaint.

C. If a respondent responds to a complaint, the Board shall send a copy of the response to the complainant and provide five days for the complainant to submit a rebuttal.

D. When the times provided under subsections (B)(2) and (C) expire, the Board shall conduct an investigation and prepare a report that summarizes the complaint and results of the investigation. The Board shall:

1. Provide a copy of the investigative report to the complainant and respondent; and

2. Provide written notice to the complainant and respondent of the date, time, and location of the Board meeting at which the complaint will be considered.

E. Both the complainant and respondent may be represented by an attorney at the Board meeting at which the complaint is considered.

F. At the Board meeting at which a complaint is considered, the Board shall:

1. Provide the complainant and respondent with an opportunity to address the Board, present evidence, and cross-examine witnesses; and

2. Negotiate an equitable and just resolution of the matters asserted in the complaint; or

3. Forward the complaint to a formal hearing.

R4 - 8 - 603.　Hearing Procedures

The Board shall conduct any hearing required by law according to the procedures in A.R.S. Title 41, Chapter 6, Article 10.

R4 - 8 - 604.　Rehearing or Review of Decision

A. The Board shall provide for a rehearing and review of its decisions under A.R.S. Title 41, Chapter 6, Article 10.

B. Except as provided in subsection (I), a party is required to file a motion for rehearing or review of a decision of the Board to exhaust the party's administrative remedies.

C. A party may amend a motion for rehearing or review at any time before the Board rules on the motion.

D. The Board may grant a rehearing or review for any of the following reasons materially affecting a party's rights:

1. Irregularity in the proceedings of the Board or any order or abuse of discretion that deprived the moving party of a fair hearing;

2. Misconduct of the Board, its staff, or an administrative law judge;

3. Accident or surprise that could not have been prevented by ordinary prudence;

4. Newly discovered material evidence that could not, with reasonable diligence, have been discovered and produced at the hearing;

5. Excessive or insufficient penalty;

6. Error in the admission or rejection of evidence or other errors of law occurring at the hearing or during the progress of the proceedings; and

7. The findings of fact or a decision is not justified by the evidence or is contrary to law.

E. The Board may affirm or modify a decision or grant a rehearing or review to all or some of the parties on all or some of the issues for any of the reasons listed in subsection (D). An order modifying a decision or granting a rehearing or review shall specify with particularity the grounds for the order. If a rehearing or review is granted, the rehearing or review shall cover only the matters specified in the order.

F. Within 30 days after the date of a decision and after giving the parties notice and an opportunity to be heard, the Board may, on its own initiative, order a rehearing or review of its decision for any reason it might have granted a rehearing or review on motion of a party. The Board may grant a motion for rehearing or review, timely served, for a reason not stated in the motion. An order granting a rehearing or review shall specify with particularity the grounds on which the rehearing or review is granted.

G. When a motion for rehearing is based upon affidavits, they shall be served with the motion. An opposing party may, within 15 days after service, serve opposing affidavits. This period may be extended by the Board for a maximum of 20 days for good cause as described in subsection (H) or by written stipulation of the parties. Reply affidavits may be permitted.

H. The Board may extend all time limits listed in this Section upon a showing of good cause. A party demonstrates good cause by showing that the grounds for the party's motion or other action could not have been known in time, using reasonable diligence, and a ruling on the motion will:

1. Further administrative convenience, expedition, or economy; or

2. Avoid undue prejudice to any party.

I. If, in a particular decision, the Board makes a specific finding that the immediate effectiveness of the decision is necessary for preservation of the public health, safety, or welfare and that a rehearing or review of the decision is impracticable, unnecessary, or contrary to the public interest, the decision may be issued as a final decision without an opportunity for a rehearing or review. If an application for judicial review of the decision is made, it shall be made under A.R.S. § 12 – 901 et seq.

R4 – 8 – 605. Disciplinary Action

After a Board meeting at which a complaint is considered or after a hearing that results in a determination that a licensee or certificate holder violated A.R.S. Title 32, Chapter 39 or this Chapter, the Board shall consider the following factors to determine the degree of discipline to impose under A.R.S. § 32 – 3951:

1. Prior conduct resulting in discipline;

2. Dishonest or self-serving motive;

3. Amount of experience as an acupuncturist;

4. Bad faith obstruction of the disciplinary proceeding by intentionally failing to comply with rules or orders of the Board;

5. Submission of false evidence, false statements, or other deceptive practices during the investigative or disciplinary process;

6. Refusal to acknowledge wrongful nature of conduct;

7. Degree of harm resulting from the conduct; and

8. Whether harm resulting from the conduct was cured.

Article 7.   Public Participation Procedures
(Refs & Annos)

R4 – 8 – 701. Expired

R4 – 8 – 702. Petition for Rulemaking; Review of Agency Practice or Substantive Policy Statement; Objection to Rule Based Upon Economic, Small Business, or Consumer Impact

A. A person may petition the Board under A.R.S. § 41 – 1033 for a:

1. Rulemaking action relating to a Board rule, including making a new rule or amending or

repealing an existing rule; or

2. Review of an existing Board practice or substantive policy statement alleged to constitute a rule.

B. A person may petition the Board under A.R.S. §41－1056.01 objecting to all or part of a Board rule because the actual economic, small business, or consumer impact of the rule:

1. Exceeds the estimated economic, small business, or consumer impact of the rule; or

2. Was not estimated and imposes a significant burden on persons subject to the rule.

C. To act under A.R.S. §41－1033 or 41－1056.01 and this Section, a person shall submit to the Board a written petition including the following information:

1. The name, home or business and e-mail addresses, and telephone and fax numbers of the petitioner;

2. Name of any person represented by the petitioner;

3. If requesting a rulemaking action:

a. Statement of the rulemaking action sought, including the A.A.C. citation to all existing rules, and the specific language of a new rule or rule amendment; and

b. Reasons for the rulemaking action, including an explanation of why an existing rule is inadequate, unreasonable, unduly burdensome, or unlawful;

4. If requesting a review of an existing Board practice or substantive policy statement:

a. Subject matter of the existing practice or substantive policy statement; and

b. Reasons why the existing practice or substantive policy statement constitutes a rule.

5. If objecting to a rule because of its economic, small business, and consumer impact statement:

a. The A.A.C. citation of the rule to which objection is made; and

b. A description of how the actual economic, small business, or consumer impact of the rule differs from that estimated; or

c. A description of the actual economic, small business, or consumer impact of the rule and an assessment of the burden on persons subject to the rule; and

6. Dated signature of the petitioner.

D. A person may submit supporting information with a petition.

R4－8－703.　Expired

R4－8－704　Oral Proceedings

A. A person requesting an oral proceeding, as prescribed in A.R.S. §41－1023(C), shall:

1. File the request with the Board;

2. Include the name and current address of the person making the request; and

3. Refer to the proposed rule and include, if known, the date and issue of the Arizona Administrative Register in which the notice of the proposed rule is published.

B. The Board shall make a record of an oral proceeding. The Board shall make any material submitted during an oral proceeding part of the official rulemaking record.

C. The presiding officer shall use the following guidelines to conduct an oral proceeding:

1. Registration of attendees. Registration of attendees is voluntary;

2. Registration of persons intending to speak. A person wishing to speak shall provide the following information on a form that is available from the Board:

a. Name,

b. Representative capacity, if applicable,

c. Whether the person supports or opposes the proposed rule, and

d. Approximate length of time the person wishes to speak;

3. Opening of the record. The presiding officer shall open the proceeding by identifying the rule to be considered and the location, date, time, and purpose of the proceeding, and by presenting the agenda;

4. A statement by Board representative. A Board representative shall explain the background and general content of the proposed rule;

5. A public oral comment period. Any person may speak at an oral proceeding. A person who speaks shall address the proposed rule. A person who speaks may ask questions regarding the proposed rule and present oral argument, data, and views on the proposed rule. The presiding officer may limit the time allotted to each speaker and preclude undue repetition; and

6. Closing remarks. The presiding officer shall announce the location and last day for submitting written comments about the proposed rule.

R4 – 8 – 705. Expired

R4 – 8 – 706. Written Criticism of Rule

A. A person may file a written criticism of an existing rule with the Board.

B. A person filing a written criticism of a rule shall identify the rule by its A.A.C. citation and specify why the rule is inadequate, unduly burdensome, unreasonable, or otherwise improper.

C. The Board shall acknowledge receipt of any criticism within 15 days and place the criticism in the official record for review by the Board under A.R.S. § 41 – 1056.